THE AROMATHERAPY GARDEN

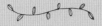

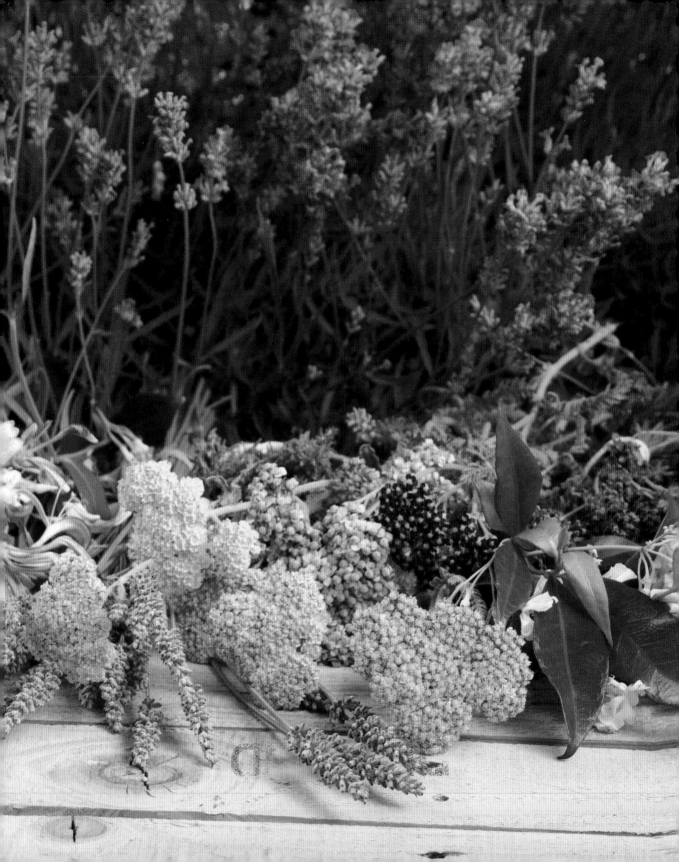

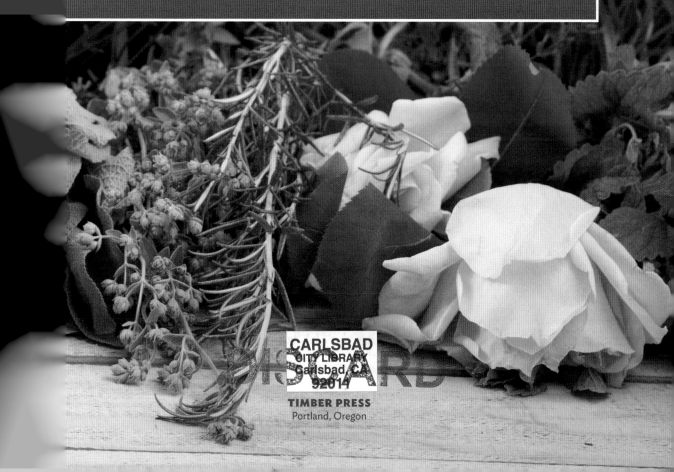

the
AROMATHERAPY GARDEN

*Growing Fragrant Plants for
Happiness and Well-Being*

KATHI KEVILLE

TIMBER PRESS
Portland, Oregon

Copyright © 2016 by Kathi Keville. All rights reserved.
Photography by Karen Callahan, Caitlin Atkinson, Skye McNeill
Kathi Keville, Mary Beth Rich, Rob Bertolucci, and Sarah Milhollin.
Detailed photo credits appear on page 267.
Published in 2016 by Timber Press, Inc.

The Haseltine Building
133 S.W. Second Avenue, Suite 450
Portland, Oregon 97204–3527
timberpress.com

Printed in China
Text design by Laura Shaw Design, Inc.
Cover design by Nina Montenegro and Skye McNeill

Library of Congress Cataloging-in-Publication Data
Keville, Kathi, author.
The aromatherapy garden : growing fragrant plants for happiness
and well-being / Kathi Keville. — First edition.
pages cm
Includes index.
ISBN 978-1-60469-549-6
1. Fragrant gardens. 2. Aromatic plants—Therapeutic use.
3. Aromatherapy. I. Title.
SB454.3.F7K48 2016
635.9—dc23   2015029697

A catalog record for this book is also available
from the British Library.

JULY 2016

To my sister Janna Buesch, who inherited the same green thumb from our gardening ancestors in England, Holland, and Bohemia. To Eduarda Amondragon, who gave me my first parsley, sage, rosemary, and thyme plants and pushed me into the garden.

contents

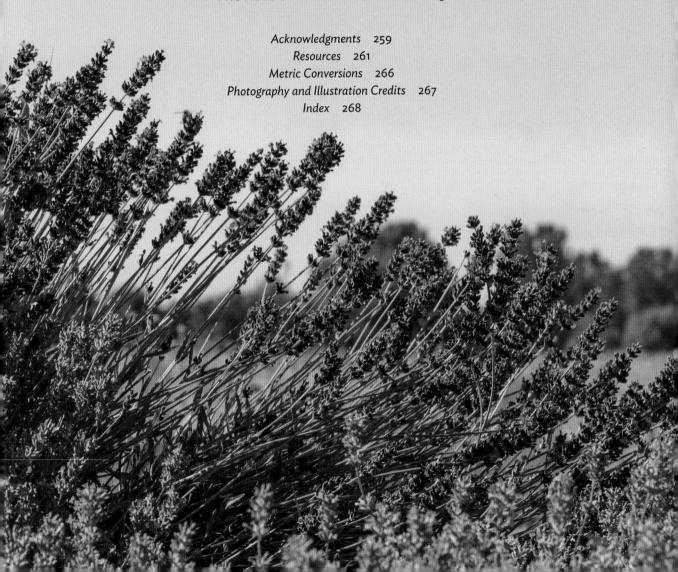

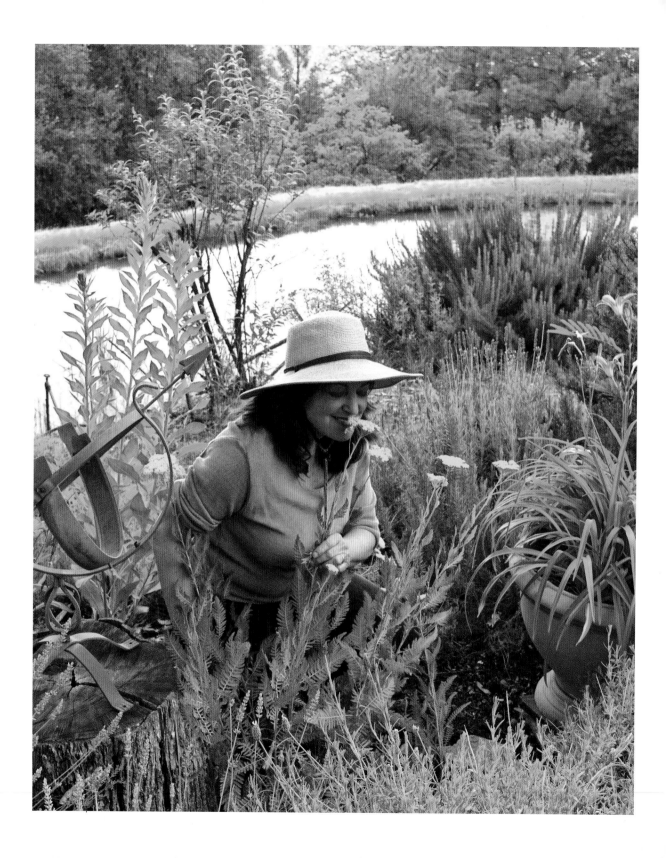

introduction

AROMAS FILL MY GARDEN AND MY HOUSE. This is nothing new. I have always loved fragrance. Since I was child, I have looked forward to the first aromatic spring flowers. There were also the outrageously fragrant roses in my grandmother Irene's porcelain potpourri jar. Her clothes were scented by the sweet lavender sachets she kept in her drawers. Grandmother Janna had a ceramic jar of freshly baked cookies. I could guess which treat was in store when she opened the lid and scents of cinnamon, almonds, or lemon floated out.

I was blessed with a good nose, but also a green thumb. I certainly developed a passion for garden plants and design at a young age. My favorite haunts were the Los Angeles County Arboretum and Botanic Garden and the Huntington Library and Botanical Gardens, where aromatic plants bloomed year-round. I became fascinated with how intriguing plants from around the world were used by different cultures. This early exploration of ethnobotany evolved into university studies in art, psychology, anthropology, and history. What really paved the way for my life's work were my first botanical books—all from the 1930s. They were Louise Beebe Wilder's *The Fragrant Garden*, Helen Fox's *Gardening with Herbs for Flavor and Fragrance*, and *A Modern Herbal*, by Maude Grieve. These are books written for a different era, but they inspired my next forty-five years of plant work as an organic gardener, herbalist, aromatherapist, and researcher.

All of this inspiration and years of gardening experience pour into my writing. In these pages I will cover some of the fascinating science and history of our olfactory sense, and the ways—subtle and not-so-subtle—that it influences virtually all aspects of our human experience. From there, we'll touch on design and cultivation ideas that will help you make the most of fragrant flora. One of the most endearing aspects of many aromatic plants is their ability to carry and impart scent and flavor long after harvest, and I will suggest ways to put those long-lasting benefits to use. Finally, I'll share some of my favorite scented plants for gardens large and small.

It is a pleasure to share my experiences with fragrance, and the stories and uses of aromatic plants with you. May it encourage you to bring more fragrance into your garden and your life.

◀ The author enjoying a noseful of yarrow. Lavender and rosemary are nearby.

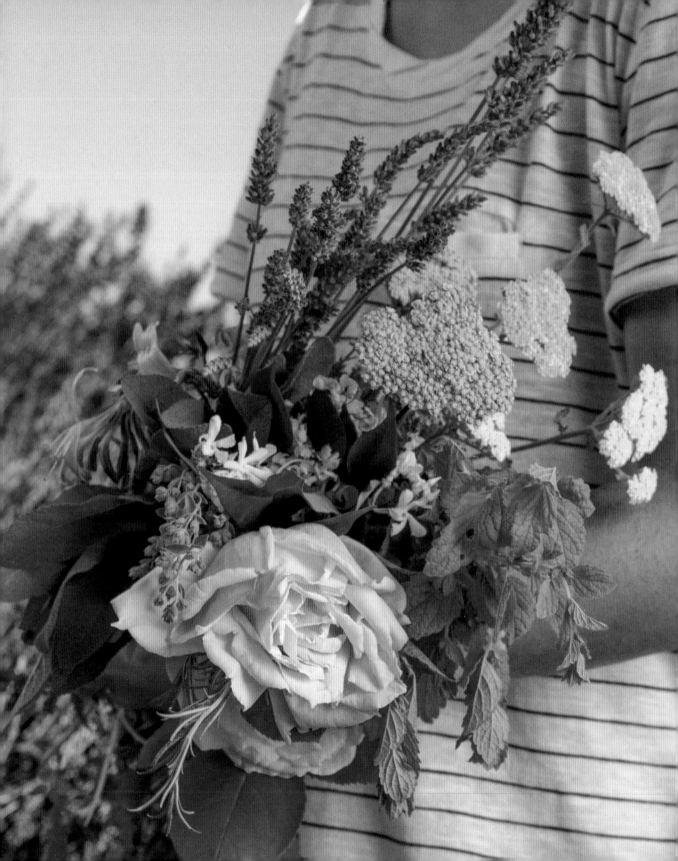

a tradition of scent in the garden

We cannot see or hear scent, making it seemingly less tangible than our senses of sight, touch, taste, or hearing. Step into a fragrance garden and it is almost magical how layers of aromas greet your nose completely unannounced. This delightful mix changes with amazing frequency walking through the garden. Some aromas dance across your senses while others are deep and exotic. There are familiar scents, while others leave you at a loss for words.

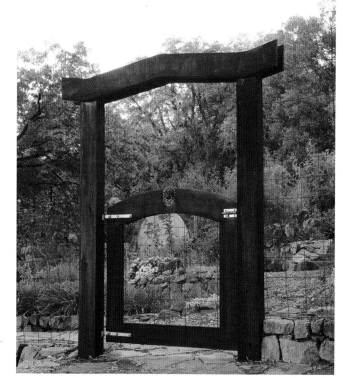

▶ A gate marks the official entry to the author's garden, but heady fragrances announce its presence long before one arrives.

▼ Some of the best paths to follow are fragrant.

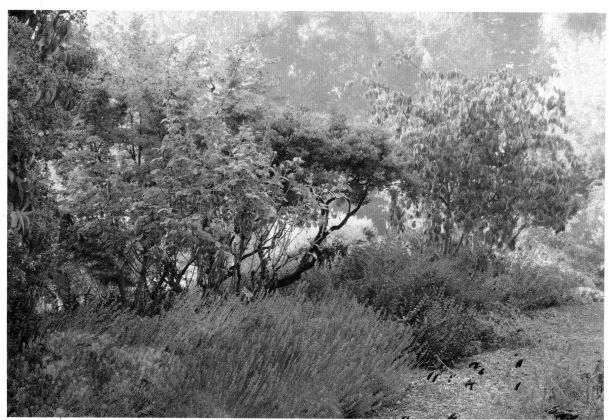

We respond to these intriguing smells with sensual delight, but while fragrant plants are enticing us, they are also hard at work, modifying our mood and frame of mind every time we inhale. Plant scientists are discovering what gardeners have always known: the fragrant garden reduces stress. Heady plant aromas make us laugh and smile more, and leave us with a sense of contentment. It's not all about the human experience, either. Scent is also important in attracting pollinators, deterring predators, and even allowing plants to communicate with each other.

what is fragrance?

A bloom in full splendor, a cup of hot herbal tea, a favorite cologne, or the earth after a summer rain—a multitude of smells enrich our lives daily. The impact is profound. Scent enhances life experiences, such as tasting and sensuality. It is also the stuff of which dreams and memories are made. It embodies poetry, mythology, imagination.

Nature's potpourri may seem enchanted, but fragrance is based on an assortment of invisible but very real aromatic compounds. They fit together like a puzzle to make up essential oils. These tiny oils easily float through the air, and can be released simply by pressing on a fragrant leaf.

Aromatic flowers, leaves, stems, fruit, roots, and bark typically concentrate essential oils in special cells. Different plant families

have characteristic places where they store the oils. For example, most members of the mint family make and keep scent in fine, glandular hairs that cover their leaves. The carrot family prefers to hold aromatic essential oils in tubes in their seeds, or sometimes in their stems and roots. You can see this in plants like angelica, coriander, dill, and fennel.

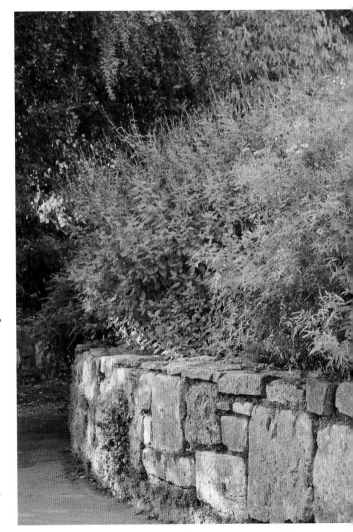

▶ The pungent aromas of Mexican marigold and sages are brought to nose level.

How we perceive aroma

Each time you inhale, tiny, aromatic molecules hitchhike a ride. Smell a rose or basil leaf, and the compounds you breathe are first greeted high in the nose by the olfactory epithelium: two small receptors that are about the size of dimes. These receptors use tiny cilia filaments to catch and identify molecules, seemingly by their shape. The information is sent to olfactory bulbs located at the base of the brain, which interpret it and send a report to the limbic system. That is where different scents are interpreted and sent to the brain, to analyze and coordinate with other senses. The limbic system also ties our sense of smell to emotions and memory. It distinguishes between aromas that draw us in and odors that fend us off. It determines when there is an emergency, such as smelling something burning. All of this happens in less than a second, making our perception and reaction to a scent instantaneous. You immediately identify the aroma as rose or basil, and think either bouquet or pesto.

Your reaction to aroma is largely based on past experiences with the scent, how a particular scent acts on your brain, and probably genetic make-up. If you are like most people, you prefer familiar fragrances that spark good memories. Sometimes past association gets in the way of fully appreciating aroma. When students at Warwick University in England took a test while smelling a certain scent and were later told they had performed poorly, they felt depressed the next time they encountered the same aroma.

Many people are attracted to lemon's clean, sharp scent, but it can also be associated with furniture polish or lemon-scented dishwashing soap. Lemon grass, citronella, and lemon-scented eucalyptus can be reminiscent of pungent insect repellent.

Putting a name to fragrance

Describing the many scents produced by plants has long fascinated botanists and perfumers. One of the first classifications of scent was by Theophrastus, a Greek botanist and herbalist from the fourth century BC. In his treatise, *Concerning Odours*, he designated aromas as simply good or evil, and categorized them as sweet, pungent, heavy, powerful, or faint. In the eighteenth century, Carl Linnaeus, who founded the system of botany we use today, divided these categories. Good scents smelled fragrant, aromatic, or like ambrosia, while bad scents were garlic, goat-like, or foul. In the next century, Eugene Rimmel identified eighteen plant-based aromas in his classic *Book of Perfumes*, defining them poetically as spicy, rose-like, anise, balsamic, and jasmine. The nineteenth-century Frenchman, G. W. Septimus Piesse, took a new approach to aroma by corresponding scents with musical "notes." Perfumers and aromatherapists still talk of high, middle, and base notes when they describe essential oils. Base notes, such as vetiver and spikenard, smell heavy. They fix scent and make the blend last longer. Middle notes—think of rose geranium or marjoram—are considered the heart of an aromatic blend, carrying and tying the mix together. Top notes like rose and lemon dance over the top of the other aromas.

Classification of plant fragrance was expanded by botanist Anton Kerner von Marilaun, a professor at the University of

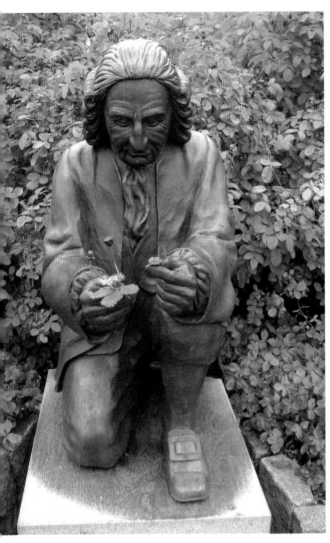

▲ Eighteenth-century Swedish botanist Carl Linnaeus created an early system of dividing scents.

Vienna, Austria, and curator of its botanical garden in 1860. He placed damask rose in a rosy, sweet-floral, almost fruity group. Violet-like orris root is paired with violets. The aromatic group lumps together the intense fragrances of clematis, heliotrope, honeysuckle, sweet pea, and Mexican orange blossom shrub. Heavy aromas that are more cloying, such as daffodil, daphne, lily, and mock orange, are in their own category. Citrus includes the obvious choices of lemon, lemon balm, lemon verbena, lemon eucalyptus, and lemon thyme. Animal scents are represented by spikenard and musk rose. Leaves are compared to mint, garlic, turpentine (such as rosemary or pine), or camphor (such as bay, sage, thyme, or wormwood). Wood-like scents are aromatic, such as cedar, or carry the turpentine scent of pine and fir.

Modern scientists organize scents according to the similarity of their aromatic compounds. If you have a good sense of smell, you will detect a common, aromatic thread. An example is the terpene group, with the diverse, green, earthy scents found in lavender and citrus. The benzoloid group includes the spicy clove of pinks and the cherry-cinnamon scent of hyacinth, as well as the cherry-vanilla fragrance of heliotrope. Scented geranium, rose, and even valerian are in the paraffinoid group.

Essential oils are the key

It is possible to capture the garden's fragrances in a bottle by extracting essential oils from plants. The most common method is by steam distillation. The tiny aromatic molecules that comprise essential oils move readily into hot steam in the same way they fill the garden with fragrance on a hot day. A steam distiller extracts the essential oils, cools the steam back into water, and separates out the pure essential oil. Most essential oils that can handle this kind of high heat are found in leaves and seeds.

The leaves of basil, bay laurel, clary sage, juniper, lemon grass, lemon verbena, marjoram, patchouli, peppermint, rockrose, rose geranium, rosemary, sage, and thyme are distilled for flavoring products including alcoholic drinks, gum, candy, and tobacco. They are also distilled to scent body care and other products. Other, less-known plant leaves, such as anise hyssop, can be distilled (I've done it myself with my steam distiller), but they are rarely commercially available due to low demand.

Aromatic flowers are a different story. Many of the essential oils responsible for flowers' fragrance are fragile and altered by the high heat of distillation. Heat changes the aromas of clematis, daffodil, daphne, gardenia, hyacinth, freesia, lilac, lily-of-the-valley, and sweet pea flowers. Most of these floral essential oils are produced synthetically in a lab and labeled as fragrance oils. The best way to think about synthetic essential oils is to compare them to cloying, cheap cologne that sticks to the back of the nose. Synthetics are commonly used in perfume, cologne, and scented body care and household products, including many labeled as aromatherapy. However, they never smell like the real thing. Some of the chemicals used to create them have questionable health effects. Aromatherapists like myself use only plant-derived essential oils.

A few flowers, such as chamomile, lavender, orange blossom, and rose, are steam distilled. Some floral essential oils are also extracted without heat using chemicals or a carbon dioxide process. These expensive oils mostly go into high-end perfume. Jasmine and tuberose are available only as "absolutes," which means their essential oil is extracted with solvents, then the chemicals are removed to leave just the essential oil. It is an investment, but you can purchase a steam distiller to produce essential oils from your fragrance garden. It requires a vast amount of plant material, which is more than most gardens can supply. However, small amounts of plant material will give you a quantity of scented water, called hydrosol, as a by-product of distillation. This aromatic water is dilute enough for use in sprays, to splash on the skin, or for use in cooking.

Pure essential oil is so concentrated that it smells much stronger in a bottle than the plant itself. In fact, it is so strong that it should be used with care. Although many people think problems with essential oils are due to extenders that are added to some inexpensive brands, even pure essential oils have the potential of being toxic. After all, one of their primary roles in plants is to deter predatory insects and animals from eating them. Undiluted essential oils such as oregano, thyme, and the citruses can burn skin. Essential oils also absorb into your skin and reach the bloodstream, and even small

▸ Tabletop distillers are a good way to capture fragrant hydrosols and a bit of essential oil from your garden.

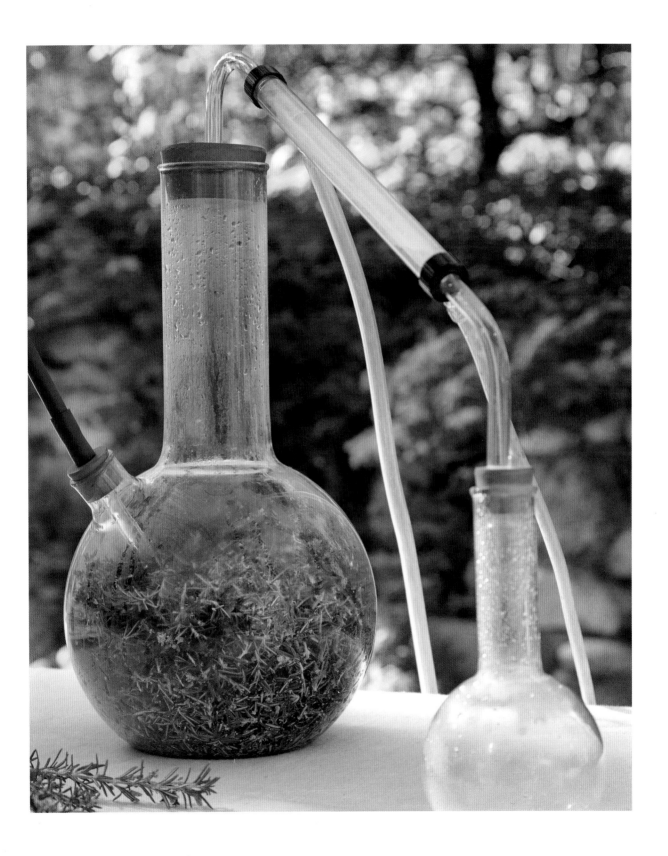

amounts can tax the liver and kidneys. Some essential oils, such as camphor, are also rough on the nervous system. For safety's sake, do not use essential oil directly on your skin without diluting it, and do not ingest oils. It does little good, since ingesting pure essential oils causes them to be absorbed mostly in the throat. Better to add oils to lotion, cream, or salve so they can penetrate into and benefit underlying tissue. Cats and dogs do not process ingested essential oils well, so can be easily poisoned by them.

why plant aromas vary

With seventeen hundred known aromatic compounds from more than ninety plant families, there are a lot of possibilities for making one plant smell different from the next. Some essential oils, such as orange, have a simple chemistry based on a few specific aromatic compounds that give them a straightforward smell. Orange is pleasant enough, but compare it to the deeply complex rose, which contains around two hundred seventy-five scent molecules. That complexity is why the captivating fragrance of rose finds its way into the imagination, poetry, and perfume.

When several plants share some of the same compounds—such as lemon verbena, lemon thyme, lemon eucalyptus, and lemon grass—they smell similar. Yet, you can distinguish these plants from each other because their other aromatic molecules give each a unique essence.

Chemotypes

Occasionally, plants in the same species look identical to the botanist, but do not smell exactly the same. This occurs when they are growing in different regions and adapt their chemistry for better survival. A chemist refers to these variations as chemotypes, because the two plants contain different percentages of their aromatic molecules. The mint family readily develops chemotypes, with at least eight chemotypes of thyme alone. So thyme growing in the mountains of southern France smells softer because it is higher in linalool, a compound that is abundant in lavender, while its seaside counterpart contains more thymol, which gives thyme its characteristic aroma. The chemotypes of rosemary include the harsh camphor, a gentler verbenone, and eucalyptus-like cineol. Korean mint, related to anise hyssop, can have the scent of either cloves or patchouli. Other plants containing aromatic chemotypes include basil, bee balm, curry plant, lavender, myrtle, sage, scented geranium, and camphor and eucalyptus trees.

how plants use scent

As much as we enjoy the fragrances of the garden, plants produce all their wonderful scents not for our enjoyment, but for their own gain. The same essential oils that create aroma are sophisticated survival tools to help aromatic plants control their environment. Since plants are stuck in one place, they use scent to reach out and lure pollinators for reproduction, to fend off predators, and to

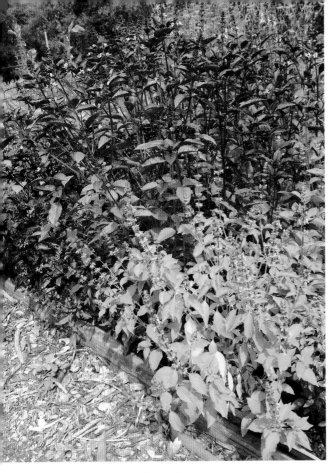

thwart competitive plants. In many cases, natural selection has favored the survival of plants with higher concentrations of scent.

DIFFERENT ROLES FOR FRAGRANT PLANTS

Aromatic flowers and leaves play different roles. Flowers broadcast copious amounts of fragrance for a just a few weeks a year, attracting pollinating creatures. Leaves generally keep their scent to themselves since they have no need for pollination; strong aroma could distract pollinators and waste precious energy. As a result, we must rub or crush a leaf to release its scent. That aroma is more pungent and "green" than floral, since it serves to keep away destructive insects and infection. Sharp-smelling leaves, such as rosemary, thyme, eucalyptus, and tea tree, are also some of the most antiseptic—not only for plants, but also for people.

Plants use scent to keep potential predators from eating them—predators that include us. We consume aromatic herbs only in tiny amounts, because their scent and flavor are so potent. Animals do not find fragrant plants such as rosemary, sage, and thyme tasty. My fragrance garden does not have to be fenced, even though deer frequent it. The aromas that are exuded into the soil from the roots of rue, wormwood, and yarrow deter neighboring plants from getting too close.

▲ Lemon, cinnamon, and purple basils each have slightly different scents.

◄ Geraniums offer a potpourri of scent and leaf textures.

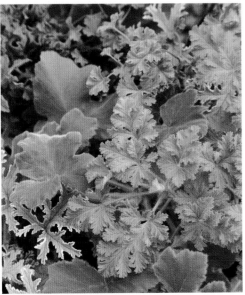

When Cornell University researchers artificially increased the scent of certain flowers, bees were unimpressed, but destructive ants were deterred by the strong scent. Flowers do not always benefit from pumped-up fragrance. Sigma Xi, the Scientific Research Society, reported that flowers with increased scent put out the welcome mat to beetles—however, honeybees were repelled, although seemingly not by the stronger fragrance, but by the abundance of beetles!

It is amazing to consider, but plants can smell. Their sense of smell is based on hormones rather than via a nose and brain neurons. They detect pheromones from their fruit to know when it is ripe. They also put out distress signals when injured or attacked. Wild tobacco that is infested by caterpillars releases a leaf scent to alert parasitic wasps that eat the caterpillars. The University of Florida and United States Department of Agriculture (USDA) found that citrus trees infected by the deadly greening disease produce a scent that attracts parasites that spread the disease, but also a wasp that is their natural enemy. Lemon tree roots exude essential oils if attacked underground. Wounded sagebrush increases its potent scent more than six times to notify other sagebrush in the area. Even tobacco plants growing downwind from the sagebrush get the message to increase their defenses—and suffer less insect damage as a result.

▶ A rich-smelling garden can offer multiple benefits.

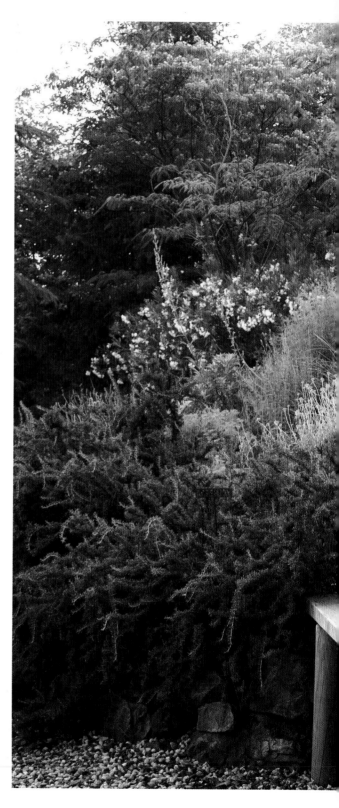

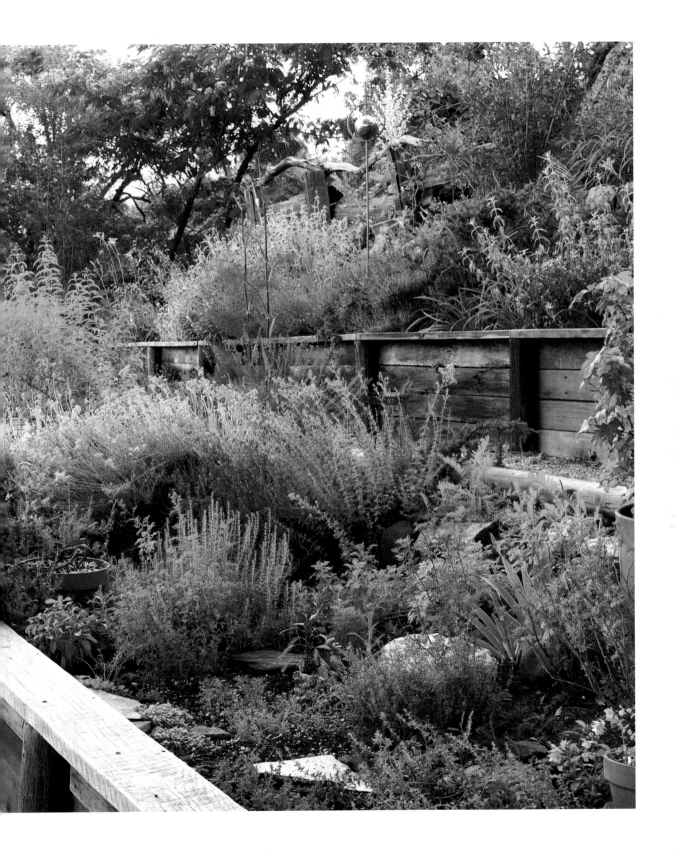

The aromatic compounds that give pine trees their well-known smell also play a significant role in reducing ground temperatures in boreal forests. The compounds react with oxygen to become aerosol vapor, rising and encouraging clouds to form in the forest canopy. The vapor-filled clouds reflect the sun's heat to cool the air below. Some scientists say that the loss of aromatic trees worldwide may be helping to warm the planet and contributing to global warming.

ATTRACTING POLLINATORS

A fragrance garden offers far more than pretty smells; it also draws an array of pollinators. Insects are nature's aromatherapists. Many of them rely on a keen sense of smell to locate the nectar and pollen that flowers advertise through fragrance. Insects and flowers have developed a mutual dependency and adapted accordingly.

Plant researchers have long said that pollinators find color more attractive than scent. However, it turns out that olfactory cues help pollinators choose the best flowers. When many flowers go into bloom at the same time, those that are most highly scented win the battle for pollinators. The Centre for Research on Ecology and Forestry Applications found that flowers in early spring in Barcelona, Spain, had much stronger, herby scents that bees love. In the summer, when far fewer flowers are competing with each other, the fragrance was less intense. This competition to attract pollinators may be why plants developed so many different scents.

Bees, butterflies, and hummingbirds demand a high-energy diet to sustain themselves and their brood. Pollen is rich in protein and flower nectar is primarily sugar water, but it does contain some amino acids, vitamins, and minerals. Most pollinators fly, enabling them to distribute pollen over a wide area. This promotes genetic diversity for the plants they visit. It's a big job: each flower requires about fifteen visits before it is fully fertilized. To ensure fertilization, flowers may rely on more than one type of pollinator.

Species that have strong daytime scents are pollinated mostly by bees and butterflies. Those that release fragrance at night are typically pollinated by moths and bats. Plants that are pollinated by bees and flies smell sweet, while those pollinated by beetles have strong musty, spicy, or fruity odors. Plants that rely on wind pollination, such as lemon grass, juniper, and wormwood, have no need to be fragrant or flashy, so they have small, greenish flowers without sepals or petals.

Different plant species have developed ways to recruit pollinators and keep them faithful, as well as ways to keep away creatures that will rob the plants of pollen and nectar. Plants often play tricks to smell or look especially attractive to an insect. Some clever flowers, especially those catering to butterflies, smell like pheromones that insects use to attract the opposite sex. Flowers signal that they are prime for pollination by increasing their scent when their potential pollinators are active. Once pollinated, they gradually lose both scent and attractiveness.

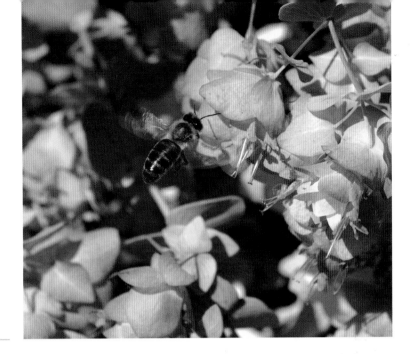

▶ A bee visits a dittany of Crete flower.

Honeybees and wild bees

Most flowers are pollinated by bees, which have specialized, furry legs to hold pollen. Honeybees are attracted to yellow, blue, and purple flowers, although they are more partial to strong, sweet scents that indicate the presence of pollen and nectar. Fragrance helps them find the correct plants. Similar to people, bees recognize aromas faster and remember them much longer than they do visual cues, according to research reported in *Functional Ecology*. We humans cannot see them, but low ultraviolet light nectar-guides on angelica, bee balm, lamb's ears, and sweet pea attract bees and help them quickly locate their target. Yarrow and tansy have a similar zone across their floral discs.

Wild bees have always been a vital part of the ecosystem. The job of plant survival fell on their wings before beekeepers kept European honeybees. Native bees prefer to pick up pollen and nectar from the native plants in their area, but they visit domesticated plants as well. Many wild bees are small with short tongues, so they prefer packed clusters of tiny flowers, such as chamomile. Ground-nesting bees are among the first to emerge to visit violets and other early spring bloomers.

Like honeybees, bumblebees form colonies with a queen, although there are fewer than fifty in a nest. Watching bumblebees maneuver into large clary sage flowers can be quite entertaining. They will also visit anise hyssop, bay laurel, clematis, honeysuckle, lamb's ears, phlox, rockrose, and wisteria. Sometimes they will pollinate smaller lavender, rosemary, and thyme flowers.

Relying on bees for pollination has become an increasing problem for many plants. The seasonal behavior of some species has been changing and natural foraging areas moving. Wild bees are beginning to emerge at different times in the year when flowering plants are not abundant. The spread of infectious colony collapse disorder has also caused a sharp drop in European honeybees. The Intergovernmental Panel on Climate Change's 2014 report warned that bees and other pollinators faced the risk of extinction because of global warming. In 2013, the European Union announced plans to restrict the use of some pesticides in the hope of slowing the decline of bee populations.

Butterfly and moth pollinators

Butterflies are particularly active during sunny days, visiting a variety of flowers. They seek out long flowers and extract the nectar with long proboscises. They have excellent vision and, unlike bees, can see red flowers. They also go for bright orange, yellow, pink, and sometimes blue. However, butterflies do not have a keen sense of smell. They rely on taste receptors on their feet to identify a host plant. Highly perched on long, thin legs, they are not able to pick up or carry as much pollen as a bee, but they still do their fair share. Flat-topped flower clusters, such as those on yarrow plants, make the easiest landing pads for large butterflies. Protective plants such as fennel and violets are used for laying eggs.

The western tiger swallowtail butterflies visit my garden to pollinate the bay laurel, dill, fennel, native honeysuckle, lavender, mint, lilac, mock orange, phlox, and wallflower. Skipper butterflies are tiny enough to pollinate the small flowers of catnip, lavender, and oregano. Phlox and rue attract the beautiful giant swallowtails, and mint and mock orange lure wood nymph butterflies. Painted ladies and sulfurs are a few of the butterflies that also feast on the nectar of phlox. Milbert's tortoiseshell butterfly visits lilacs and wallflowers and sara orangetips pollinate violets, while Baltimore butterflies flock to wallflowers.

Moths, on the other hand, are extremely sensitive to odors. They pick up honeysuckle's fragrance from half a mile away. Most are nocturnal, so the flowers they pollinate wait until dusk to emit strong scents that will carry in the night air without the sun's heat to evaporate the aroma—think flowering tobacco, gardenia, Easter lily, and night-blooming jasmine. Moths and long-tongued bees that can reach into the tubular flowers of primrose and phlox help with pollination.

Other pollinators

Other pollinators visit the fragrance garden. Hummingbirds are so sensitive to scent that they were taught to differentiate between smells at the Centro di Studio per la Faunistica ed Ecologia Tropicali del C.N.R in Santa Teresa, Brazil. For example, they could tell the difference between jasmine and lavender.

Hummingbirds are drawn to the deep red flowers of bee balm, flowering tobacco, and pineapple sage. They also go for orange, yellow, and deep pink blooms, as well as many purple and some blue-purple flowers, such as anise hyssop, hummingbird sage, Spanish sage, and wisteria. Tubular, nodding flowers with long styles and filaments—such as honeysuckle, red-flowering sage, bee balm, and some lilies—accommodate the hummingbirds' long beaks, which collect pollen as the birds drink. These flowers do not need a landing area, because hummingbirds prefer to hover while feeding.

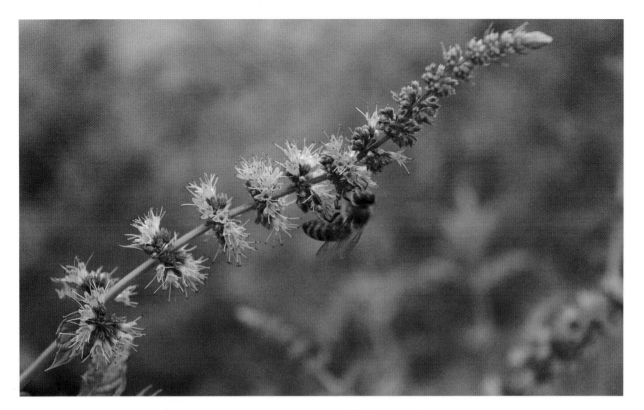

▲ Pollination of an unusual blue-flowering spearmint.

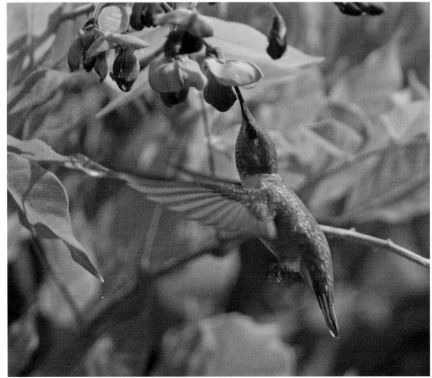

◄ Hummingbirds serve as important pollinators.

Roman chamomile is pollinated by flies, as well as by little beetles. Small wasps pollinate German chamomile and tansy. Flies gravitate toward the white and cream-colored flowers of angelica, daphne, fennel, lily-of-the-valley, peppermint, rockrose, sweet woodruff, thyme, wallflowers, tansy, and some green flowers. Flies with short tongues prefer simple, bowl-shaped flowers. Hover flies visit so many wild plants that they have been considered the next important group of pollinators after wild bees. Some even have a proboscis, to siphon nectar out of long, narrow flowers. Pollinating flies can mimic bees, but look closely and you will see only one pair of wings instead of two, as well as larger eyes, shorter antennae, and skinnier legs than bees. The larvae of nearly half the pollinating flies are laid on the plant. This helps with pest control, because the larvae prey on other insects.

How to attract plenty of pollinators, but not too many beetles, is an ongoing floral dilemma. Beetles are clumsy in flight, so require an easy entrance to the flowers. They are also messy pollinators, often chewing the plant and leaving droppings. Flowers such as Mexican marigold and rockrose have adapted ways to provide enough food for hungry, pollinating beetles, while avoiding being destroyed in the process.

Millions of years ago, when the first flowering plants began to bloom, some wasps made a switch from hunting prey to gathering pollen for their brood. Wasps are generally less efficient pollinators than bees (which descended from wasps) and lack the body hairs to trap pollen, so are unable to carry it from flower to flower. Even so, some hard-working wasps bring their young nectar and pollen.

Using aroma to deter bad bugs

The fragrant garden is fairly pest-free. Most insects in my garden are pollinators, rather than their destructive relatives. The aroma creates a built-in defense against predators that cannot pick up the scent they want through the aromatic shield. Insects rely on their acute sense of smell to locate plants to eat, with many of them flying miles to track down a meal. Night-flying moths that lay caterpillar and cutworm eggs on garden plants purposely fly upwind to detect plants.

My first garden a few decades ago was in a tightly populated beach community that still had old victory garden plots from World War II, when everyone was encouraged to grow food. My neighborhood replanted them. My refurbished victory garden held only a few vegetables that were surrounded by forty-some aromatic herbs. It was the only garden for blocks without predatory bugs— that is, my garden and the one directly on the other side of the fence. My first garden tours were to show curious neighbors the benefits of having an aromatic garden.

If your garden is invaded, peppermint, thyme, and wormwood are star players against garden pests. They remove white flies from the greenhouse. Along with basil and dill, they deter the dreaded tomato hornworm. Wormwood can almost single-handedly defend the entire garden, discouraging carrot fly, squash bug, and maggot. Along with southernwood, it also works against the cabbage looper. Peppermint deters both the ants that climb my roses and the aphids they deposit on the shrubs. Other plants to battle aphids include basil, camphor, cilantro, eucalyptus, fennel, and tansy. Use French marigold, rosemary, and rue for beetles, and tansy for Japanese and cucumber beetles and squash bugs. Catnip, cilantro, and tansy are specific for potato beetles. To deter spider mites, try cilantro, cumin, and oregano. Fennel and rosemary can be ground into a powder to sprinkle anywhere there are slugs or snails.

A plant's essential oils protect it in other ways besides just odors and aromas. Essential oils also destroy bacterial, fungal, and viral infections responsible for plant diseases. These antibiotic oils are the same ones used in aromatherapy to fight infections and heal wounds in both people and animals. Some particularly potent examples are the highly antibacterial and antifungal lavender, oregano, and rosemary. It's effective to use these aromatic plants in any combination to make a spray for infected plants or to create a powder to sprinkle around a plant's base. Simply planting them in your garden can deter pests from vegetables. French marigold roots exude an aromatic substance that repels destructive nematodes in the soil, helping prevent injury to garden plant roots.

Of course, the best way to keep your garden free of harmful bugs is to have healthy plants. Preventive health care works the same in your garden as it does for people, making the plants more resistant to disease and pests. Insects generally avoid strong plants and go after the ones that are ailing. If

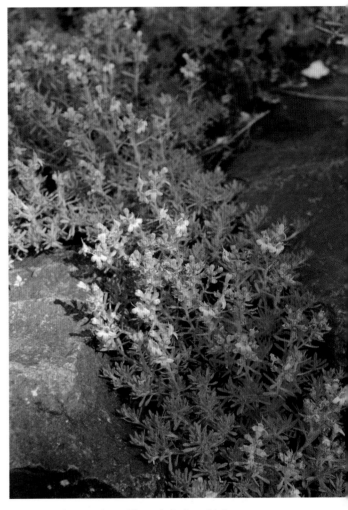

▲ The odor of caraway thyme (*Thymus herba-barona*) helps keep insect pests at bay.

you see problems in the garden, look first at the infested or infected plant itself for health problems. Pamper those plants with bug spray, compost "tea" (compost steeped in water), and sufficient water to make them more resilient.

make your own plant pest repellent

A simple, all-purpose insect spray for plants. This employs the naturally repellent qualities of plant aromas.

Approximately 1 cup fresh peppermint, thyme, and wormwood leaves

2 whole, unpeeled garlic cloves

2 cups water

blender

spray bottle

optional

1 teaspoon liquid castile soap or dishwashing liquid

2 tablespoons regular strength vinegar (any kind)

1. Place the leaves, garlic cloves, and water in a blender.

2. Blend contents into a slurry.

3. Let mixture sit overnight, then strain.

4. Use the resulting herb-scented solution as is, or add liquid castile soap or dishwashing liquid (for better adherence) and vinegar.

5. To use, pour liquid into spray bottle and apply directly onto infested plants. Dilute with water if too thick.

6. Store repellent in refrigerator, where it should keep about a week. Mark your bug spray well! When labels have fallen off, my family has eaten all sorts of herbal concoctions.

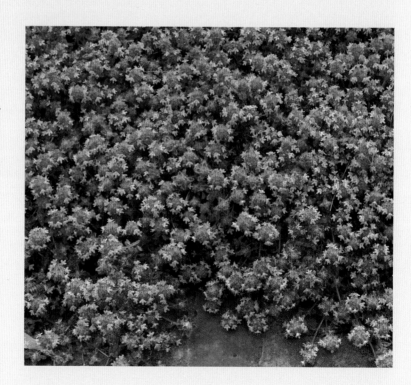

▶ Thyme is a natural pest repellent.

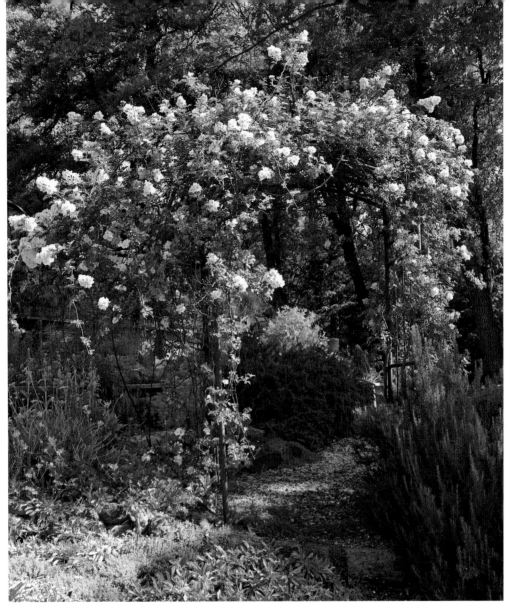

▲ A rose arbor brings cheer to visitors.

aromatherapy from the garden

At one time, it was taken for granted that spending time in a garden was healing to body, mind, and spirit. It is no wonder that gardeners love being in their gardens! They will be the first to tell you that a fragrant garden changes one's mood. Never hesitate to take an extra "dose" of garden whenever you need an emotional lift. Like many gardeners, I also bring the aromas of my healing garden into the house with fragrant bouquets, and plants such as jasmine, lilies, violets, and daphne growing outside my windows.

Scientists have been investigating the field of aromacology to discover how scent impacts us. What they found is that aromas spark areas in the brain that control emotions. One reason we respond so quickly to liking or disliking a scent is because it gains direct access to our mind. One of the ways in which fragrance alters moods is to modify brain activity. Changes are observed in brainwaves and neurotransmitters, such as serotonin and dopamine, which play important roles in regulating our emotions, anxiety, cognition, sleep regulation, and appetite. Scent also communicates with hormonal regulators in the body, especially the adrenal, hypothalamus, and pituitary glands that act as control centers to manage everyday functions.

PLANTS CAN CHANGE YOUR MOOD

Aromas impact our emotions in different ways. Calming scents help our bodies deal with stress and depression. Other aromas stimulate the mind to keep us awake or to help us work more efficiently. Most scents stir the memory, but some do a better job than others. Generally, fragrances that we find pleasant make us feel good and assist us in functioning better emotionally.

Medical science is looking into the many ways people have traditionally used fragrant plants. It's helping scientists uncover the untapped potential of aromas. Researchers are studying plants with rich aromatherapy lore, hoping to put our sense of smell to work helping us heal (as well as prevent) at least some emotional and physical diseases. As a result, we now have a selection of aromatic plants with therapeutic uses that are backed by both science and history. Aromatherapists add a number of additional fragrant plants to their pharmacy—plants that have not been scientifically investigated but have many traditional uses.

The Fragrance Research Fund, a nonprofit coalition of fragrance industry companies, began collaborating with Yale University's psychophysiology department in 1982 to investigate ways in which aroma affects personality and behavior. One program followed more than two thousand subjects over twenty years. A long list of disorders is being researched, including fatigue, migraine headaches, pain, food cravings, insomnia, depression, anxiety, schizophrenia, sexual dysfunction, and memory loss. Fragrance is certainly not as potent as its pharmaceutical counterparts, but it is non-addicting, seems to have no side effects, and can be used safely with drugs. The typical prescription for aromatherapy is simply to take a sniff every few minutes.

Relaxing, stress-relieving scents

Chamomile, lavender, lemon, marjoram, orange blossom, and other citrus scents have been shown to enhance relaxation, encourage sleep, reduce depression and anxiety, and lower the body's response to pain. It takes just a few whiffs of any one of these scents to calm the body physically and mentally. Spikenard and valerian increase the calming, meditative theta brain waves and

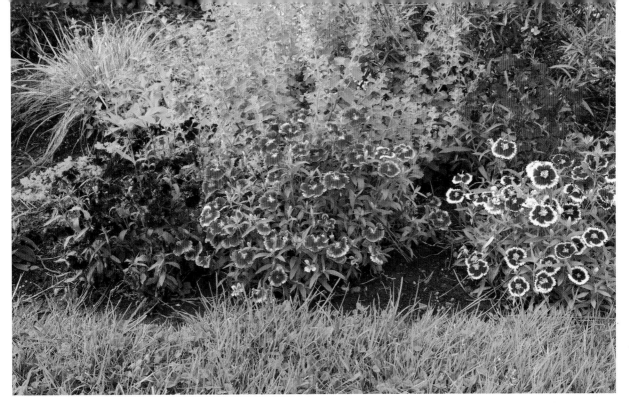

▲ Plant clove pinks to boost relaxation and happiness.

deeply relaxing delta waves, while decreasing the more stimulating beta waves. Most lemon-scented plants, such as lemon grass, and lemon itself, help the nervous system overcome stress, nervous exhaustion, and especially sleep disorders. The eleventh-century Islamic healer Avicenna recommended lemon balm to lift a bad mood.

A relaxed, happiness response is produced in the brain by clove-like scents. This may be one reason why clove-scented roses, clove pink, wallflower, and especially stocks became such well-loved garden flowers. Basil also has clove buried in its scent. The aromatic compound eugenol gives these plants their clove-like scent. University of Arizona psychologist Gary Schwartz, PhD, has had hundreds of people participate in studies on scent. He showed how clove produces relaxation and reduces stress, mental fatigue, and

nervousness, as well as memory loss. The scent does this by moderating brain neurotransmitters and reducing adrenal cortisol levels that rise when we are stressed.

Herb-like scents that are identified by perfumers as "green odors" help protect the body from the negative impact of stress. The green scents of fennel, oregano, and marjoram appear to improve feelings of general well-being by adjusting neurotransmitter activity. Many green scents, such as German chamomile, gardenia, lemon grass, rose, and sweet flag have been shown to be calming because they enhance a brain chemical called GABA that encourages relaxation and sleep, sometimes more than sleeping pills. They are thought to work through the hypothalamus and pituitary glands, which signal regulatory processes throughout the body to keep it in balance. Ruhr University researchers in Germany say that aromatherapy sprays may offer a new class of GABA modulators and "a scientific basis for aromatherapy." Sniffing jasmine may be comparable to taking sedative drugs.

Even cosmetic companies are creating aromatherapy perfumes and body care products. Research at Shiseido, the world's third-largest cosmetic company, says that stress adversely affects the complexion, but an aromatherapy facial can relax brain waves to the same extent as meditation.

Multiple research studies indicate that the scents of rose, patchouli, and orange blossom encourage relaxation and help with long-term pain and physical and emotional stress, as well as problems from the resulting high levels of cortisol and adrenaline. Orange blossom, lavender, and rosemary lower cortisol levels. Rose and patchouli seem to moderate adrenaline output and slow sympathetic nerve activity. Rose-scented geranium and lavender balance emotions by producing either relaxation or alertness. It is suspected that all of these scents help regulate the brain's neurotransmitters.

Nurses in a 2014 study from Australia's Griffith University found that the high stress and anxiety of working in the emergency room decreased after an aromatherapy spray containing lavender, lime, patchouli, rose, ylang ylang, and bergamot was misted over them and briefly massaged into their shoulders. They experienced an "immediate and dramatic" difference. Stress indicators, such as blood pressure and cortisol levels, dropped when volunteers in a 2012 study at Eulji University's College of Nursing in Korea repeatedly inhaled a blend of lavender, marjoram, orange blossom, and ylang ylang over twenty-four hours.

The relaxing and comforting scents of India's vetiver and daphne (which the Chinese called the sleeping scent) have yet to be examined by science, but both have long historical use. Research may also find potential in primrose, orris root, and violets, which English herbalists once commonly used to treat nervous disorders such as anxiety and insomnia. Even dill seeds were tucked into potpourri pillows to encourage fussy babies to sleep.

Antidepressant, feel-good scents

According to Dr. Jeanette Haviland-Jones of Rutgers University, fragrant flowers have an immediate positive effect on our emotional well-being, with the ability to "trigger satisfaction, happiness, emotional bonds with others, and alleviate depression and anxiety." She calls peonies, roses, and other fragrant flowers fabulous mood-boosters. Scented blooms even increase innovative thinking and productivity in the workplace.

Stimulants and memory scents

Aromatherapy studies from Toho University School of Medicine in Tokyo determined that basil, clove, jasmine, and peppermint are very stimulating. Next in line are lemon grass, patchouli, rose, and sage. These scents prevent the sharp drop in concentration that typically occurs after thirty minutes of concentrated work. They are not as strong as

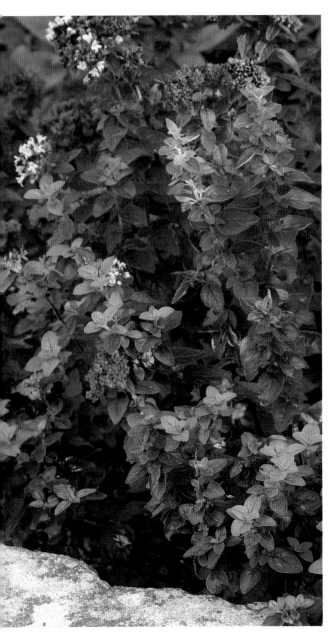

▲ Oregano may enhance feelings of well-being by affecting neurotransmitter activity.

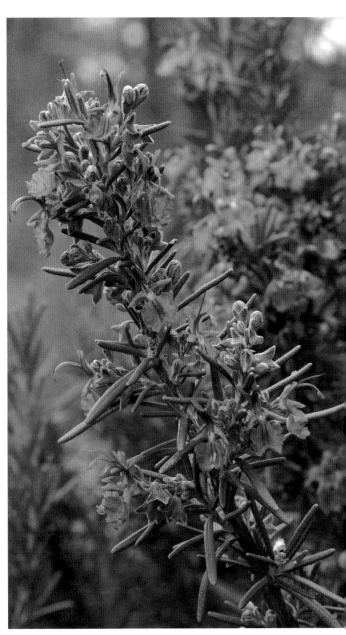

▲ "There's rosemary, that's for remembrance," said Ophelia in *Hamlet*.

drinking coffee, but also don't overstimulate adrenal glands.

The uplifting fragrances of basil, jasmine, peppermint, and rosemary appear to stimulate the brain's beta waves that focus mental activity, awareness, and alertness, and simply make a person feel good. They reduce stress and slow breathing by blocking stress-related nerve responses, but without depressing the nervous system. Mae Fah Luang University in Thailand and several other institutions found that air traffic controllers were more alert and computer operators made fewer errors and worked faster when workrooms were scented with either peppermint or eucalyptus.

The brain is imprinted with hundreds of specific scents that are attached to our personal memories. Events that are associated with our sense of smell are retained far longer and come back much quicker than memories that are connected to either sight or hearing. You probably have had at least one déja vu experience after taking a whiff of some familiar plant that whisked you back in time. You may vaguely remember your grandmother's house without prompting, but smell lilacs that she grew in her garden, and the memories come flooding back. Since memory is so tied to our sense of smell, past experiences also greatly influence whether we like or dislike a particular scent.

Psychologists call our association of smell with memory the Proust phenomenon, from Marcel Proust's novel *Remembrance of Things Past*. When the French novelist dipped a madeleine cookie in his lemon-blossom tea, the aroma brought back a flood of childhood memories, filling him with inexplicable happiness. Researchers hope to use this association to treat memory problems, even dementia and Alzheimer's disease. Strong, sharp scents such as bay laurel, jasmine, rosemary, and sage sharpen memory. Sage seems to slow short-term memory loss by blocking a brain messenger associated with memory loss. Sweet flag helps with learning and recalling facts by improving the functions of the central nervous system. Peppermint and lily-of-the-valley improve sustained concentration. In a 1992 study at the Bishop's University Department of Psychology in Lennoxville, Canada, volunteers memorized a list of words more easily if they smelled jasmine. When a study at Tottori University in Yonago, Japan, asked elderly individuals to sniff rosemary and lemon every morning and lavender and orange in the evening for one month, they had less memory loss. In aromatherapy lore, juniper counters mental fatigue, physical debility, and insomnia. The ancient Greeks found hyacinth and thyme to be invigorating and to improve memory. Europeans said that lilacs make you reminiscent. To help remember some important fact, sniff one of these plants while you memorize it. When the time comes to recall that information, smell that scent again.

▶ A brick entry greets visitors with a riot of roses and other blooms.

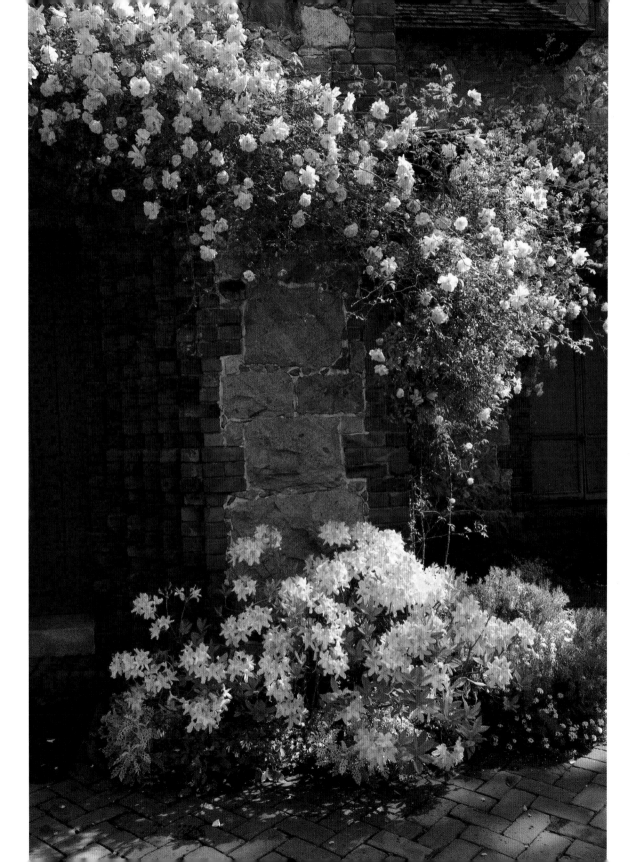

THE PASSION BEHIND SCENT

The sense of smell is not the same in both sexes. Women will usually recognize a scent more readily than men, especially food aromas. They take more time to consider scents that they prefer and can readily describe them. Men, on the other hand, do not pick out scents as easily and have little to say about them.

Aroma can definitely alter an attraction to another person. Men see women differently if the males smell a perfume they like. For one thing, they will estimate a women's weight around four to twelve pounds lighter. Researchers say that the reaction of both sexes to scent is probably hormonal, since the sense of smell declines in women taking testosterone shots.

Fragrant aphrodisiacs

Men and women are attracted to different scents. Studies show that what turns on women are licorice and cucumber scents, followed by lavender. Men are also responsive to licorice and lavender, and in much higher numbers than women. Licorice-scented plants in the fragrance garden are anise hyssop and fennel, which are added to some perfumes and colognes in small amounts. It is no surprise that chocolate is also on the list for women, bringing to mind the chocolate-scented clematis, geranium, and peppermint plants. By the way, what women do *not* care for is the scent of cherry.

Men found pumpkin pie spice to be the most stimulating aroma of all. Its overriding scent is cinnamon, a well-known aphrodisiac historically. The strongest cinnamon scents in the fragrance garden are found in cinnamon

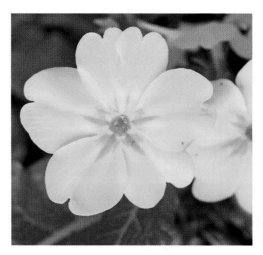

▲ Primrose contains a trace of cinnamon scent, which is favored by men.

basil and sweet flag, both aphrodisiac fragrances that are used in perfume. Garden plants that hint at cinnamon are primrose, some scented geraniums, and the white-flowering wisteria cultivar 'Alba'. Men like their cinnamon, licorice, lavender, and cola scents combined with the smell of doughnuts, but it's not entirely clear how one would match that in the garden! Pumpkin pie spice also contains clove, which was discussed earlier as a known relaxant, and is a popular scent in men's colognes.

Older men and women of any age favor vanilla scents. Women particularly find the vanilla-like scent of baby powder appealing. Vanilla-scented plants are clematis, dried sweet woodruff, oleander, and the softly fragranced, modern-day wallflower. Wisteria flowers also carry a note of vanilla. Women are generally more receptive to men's advances if there are aromatic flowers nearby, say University of South Brittany psycholo-

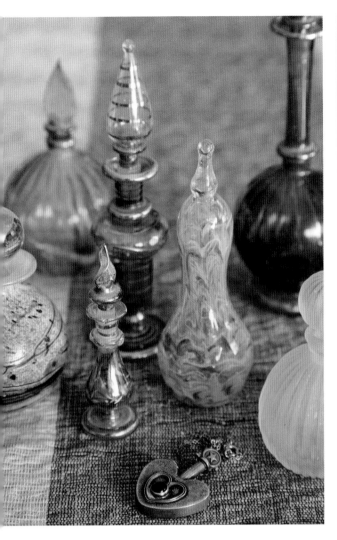

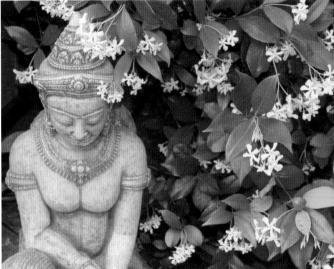

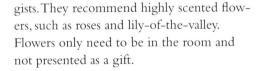

gists. They recommend highly scented flowers, such as roses and lily-of-the-valley. Flowers only need to be in the room and not presented as a gift.

Plant-inspired perfume

It is no secret, with perfume brand names such as Tabu, My Sin, Opium, Perhaps, Shocking de Schiaparelli, Poison, and Sexual, that personal fragrance has long been all about sex appeal. Like most perfume, these well-known scents are based on plants that have age-old reputations as aphrodisiacs. Jasmine, labdanum, orange blossom, patchouli, rose, sweet flag, tuberose, and vetiver were originally made into exotic, solid perfumes that predated the modern alcohol-based products. Coriandre perfume by Jean Couturier for Women is based on the spicy coriander seed, which was an aphrodisiac mentioned in *The Arabian Nights*. Cardamom is another well-known aphrodisiac spice that finds its way into modern perfume. It was a key ingredient in ancient Egypt's once-famous *kyphi* perfume, as well as another traditional fragrance from India in which it is blended with coriander, jasmine, basil, and cloves. Many perfumes have been inspired by lily-of-the-valley, or *muguet* in French, including Christian Dior's Diorissimo. Gardenia is the foundation for at least fifty perfumes. Popular for nearly one hundred years, My Sin and Arpege are a few of the many perfumes based on jasmine.

Today, in addition to all the traditional plants used for fragrance, fruity-violet mignonette, daffodils, and a few strongly scented bee balm species are also cultivated for the perfume industry. A small hint of a potent scent (such as clary sage, curry plant, lemon marigold, or santolina) give high-end perfumes a fragrant boost. Among contemporary popular scents, lavender is the star of Chanel Jersey; orange blossom is integral to Dolce & Gabbana Velvet Sublime and Elie Saab Le Parfum; and Roberto Cavalli Paradiso combines notes of bergamot, jasmine, and cypress.

Cologne is a lighter version of perfume. It often contains at least one aphrodisiac aroma, but it tends to be less floral than perfume and more herbal, spicy, or woodsy. It often contains cloves, cedarwood, or juniper. The original eau de cologne from the seventeenth century was orange blossoms, bergamot, lavender, lemon balm, and rosemary. The tuberous earthnut sweet pea is sometimes used in cologne. Tobacco gives cologne a dry, masculine scent with a heavy base note, for its musty appeal.

fragrance garden history

The gardens of antiquity were heavy with fragrance. Persian palaces, Egyptian temples, Roman villas, and European estates and monasteries were all based on formal garden design. A garden that was constructed with a geometric design and filled with aromatic plants was considered especially tranquil. Tall walls surrounded the gardens, creating a retreat from the outside world and inspiring inward reflection. The walls also served to capture the fragrance of the plants contained within. Aromatic trees were an important source of medicine, spiritual inspiration, and shade, so they were often grown in the fragrance garden or an adjoining area. Through most of garden history, fragrant gardens were thought able to ward off illness. A sixteenth-century poem tells of a walled garden with benches and arbors; it is so sweetly fragrant, it counters disease.

The fragrance garden was a place to seek peace and contemplation. Throughout Europe, the Middle East, and India, gardens were considered a perfumed heaven on earth where one could purify the soul. The plants in these gardens held important religious symbolism that was often associated with their aromas. Their fragrance was said to be able to transform raw emotion into religious passion. This transference was considered possible in the garden because passion for both worldly desires and spiritual development were associated with scent.

Aromatic gardens for love and beauty

Scented gardens also have their secular side. Most often the garden's theme turned to love, romance, and even passion. The plants grown in a fragrance garden were often the same ones found in a religious garden, but their scents carried new symbolism. Favorites, such as the rose, were able to span the

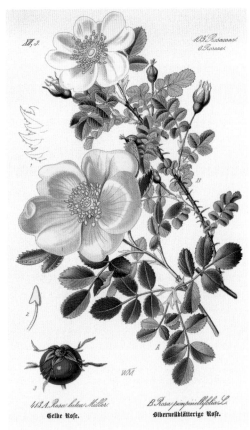

III. 3.

103. Rosaceae.
6. Roseae.

B

A

413.A. Rosa lutea Miller.
Gelbe Rose.

B. Rosa pimpinellifolia L.
Bibernellblätterige Rose.

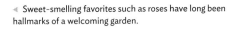
◄ Sweet-smelling favorites such as roses have long been hallmarks of a welcoming garden.

wife in the seventh century BC. Sennacherib described the highest platform that imitated the Amanus Mountains, with "all kinds of aromatic plants, orchard fruit trees, trees that enrich not only mountain country but also Babylonia."

Fragrance captivated ancient Greece and Rome. Sailors said they knew when they were approaching the Greek isle of Rhodes because the fragrance of rose wafted over the sea. An entire street in Capua, Italy, devoted to manufacturing scented products like rosewater was said to be thick with heady fragrances. Greek and Roman gardens were dedicated to their gods and goddesses, so they contained the bay laurel, lilies, myrtle, and narcissus that were associated with such mythology. Their gardens were also scented with chamomile, oleander, violet, and roses. The fragrant herbs they grew were hyssop, juniper, lemon balm, mugwort, orris root, mint, pennyroyal, and rue for use as culinary herbs and medicine. The many aromatic spices cultivated in these classical gardens included basil, coriander, dill, fennel, marjoram, oregano, sage, wormwood, and thyme. Pliny the Younger chose aromatic rosemary hedges to surround his garden at his coastal villa because they tolerated wind and sea exposure better than the common boxwood hedge.

It seems that gardeners have always been fascinated with acquiring new plants. Botanical exploration for fragrant plants led Egyptian queen Hatshepsut to send an expedition

spiritual and common nature of the individual, so they found a welcome home in both types of gardens.

Perhaps the most famous ancient gardens that were constructed for love are the Hanging Gardens of Babylon. They are usually credited to Nebuchadnezzar II, but according to Oxford scholar Stephanie Dalley, they may have been the gardens that surrounded the Nineveh palace in modern-day Iraq. These elevated gardens were built by Assyrian king Sennacherib for his beloved to Punt—possibly Somali—around 1500 BC. Her boats carrying fragrant myrrh trees for her garden are depicted on a wall relief at her temple on the Nile's west bank at Deir el-Bahari. These trees were said to have eventually grown to a good height, thanks to their roots being carefully wrapped for the voyage. As the collection expanded, Egyptian gardens became botanical showplaces. A mural in the Botanical Garden room at the fourteenth-century temple of Amun at Karnak in Egypt illustrates two hundred fifty species that were grown in that temple's twenty-six gardens. They included all kinds of beautiful flowers and aromatic spices, such as cumin, marjoram, anise, and coriander.

Much of garden history corresponds with the conquest of new territory. King Ramses III had pots of exotic trees and flowers shipped back to Egypt from his army's twelfth-century BC conquests in Libya, Syria, and Cyrenia. Alexander the Great sent plants from lands that he conquered in the fourth century BC to his tutor, Aristotle, to establish a botanical garden outside of Athens, Greece.

Monastery gardens

The Romans brought fennel, rue, rosemary, southernwood, sage, and thyme to British gardens during their conquest. When they left Britain, the aromatic herbs remained. The Damask rose, and probably jasmine and lilac, are fragrant plants that arrived in medieval Europe when crusaders returned from the Middle East. Roman emperor Charlemagne decreed around AD 800 that all of the monasteries and estates under his extensive reign in Europe should grow eighty-nine herbs and trees listed in the *Capitulare de villis vel curtis imperialis*. This list was likely compiled by the French abbot Benedict of Aniane, who was already exchanging garden plants with Alcuin, the abbot of Tours and one of Charlemagne's advisors. Alcuin was known for his beautiful lilies and gallica roses, which were included on the mandatory list, along with other aromatics such as coriander, dill, fennel, juniper berries, mint, pennyroyal, and rue. The *De naturis rerum* by Alexandri Neckam notes in 1210 that Londoners were growing fragrant flowers such as heliotrope, lilies, roses, and violets in their private gardens.

Dominican monk Albertus Magnus specified in 1260 that gardens should have "a great diversity of medicinal and scented herbs, not only to delight the senses by their perfume, but to refresh the sight with their flowers." He described gardens containing "every sweet smelling herb such as rue, and sage, and basil, and likewise, all sorts of flowers, as the violet, columbine, lily, rose, iris, and the like . . ." German herbalist Hildegard von Bingen (1098–1179) grew all of these in her cloister garden, plus catnip, chamomile, clary sage, myrtle, oregano, tansy, thyme, valerian, and yarrow. She recommended the scents of fennel, rose, violet, and wormwood to counter depression, and spike lavender to improve one's disposition.

The medieval monastery herb gardens, or herbaries, contained aromatic plants intended to nurture the soul and provide

▶ A Celtic garden of fragrant herbs and flowers. Stone carving by Martin Akerstone.

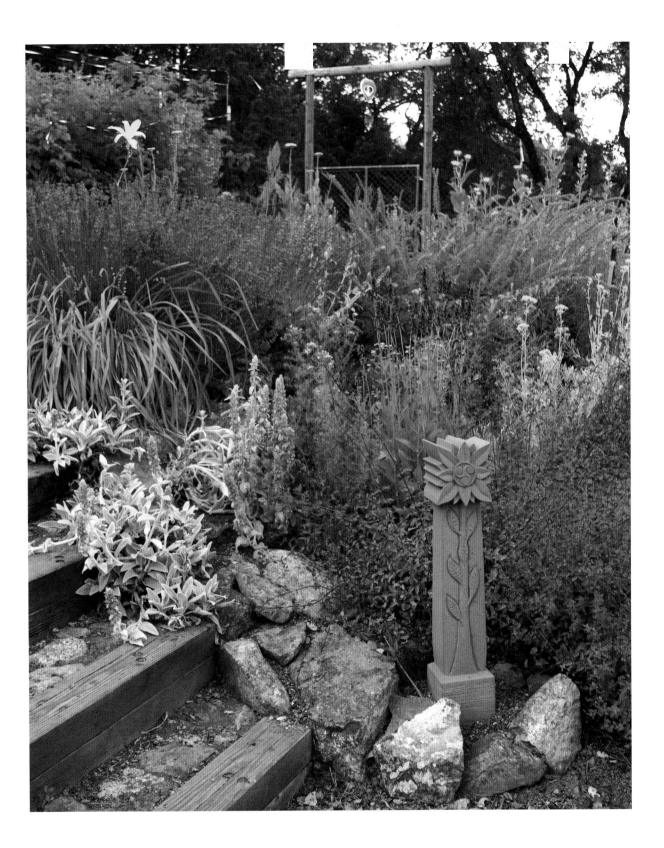

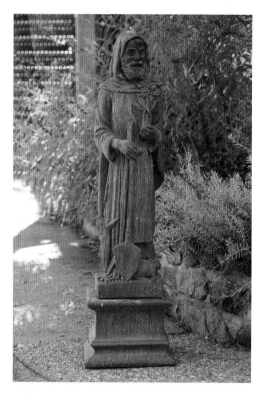
▲ Saint Fiacre, patron saint of herb gardens.

European tapestries made around 1500 hang at The Cloisters museum. In the most famous panel, a unicorn is portrayed in the middle of an informal meadow filled with highly scented flowers. Such fields were referred to as millefleurs, or "a thousand flowers." Eighty-five of the plants on the tapestries were identified by two botanists. These include the fragrant flowers of clove pink, Madonna lily, and violets.

Gardens of delight

The late Middle Ages saw spirituality give way to pleasure and sensuality in the European garden. Arbors of fragrant roses, representing both love and religious devotion, concealed intimate seats where one could play music, embroider, contemplate, or be romantic amidst the fragrance. Part of the medieval love poem *Roman de la Rose* by Guillaume de Lorris takes place in a walled garden like this. He describes lovers meeting where "the earth was very artfully decorated and painted with flowers of various colors and sweetest perfumes." The garden's design stayed formal, but the walls surrounding it were lowered to see the world beyond. Boccaccio, in his book of tales, *The Decameron*, describes a fourteenth-century garden in which "the sides of these walks were almost closed in with jasmine and red and white roses, so that it was possible to walk in the garden in a perfumed and delicious shade." The inner lawn, which was bordered by orange trees, "pleased the sense of smell."

The New World had its own spectacular fragrance garden. In 1519, Bernal Diaz del Castillo arrived from Spain to the Aztec capital of present-day Mexico City as a Spanish

herbal remedies. Benedictine, Chartreuse, and similar liqueurs were flavored with dozens of aromatic medicinal herbs that were grown by the monks. Monastery gardens were filled with symbolic plants. They often had an alcove dedicated to the Virgin Mary that was overflowing with the fragrant flowers associated with her, such as lily-of-the-valley, roses, and violets.

Fifty of the plants in the Trie Cloister garden—at The Cloisters museum, part of the Metropolitan Museum of Art in New York—were chosen from those displayed on famous tapestries titled "The Hunt of the Unicorn." These lavishly woven, plant-dyed

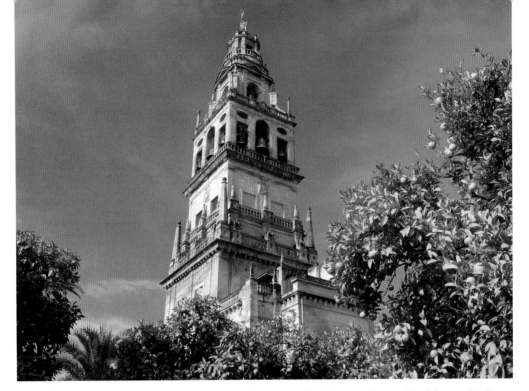

foot soldier. He was amazed to see the city covered in beautiful floating and rooftop gardens. In *The True History of the Conquest of New Spain*, he wrote, "I was never tired of looking at the diversity of trees, and noting the scent each one had and the paths full of roses and flowers."

Zahir-ud-din Muhammed, a descendant of Gengis Khan known as Babur, was interested in literature, art, music, and gardening. He established gardens in every Central Asian city he conquered in the early sixteenth century. Babur was greatly influenced by the Persian culture and its love of fragrant flowers, so he made sure that every garden in the Mughal dynasty that he established in India was filled with "sweet herbs and flowers of beautiful color and scent." One of his first acts as emperor was to have several gardens created in the city of Agra, which were followed by more gardens in other Indian cities. He personally designed landscaping for ten gardens in Kabul, Afghanistan. The most famous example of Mughal architecture, the Taj Mahal, was once surrounded by extensive gardens.

The Moors brought their passion for fragrant flowers, shade, and garden pools with them when they conquered Spain. Roses, carnations, jasmine, lilacs, lilies, narcissus, wallflowers, and orange tree flowers perfumed their gardens. A fragrant, trimmed myrtle hedge surrounds the Court of the Myrtles, at the medieval Alhambra palace and fortress in Granada, Spain. The tenth-century Mosque of Cordoba was renowned for its fragrant gardens. A well-known twelfth-century writer, Al-Fath Ibn Khaqan, described the breeze "blowing day and night over the garden loaded with scents." The Court of Oranges had orange trees planted in a sunken garden that was fifteen feet below the walkway. This allowed visitors to smell the pure aroma of neroli orange blossoms as it floated off the treetops.

In the seventeenth century, many women who had the means to do so put aside their embroidery and began botanizing and designing gardens as a hobby. The 1617 *Country Housewife's Garden* by William Lawson presented them with ideas for kitchen and flower gardens. He suggested that they plant rosemary, roses, and sage, among other plants. Even Josephine, the wife of the French emperor Napoleon Bonaparte, was an amateur botanist who brought nearly two hundred plants to France for the first time. Through France's conquests, she acquired rare species to grow in her garden. She commissioned Belgian botanical artist Pierre-Joseph Redouté to illustrate the flowers at her Chateau de Malmaison. He painted marvelous renditions of five hundred lilies and two hundred roses. Known for her beautiful roses, Josephine had several varieties named after her and properties, including the fragrant 'Souvenir de la Malmaison'.

Under the influence of Louis XV's Marquise de Pompadour, plants in her eighteenth-century garden at the rustic hermitage at Versailles were arranged by scent, so that one heavenly smell led to another. An avid gardener who loved fragrance, the Marquise had lemon trees, gardenias, jasmines, myrtles, tuberoses, oleanders, lilacs, and fifty orange trees planted in straight avenues with trellised walkways leading to the rose bowers.

Fragrance gardens enter the modern world

The expanding imperialism of nineteenth-century Britain brought exotic plants from the far reaches of the world into British gardens. The country style garden took off and gentry who had the time and money to garden raised splashy displays of fragrant flowers. Scented geraniums and orchids were kept in large, glass houses that were made possible by advances in steel and glass manufacturing. Thanks to the invention of cast plate glass in 1848, large sheets of inexpensive, strong glass were used to build the Crystal Palace for the 1851 World Exhibition in London. My great-great-grandfather, Jesse Keville, was a gardener in London at that time. In his memoirs, he recounted how impressed he was by the advancements in gardening technology that were displayed at the exhibition.

The home gardener needed a supply of seeds, and the R. K. Bliss & Sons seed company led the way, offering nearly seven hundred varieties of flowers in their full-color seed catalog. By the turn of the twentieth century, there were about eight hundred seed companies in the United States alone. A growing middle class rolled up their sleeves, grabbed shovels, and set to work planting colorful, fragrant gardens. A renewed appreciation of flowers developed as more potted plants and bouquets were brought into the house. Specially designed pots for tuberose plants, which grow in low light conditions, became popular in Victorian parlors. Books were written about the symbolic folklore of fragrant flowers.

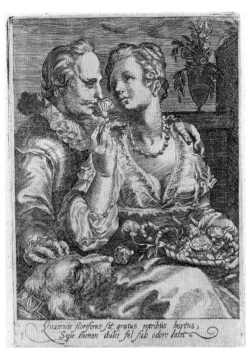

◄ A sixteenth-century depiction of the importance of floral fragrance.

▼ Scented geraniums were kept in glass houses (early greenhouses) in the nineteenth century.

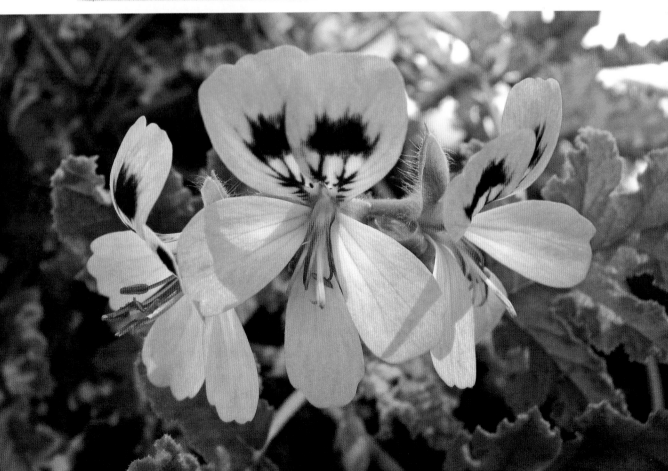

designing with the nose in mind

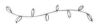

Your fragrance garden deserves to look as beautiful as it smells. Why not create a paradise that is a sensory feast; a work of art in which nature becomes your canvas? A garden is a three-dimensional environment. The angles, views, and scents change from one moment to the next as you walk along, experiencing everything from different perspectives. Colors and scents provide constant variations for never-ending interest.

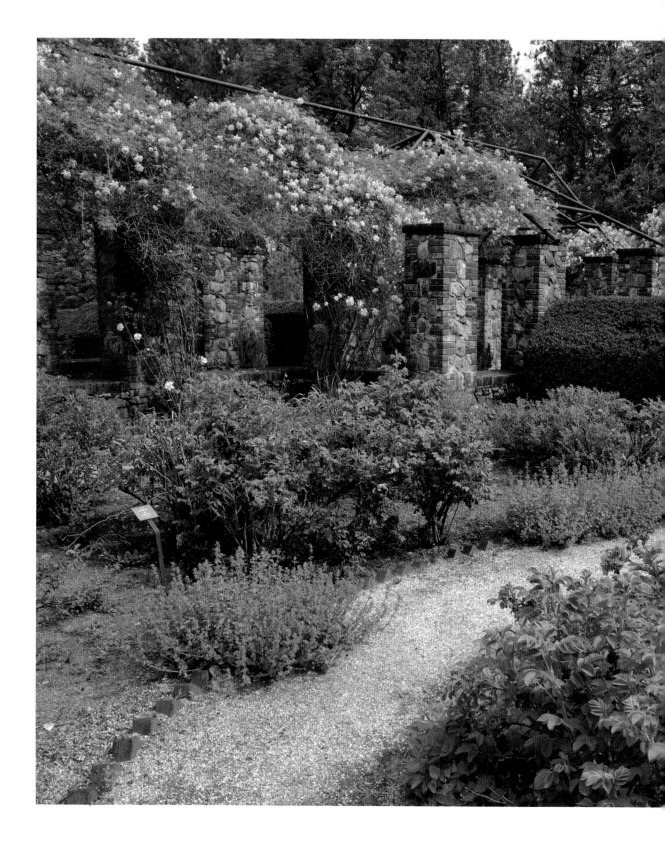

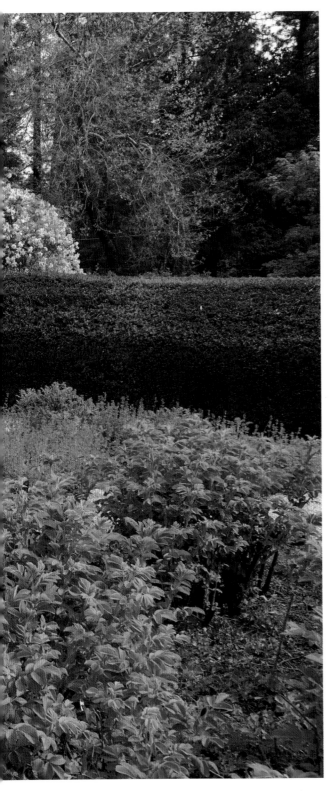

Design inspiration for a fragrance garden can come from many sources: gardens you visit, an idea in a book, garden societies, artwork, and nature herself. The time spent visualizing details for a new garden is worth it. Although most plants flower for only a limited time each year, your garden can be designed to present color and scent through the seasons. The result is a haven that touches all the senses with color, texture, aromas, and the songs of birds that can't resist your garden any better than the humans it delights.

As you think about design, try to visualize what the garden visitor will encounter from the pathway in different seasons and times of day. Plants do not bloom all at once, so pay attention to their blooming cycles when mixing, matching, and contrasting color and scent. Keep it fun. After decades of gardening, I am still experimenting with new ideas; moving and replacing plants.

Fragrance gardens have a way of looking and smelling good no matter how they are planted, although a few design rules can be helpful. I rely on design concepts that I learned in art school. The approach is the same whether it is applied to painting, sculpture, photography, or gardening. It is about contrasting or blending colors, shadows, forms, and depth of field. The goal is to have these elements play off each other so that the eye is constantly engaged.

◄ A well-designed fragrance garden is one that beckons all the senses.

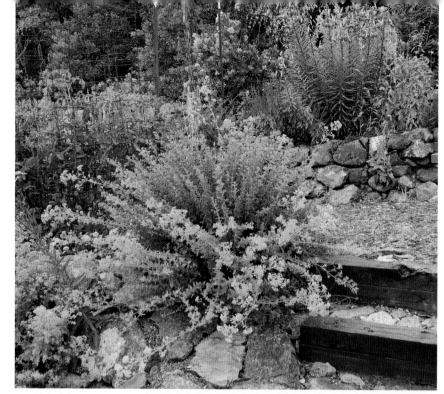

▶ Oregano fans over a wall and steps; lilies
bloom in the background.

▼ Artemisia ground cover and rosemary
line a pathway.

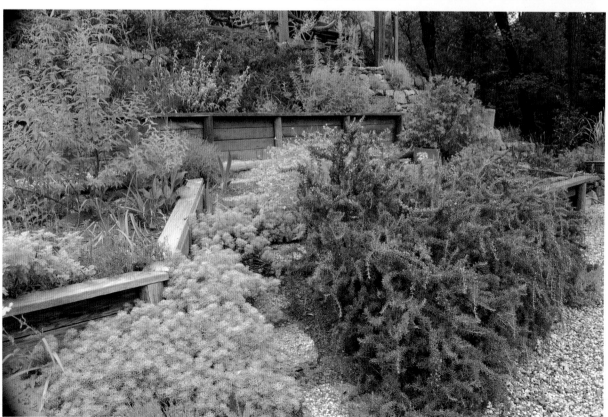

garden styles

A garden's style gives it personality. The placement of color, form, texture, and scent can make it seem orderly or random. Think of these style concepts as guidelines. Feel free to mix and match by borrowing your favorite elements from different garden styles. One of my gardens has a central pathway going up a hill with stone wall terraces on either side. This is a formal design, except that the width of the beds varies and the rounded corners of the walls slope down to blend into the ground. The result is an organic feel that still maintains a sense of order. My informal garden has two pathways running somewhat parallel to each other. A border of tall plants along the pathways makes it unclear where you are headed. Although you can hear the waterfall from everywhere, it is a surprise when you reach it.

The formal fragrance garden

A formal garden design divides beds into a symmetrical grid that is composed of geometric shapes. It uses squares, rectangles, triangles, or circles, or any combination of these. These shapes can also intersect with each other into a more complex garden design. This is the easiest type of garden to design because it follows simple, repeating patterns. The plants are well-spaced. In the most elaborate versions, they are tightly trimmed into geometric forms. There is often statuary or a large, potted plant at the center to catch the eye.

Here, scented plants are carefully positioned so that each one is encountered individually while walking along a pathway or sitting on a bench. Historic gardens in Europe, India, and the Middle East are based on this type of formal design. The orderliness of a formal garden is considered to be very peaceful and meditative; thoughtful placement of fragrant plants can enhance that experience. It is all easily comprehended and offers no surprises.

The fragrant cottage garden

At the other end of the spectrum is the more organic cottage garden. In this informal style, pathways meander about. Fragrance comes into play by placing a scented surprise around a bend, such as a spectacular angelica plant. Art, bird feeders, and hanging planters are placed wherever space allows. Plantings are tight, with groupings of mixed flowers to produce a riot of scent and color that indulges the senses. This style is more outgoing than a formal garden. It feels energizing and exciting and inspires creativity and accomplishment. Claude Monet's famous garden at Giverny is a cottage-style garden.

The fragrant Asian garden

In the classical Asian garden, form is paramount. Rocks, stones, sand, and nature-inspired artwork are positioned with intent. Aromatic plants are separated to make sure each individual fragrance is appreciated. Flowers are greatly prized, especially in Japan, but Asian gardens favor longer-living, scented shrubs to represent permanence and stability. Ancient China devoted entire gardens solely to cultivating jasmine, for scenting perfume, wine, tea, food, and garlands.

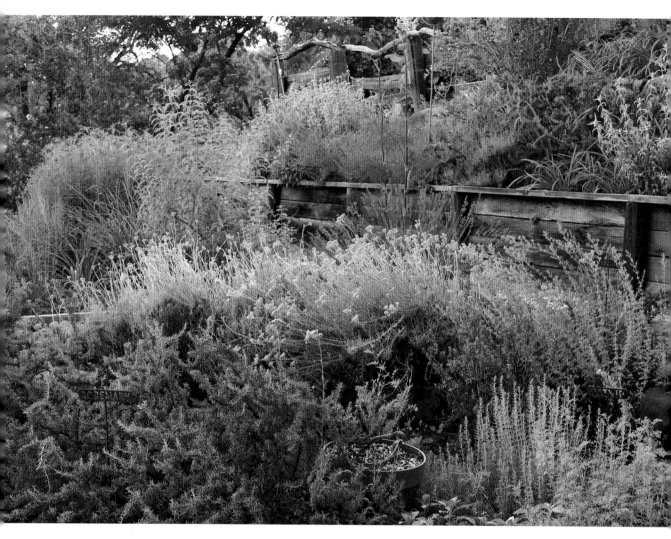

The Japanese garden flows in a free-form style, yet is very orderly and clean, with large expanses that highlight each feature. Rather than being symmetrical, repeating patterns of color and form create a sense of formality and peace. You can find Japanese gardens at a number of botanical gardens. Some beautiful examples in the United States are at the Huntington Botanical Gardens in Pasadena, California, and the botanical gardens in Brooklyn and Denver.

The fragrant border garden

Border gardens are mainly used to edge a main path, driveway, lawn, or patio. They can also be borders for other gardens; for example, bringing color and scent to the perimeter of a vegetable garden. Since these borders are often closest to visitors, they offer an ideal location for fragrant plants. Plants are typically tightly planted, creating a wonderful blend of fragrance.

◀ Raised beds filled with rosemary, curry plant, wormwood, lavender, lemon verbena, and a selection of salvias.

▼ Freesia lends bold spring fragrance.

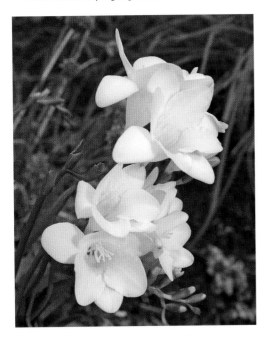

planning for scent

A garden that is filled with fragrant plants creates a complex aromatic blend that becomes the garden's own signature perfume. Scent is as much a part of the design as visual appeal. Fragrances can be contrasted or mixed much like colors. In a garden, the nose is attracted by a scent and lingers on it, then a breeze picks up another fragrance or you brush against a different plant that delightfully distracts you with another aroma. At other times, it seems like the entire garden chimes in to create a symphony of fragrance.

Mixing and matching

Fragrant plants that are grown closely together merge into a potpourri of scent to delightfully overload the senses. However, try to place strongly aromatic plants that have similar fragrances and bloom around the same time in different areas of the garden. That way, the scent of plants like jasmine, honeysuckle, and tuberose can be appreciated individually.

Strongly fragrant flowers

The most potent garden aromas come from flowers that call out to pollinators to pick up their scent. These flowers broadcast intense fragrance throughout the garden and beyond. You can create a succession of blooms that drench the garden in scent for months; to do so, plant wintersweet and daphne for their winter flowers, and violet, freesia, and lilac to follow. Early summer bloomers are jasmine, lilies, tuberose, and flowering tobacco. Late summer brings trumpet flowers, which are followed by lemon and orange trees. Clematis and honeysuckle flower in spring, summer, or fall, depending upon the species, to fill in any aromatic gaps. It makes a heady combination, but these plants could be planted together in the same spot to create an aphrodisiac-themed garden.

Blooms with a less-intense scent

Many flowers are not so overbearing, but still create an aura of fragrance around them. They blend together, but the blend is subtle and the predominant scent shifts as you move from plant to plant. Even when these plants are in the same area of the garden, it is still possible to detect the distinct aroma of each. To have a succession of light fragrance, begin with the well-matched scented blooms of daffodil, hyacinth, and lily-of-the-valley in early spring. Next come the sweet peas, phlox, stocks, and wallflowers of midspring; this is a traditional combination in the cottage-style garden. Carnation and gardenia bloom in early summer. The midsummer scent of clary sage and Mexican marigold in late summer join this mix, although their topmost leaves smell stronger than their flowers. Just lightly brushing against these plants on a hot day releases their aromas.

Fragrant leaves

Most aromatic leaves are much more private than flowers about their fragrance, preferring to keep it to themselves unless they are lightly rubbed. They only scent the air around them on a very hot day. Many plants that have fragrant leaves are in the mint family, including lemon balm, marjoram, oregano, peppermint, spearmint, sage, and thyme. They are joined in the fragrance garden by anise hyssop, bee balm, lemon verbena, scented geranium, and wintergreen. Since these scents do not interfere with each other, the entire group can be planted together as an aromatic herb garden. Trees and shrubs often have fragrant leaves that need to be broken, rather than rubbed, to fully enjoy their scent; examples are rockrose and juniper shrubs, and the bay laurel tree. Plants that have aromatic leaves are fragrant far longer than the few weeks allotted to most flowers. Leaf scent peaks as the plant goes into bloom, but

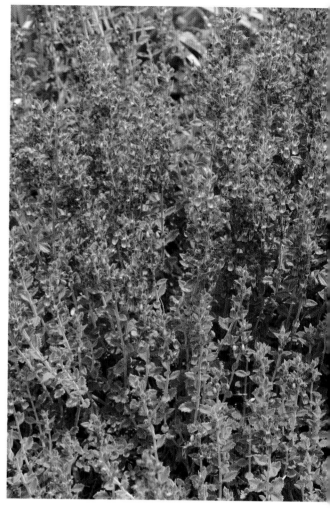

▲ Marjoram's leaves offer a spicy scent.

leaves typically keep their fragrance throughout the growing season, and in the warmest regions, throughout the year. They also tend to smell herby instead of floral. This is because their aroma performs a different job, deterring bugs rather than attracting them as pollinators.

plants as design elements

A fragrance garden delights the eye as well as the nose. The colors and visual textures of flowers, leaves, and hardscaping materials can be contrasted to better define an area, or closely matched so they seem to blend together.

Color in the fragrance garden

Flowers offer the brightest garden colors, managing to successfully pull off combinations that most of us would never dream of combining in our wardrobe. This makes the job of landscape design easier, since there are few bad color combinations in nature. Like scent, color creates different moods. The way we see color is also influenced by fragrance. For example, the University of Montpellier in France discovered that lemon-yellow color appears warmer when a lemony aroma is smelled at the same time.

Green represents tranquility, balance, and healing. When your eyes are strained, take a break in the garden to focus on green. If you are creating a fragrance garden devoted to healing, choose green plants used in aromatherapy and herbal medicine, such as angelica, holy basil, bay laurel, fennel, lemon balm, lemon grass, oregano, peppermint, rosemary, and thyme. These can be accented with the soothing scents of roses, rosemary, scented geranium, and perhaps a lemon or orange tree.

Light-colored flowers and leaves Flowers and leaves in hues of white, silver, and gray pop out, especially against deep green foliage. They produce a peaceful feeling of coolness.

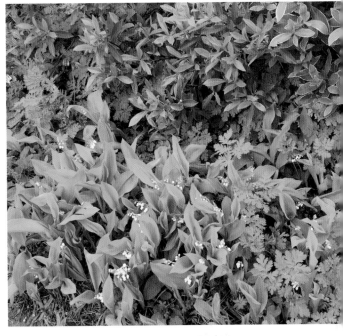

▲ Lily-of-the-valley and daphne offer their tranquil green hues.

They seem to glow in low light, making them ideal for an evening garden that is viewed under the moonlight—or a peace, prayer, or meditation garden scented with the calming fragrances of white-flowering lavender and white lilies. Or choose the stark white flowers of angelica, chamomile, flowering tobacco, gardenia, jasmine, orris root, rockrose, or tuberose. Gray catnip, curry plant, lamb's ears, lavender, santolina, and wormwood can provide additional soothing scents. Yellow flowers, such as those of Mexican marigold and yellow freesia, lilies, roses, and wallflowers stand out in the garden during the day and at dusk. So do the yellow-green leaves of lemon balm, lemon verbena, and lemon tree. Variegated daphne,

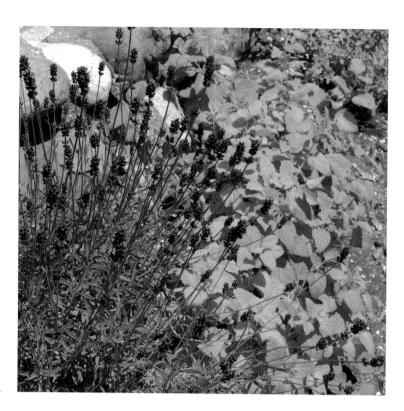

▶ Lavender flowers and leaves are contrasted with the yellow-green of lemon balm.

lemon balm, myrtle, orange mint, rue, sage, scented geranium, thyme, and the multi-colored leaves of southernwood provide their own contrast, which is enhanced next to any solid-colored leaves. Yellow and green colors make an ideal combination for a fragrance garden that is devoted to relaxed focus and concentration, as do the aromas of lemon-scented plants and bay, rosemary, rockrose, sage, peppermint, and lily-of-the-valley.

Bright-colored flowers Bright orange, red, and pink are showy colors found mostly in flowers and berries. The flowers of pineapple sage, red-flowering freesias, pansies, flowering tobaccos, roses, and scented geraniums all brightly decorate the garden. Sunlight highlights vivid colors, while dappled light creates flashy patterns. In fact, bright

summer sunlight can wash out all but red and orange colors. If you spend much time in your garden, these colors remain high-profile until dusk, when they blend into the green foliage. Lively colors give the garden warmth and a sense of energy, motivation, well-being, and even passion. They are perfect for a lovers' garden, with plenty of fragrant red roses—perhaps on an arbor covering a partially concealed bench. They could also surround an art studio or a patio that is intended for daytime garden parties. For energetic aromas, plant fennel, peppermint, or eucalyptus next to plants with intense colors.

Flowers and leaves with deeper hues Dark blue flowers tend to not be as fragrant as those from the other side of the color wheel. The deeper blues and purples are

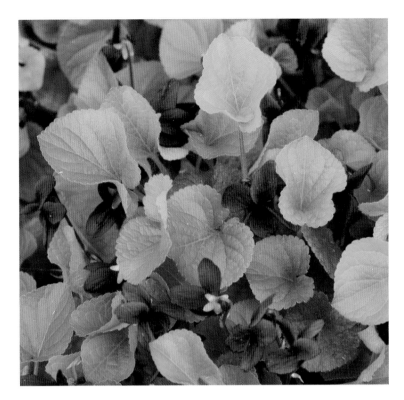

◀ Richly colored violets delight the senses of sight and smell.

more visible in mixed plantings when contrasted with white, pink, or vivid colors. Blue, purple, and deep blue-gray colors easily lose their definition and clarity, especially from a distance or in the low light of a cloudy day or the evening. Purple and especially blue flowers and leaves evoke a cool, relaxed feeling. The purples of the flowers of anise hyssop, lavender, lilac, violets, and pansies are not as vivid as red-flowering plants, but they still look dramatic and have relaxing fragrances. The leaves of purple basil, bronze fennel, honeysuckle 'Repens', and blue-green rue make bold statements. Violets and lavender, with their purple flowers, could surround a bench set into an alcove and covered with honeysuckle or a small chamomile lawn. A hammock could be tucked in among the

lilac shrubs with violets and pansies planted underneath.

Shadows and texture in garden design

Texture and shadow also shape a fragrance garden. The flat, shiny leaves of bay laurel, lemon, and myrtle are noticeable because they reflect light, especially when they seem to be wet.

Dark shadows absorb light. The crinkled leaves of patchouli and scented geraniums as well as the feathery leaves of dill, fennel, and yarrow create small shadows that define them. Angelica, clary sage, and trumpet flower provide contrasting shadows with their impressively large leaves. They make the garden seem more expansive, while highlighting brighter plants. Shrubs and trees in and around the garden can be

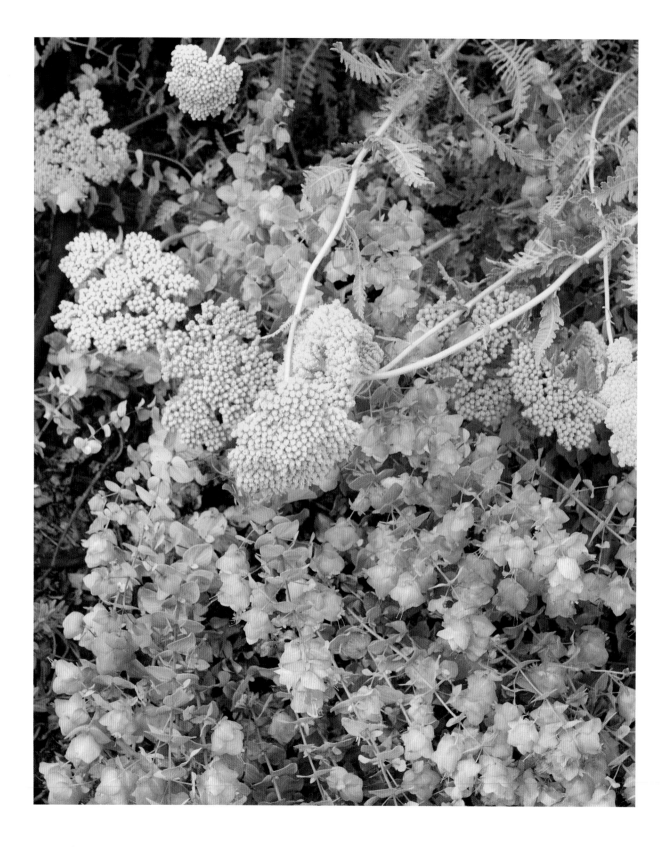

thinned to create more shadows that increase this effect.

Shapes contribute to garden design, such as the heart-shaped leaves of spikenard and violet, the interesting whorled leaves of sweet woodruff, and a variety of maple shapes on scented geraniums. There are the spear-shaped leaves of lemon grass, orris root, palmarosa, sweet flag, vetiver, and lily for contrast. Another way contrast can work in design is to set off an airy plant structure (such as that of lemon verbena) from a tightly formed habit (as with the bay laurel tree).

Highs and lows

Plants also make a presence with height. Anything that rises above other plants draws attention. This can be achieved with shrubs, trees, trellises, raised beds, tall pots, and pots that hang or are elevated on stands. Formal gardens often surround a tall plant, such as a potted bay laurel, with much shorter plants. They also use topiaries, in which shapes are sculpted out of tight-growing shrubs. Topiaries make striking design elements, but they require a lot of maintenance.

Hedges add a band of height in the garden to create visual interest. They can surround the garden or divide it into portions. They can be allowed to grow loosely or be trimmed and sculpted once the plants are a few years old. Daphne and gardenia can create low-growing, fragrant hedges that allow you to see over the top. A short, informal hedge for the summer can be composed of curry plants, lavender, wormwood, or some

◄ Golden yarrow overlaying dittany of Crete.

sages. Juniper and large roses make taller barriers. A line of fennel will grow into a seasonal living fence that lasts from midsummer into autumn.

hardscaping your fragrance garden

The foundational element of hardscaping gives a garden character. It provides a framework for plants. Raised beds, walls, paths, sculptures, stone formations, and other landscape features define the placement of plants and allow you to create special, fragrant areas or theme beds. Mints, tansy, and other invasive, aromatic ramblers can be given their own small, contained beds or planters. Interesting additions such as birdbaths, sundials, or reflective gazing balls can lead the garden visitor to an especially fragrant grouping. A bench provides the opportunity to sit back and enjoy the garden's fragrance and design. Hardscaping also helps defines the garden throughout the year—even in winter, under a blanket of snow, the outlines of terraces and raised beds can be seen as a reminder of pleasant scents to come.

Thinking ahead

Start planning your garden by evaluating what is already on the site, to see what you need to work around and what can be altered. Ask yourself a series of questions. Do buildings, driveways, or other structures need to be camouflaged with plants? Does poor soil need to be replaced with healthy soil so that plants will be more lush and fragrant, or does a marshy area require drainage? Would a dirt mound, a sunken area, or a pool add interest? Can pathways and stepping-stones allow better access to fragrant plants? You do not have to know exactly where every plant will be placed, but it helps to have a basic game plan. Make sure the larger plants have deep enough beds. Determine how wind, sun, and shade from trees or buildings will affect plantings, and how hardscaping could be adjusted to accommodate plant needs.

It helps to at least loosely sketch design ideas. There are computer garden design programs and kits in which plants, beds, and garden features can be moved around to alter the design. To help visualize where pathways, raised beds, and walls should go, place strings between stakes of various heights. Use whatever props are on hand—pots, buckets, garbage cans and such—to designate spots for tall plants, garden features, and garden art. Once the hardscaping design is established, walk through it to envision it before making final decisions.

If your garden needs to be irrigated, decide where to place the water system. It is better to bury irrigation and electrical lines for watering, timers, lights, or greenhouse heating than to end up with a maze of hoses and wires. Consider lighting for special effects if you entertain in your garden at night or enjoy flowers that put on a show after dark. Use lights to showcase evening stars such as fragrant tobacco and night-blooming jasmine.

Terraces, walls, and raised beds

Raised beds elevate aromatic plants closer to nose level so you can better appreciate their fragrance. They also make cultivation and harvesting easier for gardeners who are in wheelchairs, are blind, or have trouble bending over. Raised beds provide better drainage and can be filled with improved soil that will provide more fragrant plants. They protect against gophers and moles if you place a barrier (hardware cloth, plywood, or other) underneath the bed.

Terraces, garden walls, and garden stairs can be built of wood, brick, natural or imitation stone, or poured cement; these design features make it possible to garden on a hill. They can highlight plants such as fragrant thyme and oregano that like to trail off the edge. Rock walls can curve and dip, and can have a seat or a recessed niche to hold an aromatic plant or artwork. Dry stack rock walls, which fit together without cement, can be built with small gaps between the rocks—perfect for inserting plants like thyme and mints.

Similar construction materials are generally used throughout a garden so that everything matches. Gray, white, pale yellow, and cream colors strongly contrast against the green hues of plants and give a garden more definition. Dark materials like black lava stone recede into the background, so are used against light plants or to cause an area to recede into the background. Green gravel and rock blend into the garden.

Down the garden path

Pathways define garden beds and make it easier to garden and get close to a particularly aromatic specimen. They can be designed in a formal grid, radiating from a center, or rambling through the garden. Place plants far enough from the pathway to

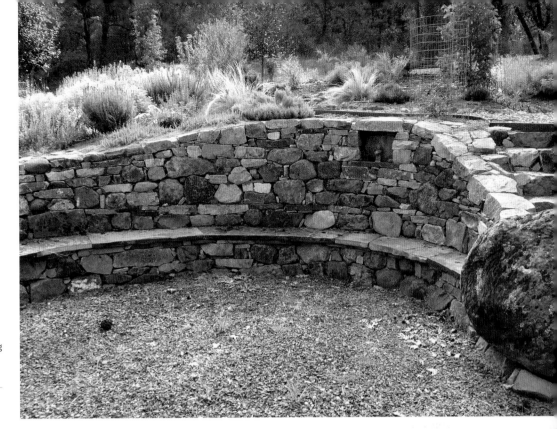

▶ Rockwork landscaping constructed by mason Ron Bertolucci.

▼ Thyme decorates a garden wall.

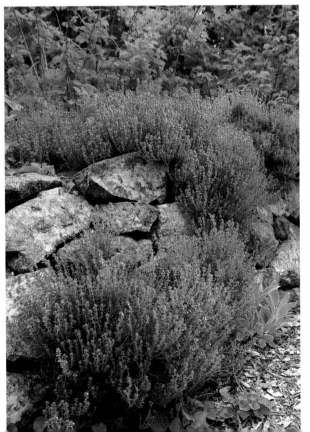

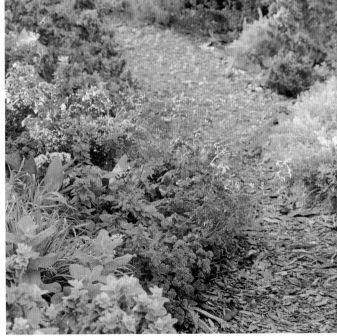

▲ Pathways can lead you from one garden fragrance to the next.

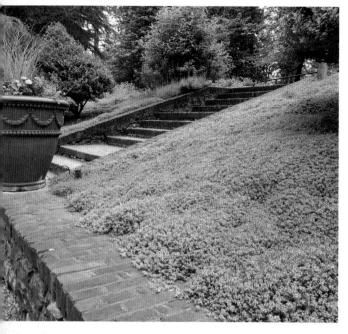

◁ A bank of flowering thyme.

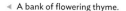

▷ This medieval-style bench has a seat of relaxing Roman chamomile. Bench designed and constructed by mason Ron Bertolucci.

allow unencumbered passage, unless you are going for an informal, jungle look. Stairs provide ease of access when a pathway has an elevation change. They can look artsy, but they need to have the same comfortable distance between each step to accommodate where the foot expects to land. Take the opportunity to edge stairs with low-growing aromatics like thyme and oregano. These have beautifully self-seeded among rocks that line stairs in my garden. Roman chamomile and other scented ground covers can also be grown on the stairs themselves, where they will scent the air with every step.

Gravel, sand, and wood chips make the easiest pathways. Brick, stone, cement forms, and poured cement are other choices. Avoid slippery or uneven materials that could cause someone to lose their footing. Take time to construct a pathway correctly. The area first needs to be flattened. Putting landscape cloth down greatly reduces weed growth. Do not use plastic sheeting; rain and irrigation water can pool and make the pathway muddy. A layer of fine, rough-edged gravel can be held in place by bricks, stones, or landscape edging. This border keeps gravel and wood chips from being kicked into the garden and looking unsightly (wood chips also make soil more acid, which can be a problem for alkaline-loving plants). The fine gravel is tamped in place to make a flat base on which to set final pathway material.

Scented lawns and ground covers Low-growing thyme, chamomile, and yarrow make wonderful scented pathways and lawns. These plants tolerate being walked on, although they do not do well in high-traffic areas. The best method is to place them around stepping-stones, where a few sprigs will be stepped on and the plants' scent will be released. Stepping-stones nicely accent plants. There are also driveway bricks with large holes designed to hold turf—these can be planted instead with herbs, for use as a pathway.

Benches

A bench is a thoughtful addition, providing the visitor or hard-working gardener a place to stop and smell the roses—and all the other wafting scents. Think about not only how seating looks in your garden, but the view from the seat. A strategically placed bench can showcase a particularly attractive view. Almost every fragrance garden has space for seating. In a small backyard garden, place a bench along a fence backed by flowering

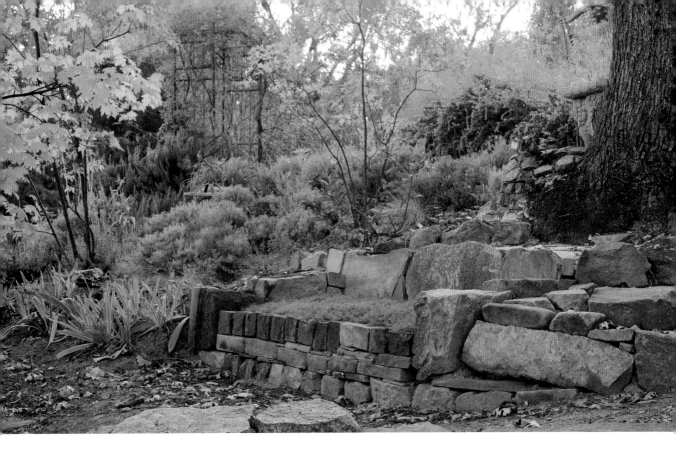

honeysuckle vines or climbing roses. Garden seats can also offer privacy when placed under an arbor or behind a garden screen.

    The scented bench A fragrant bench is made from stone to imitate a wooden bench. The seat itself is filled with garden soil and planted with a fragrant ground cover of Roman chamomile or mother of thyme, both of which are fairly tolerant of being sat upon. The plant's aroma surrounds those tarrying awhile on the bench. Such fragrant seating was once popular at European estates and monasteries, but few still exist. Chamomile was considered a relaxing scent, as well as a general healer of mind and body. The aroma of thyme was used to increase mental focus, reflection, and fortitude. I have a chamomile bench in my fragrance garden that overlooks plants and the pond beyond—a perfect location for reflection.

Garden backdrops

Fences, walls, and existing structures can be incorporated into landscaping to become deliciously scented backdrops. Honeysuckle, jasmine, roses, sweet peas, or wisteria can climb on trellises; large shrubs such as lilacs can form hedges. Fences can support potted plants or display artwork. Privacy screens made of lattice, a wall, or tall plants enclose the garden or break it into sections.

    Many aromatic plants actually need no fence at all. My fragrance garden contains sixty species that are untouched by deer. The plants in it, such as lavender, bay laurel, lemon verbena, and wormwood, taste too strong for a deer's palette. They have not touched the jasmine or honeysuckle, either. Arbors place the roses above a deer's reach. Aromatic plants whose leaves are less-intense smelling or tasting—such as phlox, stocks, violet, wallflower, and basil—are in a fenced garden, as deer do eat them. Deer also snip off flowers of lilies, and sometimes the blooms of Indian valerian.

themes in the fragrance garden

Sub-themes can be tucked into sections of your fragrant plot, or your entire garden may be made up of various fragrance themes. See the reference section of this book for a list of public fragrance-related theme gardens you can visit for inspiration.

A culinary treat of smells and tastes

The kitchen herb garden is harvested often, so it needs to be as practical to use as it is aromatic. Make the plants accessible with narrow beds or place stepping-stones to enter the garden without disturbing plant roots. You may want it close to your kitchen for easy access to fresh herbs, and to have spaces to set a harvest basket. The most important plants for a culinary garden are basil, bay laurel, coriander, dill, fennel, marjoram, oregano, rosemary, sage, and thyme. For more adventure-some dining, include lavender and at least one of the scented geraniums. These plants can be used fresh, or dry them for wintertime culinary delights.

Scented tea garden

Traditional Japanese and English tea gardens were designed for serving black tea, but why not have an herbal tea garden? It creates the perfect aromatic setting to entertain a friend or enjoy a good cup of tea made from herbs grown in your own garden. A tea garden does require a seat and a small table. Situate this garden close to your kitchen or a garden kitchen for convenience. Plant it with bee balm, lemon balm, lemon verbena, lemon grass, peppermint, rose, and wintergreen. You might also add jasmine, lavender, rose, and violet for their flowers, and a lemon tree for the fruit's peel. All of these plants make delicious, flavorful teas, as do combinations of them, so feel free to experiment with making your own garden blends. Equal parts works with most. I name my favorite aromatic tea blends—for example, "Naturally Glad" contains anise hyssop, lemon balm, lemon grass, peppermint, and rose petals.

Aromatherapy healing garden

This themed fragrance garden contains plants that are used therapeutically in aroma-therapy. The scents alone have beneficial effects on one's mood. Plants whose leaf scents are thought to create positive feelings include bay, coriander, clary sage, curry plant, juniper, lemon balm, lemon verbena, lemon grass, palmarosa, patchouli, scented gera-nium, and rosemary. Flower scents with such effects include jasmine, lavender, and rose. Seeds are also used, including angelica, dill, and fennel. Even roots get into the act, such as those of spikenard and vetiver, as well as the rhizomes of valerian. All of these plants

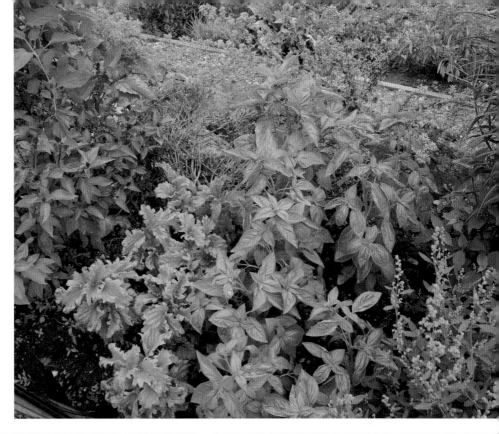

▶ Basil and other herbs thrive in this border bed.

▼ Lime thyme planted in a strawberry pot.

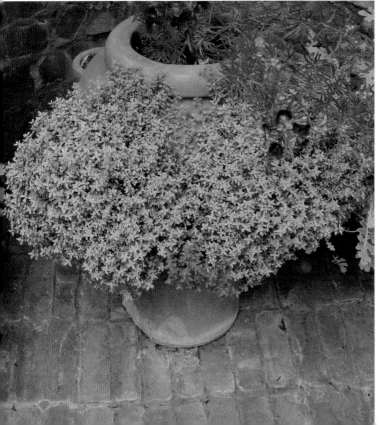

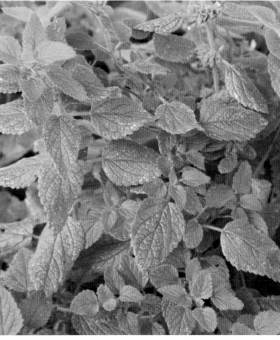

▲ Lemon balm makes a tasty cup of tea.

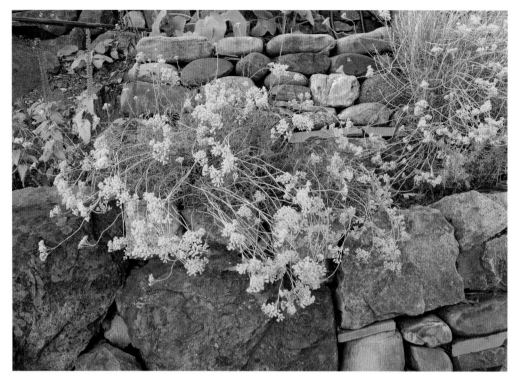

▲ The scent of curry plant can be used for aromatherapy.

are distilled into a selection of essential oils that are sold in natural food stores and online to make aromatherapy products. However, the good news is you do not need bottled essential oils if you have a fragrance garden—since you can experience aromatherapy firsthand.

Braille garden of smell and touch

I often visited the Braille Garden at the Los Angeles County Arboretum and Botanic Garden in Arcadia, California, with my mother Naomi Keville, who was blind, but had a wonderful sense of smell. We volunteered in their extensive herb garden, but our favorite destination was the stone terrace garden that had signs in braille to identify the fragrant plants. The tall terrace

was the perfect height to sniff the plants. The best plants for this garden are those that grow close to the ground and have leaves that easily release their scent when they are pressed between the fingers. Some of my mother's favorites were bee balm, lavender, lemon balm, lemon verbena, marjoram, oregano, scented geraniums, and all of the mints. There are several public gardens around the United States that have similar terraces designed for the visually impaired.

A child's fragrance garden

Fragrance gardens for children should inspire wonder and imagination through scent, color, touch, and form. A multicolored pathway and some whimsical artwork, such as a colorful wind flag or spinner, will add a

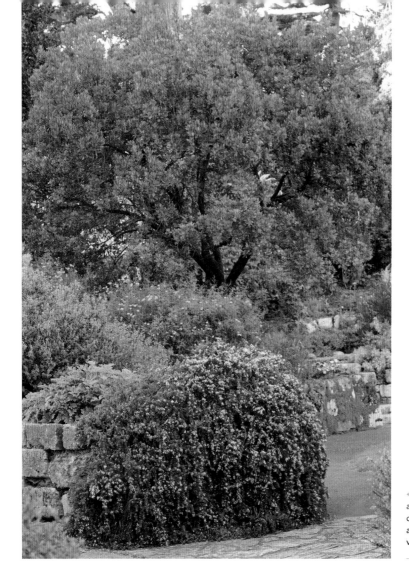

◄ The Garden of Fragrance at the San Francisco Botanical Garden, with terraces for access to those who are visually impaired.

fun touch to the child's garden. Children like to see different heights and small pots in various shapes and colors in a garden. A reflective pool with goldfish can be created from a large pot. If there is enough space, consider adding a garden swing.

Lamb's ears is often a child's favorite fragrant plant. It has a very light scent, but is extremely soft to the touch. Children are equally delighted to learn its name. They also like any of the sages that have fuzzy leaves. Pansy's face-like flower and sweet pea's shape and colors also delight. Children love the small, daisy-like flowers of chamomile, as well as Corsican mint's tiny leaves. Tell them lily-of-the-valley's nickname from days gone by: "fairy bells." Peppermint, spearmint, lemon balm, and chocolate mint are all favorites because they smell like candy. Children could also be encouraged to grow their own garden or to try an herb tea. A recipe of equal parts chamomile, lemon

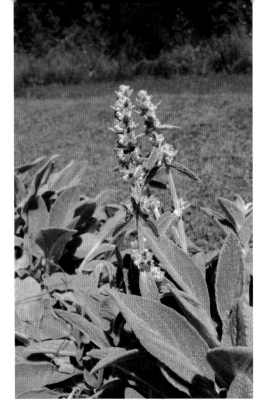

▲ Lamb's ears, a favorite with children.

balm, and peppermint makes a tasty children's tea that is very calming (either warm or iced). Don't forget to include plants that attract butterflies.

Moon garden: a reflective paradise

Gardens filled with gray, white, and yellow colors seem to be magical as they glow under the moonlight. Plants that reflect moonlight are curry plant, lamb's ears, santolina, woolly thyme, yellow yarrow, wormwood, and any of the gray sages. The white and yellow flowers of yarrow and trumpet flower also seem to shine in moonlight. Add white night-blooming flowers to scent the night air, such as those of jasmine and flowering tobacco. The effect can be increased with white gravel or other lightly colored landscaping material on pathways and around plants. To best enjoy the fragrant evening and the stars, find a spot for a lounge chair or place this garden within easy distance from the house.

Popular fragrant regional natives

Bringing native plants into the garden helps maintain wild plant diversity and sustain wildlife at a time when native habitats are quickly dwindling. These plants help attract birds and pollinators. Native plants are adapted to your climate, but still need an initial boost with slightly improved soil and watering when they are young or newly transplanted. They may need protection from predators. United Plant Savers, an organization that promotes the cultivation of native medicinal plants, advises gathering seeds or purchasing plants from a native plant nursery rather than uprooting them from the wild.

I asked a dozen well-known herbalists, avid gardeners from across North America who are mostly authors of gardening books, to suggest their favorite fragrant natives. Their responses are shown in the accompanying table. Suggestions came from Tim Blakely, Susan Belsinger, Juliet Blankespoor, Richo Cech, Bevin Clare, Doug Elliot, Steven Foster, Erika Galentin, Rosemary Gladstar, Mindy Green, Kathleen Maier, and Emily Ruff. They recommended regional species of anise hyssop, bee balm, wild rose, sage, sweet flag, and yarrow, as well as cypress, mock orange, and juniper trees. Other favorites were anise-scented sweet cicely (*Osmorhiza*), and spicy-leafed sweet shrub (*Calycanthus*), which grow in moist, loamy soil in partial shade, and prefer zones 4–6.

fragrant regional natives

EASTERN NORTH AMERICA WEST TO THE MISSISSIPPI RIVER (ZONES 4-6)

American dittany (*Cunila origanoides*) is a marjoram-scented mint.

Anise-scented goldenrod (*Solidago odora*) is a particularly fragrant species that makes a good herb tea.

Horsebalm (*Collinsonia canadensis*) has citronella-like scented foliage.

Milkweed (*Asclepias syriaca*) has a scent that resembles violets.

Sweet bay magnolia tree (*Magnolia virginiana*) has flowers that combine the scents of bay laurel and light lemon.

GULF COAST (ZONES 9-12)

Florida water mint (*Clinopodium brownei*) leaves have a strong peppermint-like flavor and fragrance.

Gumbolimbo (*Bursera simaruba*) has a resinous aroma that resembles frankincense.

MIDWEST (ZONES 4-8)

Clove currant (*Ribes odoratum*) produces clove-scented flowers in midspring.

WEST (ZONES 5-9)

Mountain mint (*Pycnanthemum virginianum*) is known as wild basil for its potent, mint-like aroma. It makes a tasty tea.

Wild azalea (*Rhododendron canescens*) flowers have a pungent, sugary sweet scent.

Wild pennyroyal (*Monardella odoratissima*) has the same fresh, minty scent as European pennyroyal. It wants moist, well-drained soil in full or partial sun.

Woolly blue curls (*Trichostema lanatum*) has an overwhelmingly sour aroma, earning it the nickname vinegar weed.

SOUTHWEST (ZONES 9-11)

Chocolate flower (*Berlandiera lyrata*) flowers smell and taste like chocolate (zone 6–8).

Creosote shrub (*Larrea tridentata*) leaves are sticky with a strongly scented, turpentine-like resin.

Desert lavender (*Hyptis emoryi*) leaves and flowers resemble dusty-smelling lavender.

Desert rosemary-mint (*Poliomintha incana*) smells like a combination of rosemary and mint. Tewa and Hopi tribes use it in cooking.

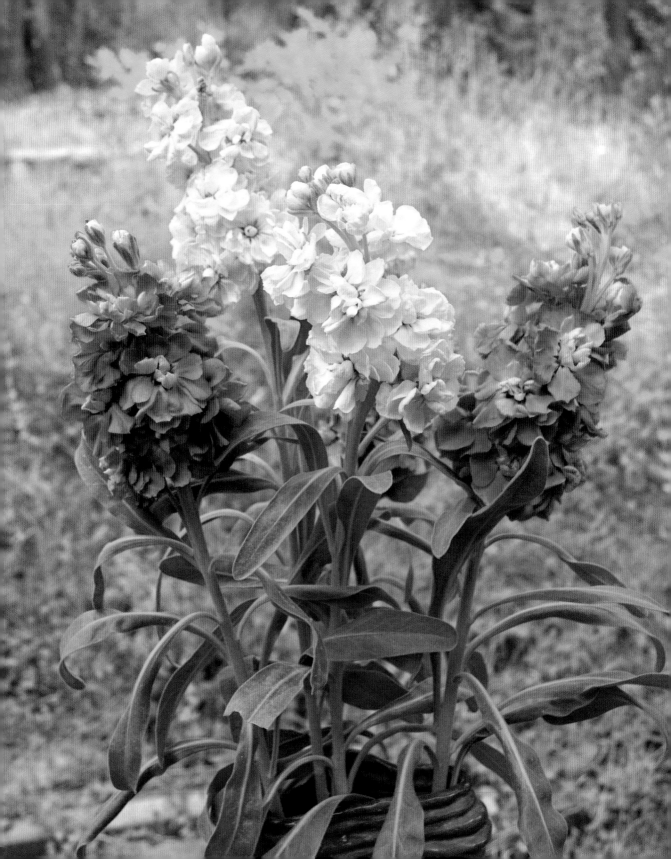

cultivating a
fragrance garden

Aromatic plants are a healthy lot, thanks to the essential oils they contain. Besides their benefits to humans (who are lucky enough to inhale their scents), these oils also deter infections and destructive insects, and invite pollinators to the garden. For the fragrance gardener, this means a concerted focus on ensuring plants receive proper soil, water, and light. All these factors affect both the quantity and quality of fragrance produced.

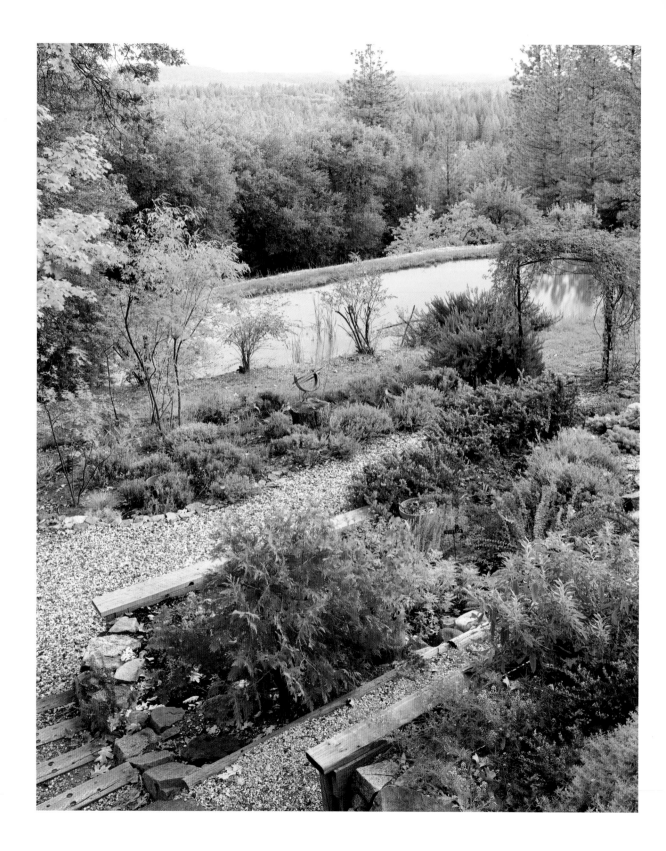

Plants have different cultivation requirements to produce the most scent. This largely depends upon the environment in which a plant originated. Thanks to the diverse selection of aromatic plants, you can enjoy a fragrant garden no matter how much sun, shade, or water there is in your garden—or how small it is.

look to a plant's homeland

Fragrant plants evolved in different environments all over the world, so their cultivation requirements for soil, water, and sunlight can vary widely. Wintergreen's shiny leaves would contrast nicely in concert with a stand of lavender—but it evolved in the shady woods of northeastern North America, while lavender originated in the hot, dry Mediterranean. A little detective work into each plant's origins reveals a lot about where it developed and how to duplicate that environment to make it feel at home, be as healthy as possible, and produce the most robust scent.

While you may not be able to re-create a Grecian hillside overlooking the Aegean Sea for rosemary, you can still roughly match the plant's native setting. I dedicated each of my twelve herb garden terraces to a different region of the world and prepared them accordingly. The eastern woodland garden has humus-filled, mulched soil, filtered

◄ The only thing better than a scented garden is a scented garden near water.

shade, and overhead watering to mimic rain, while the Mediterranean section is dry with well-drained soil. The India garden is in hot, full sun, but the China bed runs from full sun to partial shade to accommodate plants from that large region. Semi-tropical plants like trumpet flower are richly fed, watered daily, and grown mostly in pots, ready to winter over in the greenhouse or indoors.

from the soil up

One thing plant scientists agree on is that proper soil nutrition is a big factor in growing more-fragrant plants. Healthy plants grow better, live longer, produce more aromatic flowers and leaves, are disease and bug resistant, and can withstand adverse weather. Healthy does not always mean bigger, though. Gardeners who love to overfeed and overwater aromatic plants end up with oversized specimens that are visually striking. However, it takes just one sniff to discover that these pumped-up plants often have less scent and fewer flowers. Other gardeners recommend that plants be "starved" into producing more fragrance. It is true that aromatic plants tend to produce more essential oils when stressed. However, plants grown in extremely poor soil do not smell more aromatic to my nose and they certainly do not look healthy. Your best bet is to consider the needs of each plant individually. Develop the soil to match each plant's homeland. Israeli studies found good results when basil, marjoram, lemon balm, oregano, and thyme were fertilized similar to vegetables.

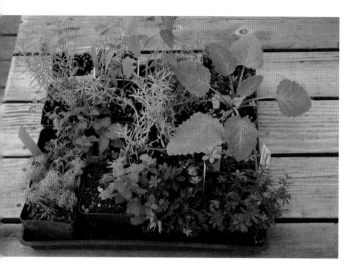

▲ Aromatic plant starts ready for the garden.

The correct alkalinity or acidity in soil also increases fragrance. It governs plant health by regulating how well the plant absorbs and utilizes nutrients from the soil. Fortunately, many aromatic plants adjust to a fairly wide range, with soil pH anywhere between a slightly acidic number 5 and a slightly alkaline number 8. Lavender, rosemary, and other Mediterranean plants lean toward alkaline soil, so they appreciate amendments such as lime, ground eggshells, and wood ashes, which are mostly calcium carbonate. Forest plants, such as gardenias, prefer acidic soil, which can be encouraged with peat moss, or pine needle or wood chip mulch.

The role of compost in fragrance

I am often called the fragrance or herb lady, but I would be just as happy being a compost queen. I view compost as a dinner party for plants. It is well documented that compost provides a balance of bioavailable nutrients, including trace minerals such as boron, copper, iron, magnesium, and zinc, to promote growth, health, and beneficial mycorrhizal fungi in the soil. It also aerates soil and makes it more friable.

Studies from the Department of Plant, Soil, and Insect Science at the University of Massachusetts Amherst and research centers around the world found that adding compost or pouring compost tea (made by steeping finished compost in water) around a plant's base makes chamomile, clary sage, fennel, and sage more fragrant, and often results in more flowers, which in turn results in more scent. Compost also enhances certain aromatic compounds, such as the geranial and citronellal found in geranium, lemon grass, and palmarosa.

Using compost or growing a legume cover crop contributes nitrogen to encourage plant growth. Scientists found that nitrogen increases the fragrance produced by chamomile, marjoram, lemon balm, oregano, peppermint, scented geranium, thyme, and *Agastache*, as well as many annual herbs such as basil, dill, and coriander. However, don't overdo the nitrogen or plants will have fewer flowers and less scent and be more susceptible to frost and fungal infection. Some plants that dislike nitrogen-rich soil are pine, juniper, and rosemary. Too much nitrogen in relationship to phosphorus will keep wisteria from flowering.

Potassium helps plants manufacture food and be more vigorous and disease resistant. It enhances the fragrance of caraway, peppermint, and scented geranium. It can make palmarosa nearly twenty-five percent more aromatic. An Italian study found that potassium helps increase the aromatic compound thuja in Dalmatian sage, making it more pungent. This may also be true for other plants that contain thuja, such as wormwood. Organic farmers recommend sulfate of potash or greensand to increase potassium in the soil. I add ashes from my woodstove.

Phosphorus improves flower, fruit, and root development. It increased the aromas of sage and some mints at the Department of Cultivation and Production of Medicinal and Aromatic Plants at the National Research Centre in Cairo, Egypt. It also enhances basil's clove-like scent. However, there was a lower output when the horticultural science department at Shiraz University in Iran added excessive phosphorus to the soil. I suggest adding soft rock phosphate in moderation.

Compost goes a long way toward improving the nutritional value and pH of garden soil. How much soil amendment to add depends on the soil's composition. Local nurseries, Master Gardener groups, and county cooperative extension services can help you determine how much is needed. You can find soil pH testers at garden supply stores. The best time to dig compost into beds is before planting. Compost placed on top of the soil, called top dressing, soaks in from rain or watering and is available to the plant's roots in a few weeks. Liquid fertilizers, such as fish emulsion, kelp, and compost tea, can be applied around the base of the plant or used as a foliar spray when plants need a quick boost. Even if a plant is drooping, wait three weeks after transplanting to apply liquid fertilizer since it can burn root endings that were damaged during transplanting.

sun and shade for the fragrance garden

The proper amount of sunlight not only improves plant health but affects growth and fragrance. As with soil and watering needs, look to a plant's origins for how much sun it prefers. When plants are not happy where they are growing, transplant them to a better location with more sun or shade. Straggly plants and stems reaching for the sun signal a need for more light. A plant is getting too much direct sun when it develops dry spots from sunburn on the leaves.

The fragrant sun garden

There are far more aromatic plants in my garden that prefer sun than those that like shade. Plus, according to plant researchers, many plants produce more fragrance when they are grown in the sun. Keep in mind that the term "full sun" does not mean the same thing everywhere, and many gardening books are written with a specific region in mind. A gardener in eastern North America or on the English coast may correctly indicate full sun for a plant like chamomile. However, try growing the same plant in the state of Arizona, and you quickly discover that the intention was full sun in a cooler, moister climate with some summer cloud cover.

The sun's UVB rays are what promote essential oil production, increasing the amount of fragrance in a plant. Sun-loving plants usually require at least five hours of full sun a day. Plant scientists have found that some plants, such as basil, lemon balm, fennel, juniper, and culinary sage, increase their scent production with even more sunlight. The aromas of marjoram, yarrow, myrtle, lemon verbena, and scented geranium are also stronger if the plants are grown in a place with maximum sunlight. Northern European natives, such as German chamomile, catnip, caraway, peppermint, and spearmint, are attuned to long, sunny summer days at that latitude. So is basil, which will not completely develop essential oil glands in its leaves without sufficient sunlight. The more daylight these plants receive, the stronger their aroma, so consider planting them in the sunniest areas of your garden. A full fourteen hours of sunshine during summer's height is optimum for peppermint. This makes the quality of the peppermint grown commercially in sunny central Oregon rival that of Michigan's famous peppermint crop. Sunlight causes some plants (such as lavender and German chamomile) to produce more flowers, and fennel to have plumper seeds. Aromatic plants that thrive under hot, full sun, even in the desert, are juniper, Mexican marigold, rosemary, rockrose, wormwood, and the thick-leafed sages. Planted together, they make an excellent fragrant border. Other choices for desert gardens are species that are native to arid regions, such as white sage and sagebrush.

Sunlight also improves the quality of fragrance. Peppermint is often grown in semi-shade, but in the sun, it develops more of the tingly menthol for which it is famous, and fewer off-smelling menthone compounds. Thyme's sharp, distinctive aroma praised by cooks increases when the plant is sun-grown. Juniper develops more of its characteristic pepper-like spiciness in sunlight. The sun also brings out sweet flag's herby fragrance while decreasing the amount of a somewhat toxic beta-asarone compound.

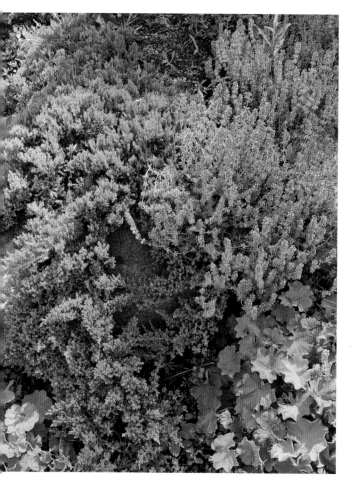

◄ Sunlight intensifies the aromas of juniper and thyme.

If your garden is too shady, bring in more sun and open crowded areas by trimming back or removing plants, so plants seeking more light are farther apart. Even reflected illumination from light-colored gravel paths, rocks, sand, and structures brightens a garden. Tall planters, platforms, and hanging pots can position plants in sunny spots. Potted plants on wheels can be moved around a patio as the sun pattern changes during the year.

The fragrant shade garden

It is easier to create shade in the garden than to bring in more sun. Garden structures, such as rose or honeysuckle arbors, offer shade for part of the day. Nursery shade cloth suspended on frames can be incorporated into garden design. Deciduous plants offer summer shade and then allow the sun to shine through after their leaves fall in autumn. If your garden is large enough, shrubs or trees can shade shorter plants, although it can be difficult to grow anything under sizable plants if they produce surface roots or dense shade.

My shade garden is filled with fragrance from February to July. The wintersweet blooms in late winter, followed by a lovely combination of daphne and violets. Then comes a succession of spring blooms from short plants that line the pathway: primrose, lily-of-the-valley, sweet woodruff, and wintergreen. Finally, gardenia blooms step in to scent the early summer air. Conveniently, all of these plants want the same

shady, woodsy conditions with mildly acidic soil that is rich with humus and never quite dries out. They do not bloom together, but their interesting leaf formations make a stunning combination when they are planted next to each other. Add a bench or hammock to this shady garden setting and it invites you to relax in the richly scented shade. My hot tub is in the shade garden so that I can relax while surrounded by the aroma of plants.

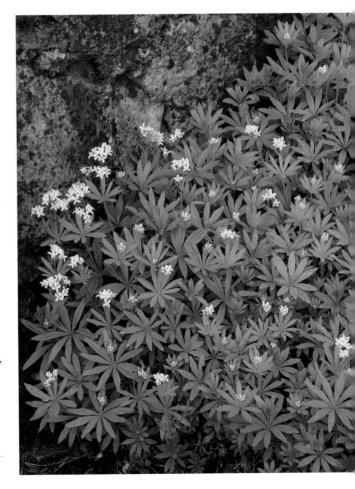

▶ Sweet woodruff brings spring scent to shady spots.

If your garden is shady, you can still grow sun-loving angelica, bee balm, clary sage, fennel, lemon balm, and orris root. They may not be quite as fragrant, but they do tolerate dappled light, especially where they receive reflective light. In hot, arid, desert climates, these same plants actually benefit from being grown in partial shade. An east-facing wall that only gets morning sun protects them from intense sunlight, as well as wind. You may want to keep them trimmed back so they do not become leggy reaching for the sun. All of these plants favor slightly alkaline soil that dries out between waterings, so they can be grouped together. The tall clary sage and fennel make an attractive backdrop to the mid-height angelica and lemon balm, and smaller plants.

Mignonette, wallflower, and Roman chamomile are fickle about light requirements. They benefit from full sun in the north, but grow better in some shade in southern climates. These plants can be planted together in slightly alkaline soil if mignonette and wallflower receive extra water.

The semi-tropical perennials in my fragrance garden are versatile in their sun requirements. Cardamom, lemon grass, palmarosa, patchouli, Indian valerian, and tulsi basil are commercially grown under full sun in humid Indonesian and Indian fields. They all grow under my hot, dry northern California sun if planted in the ground and watered twice daily, but they are easier to maintain in pots placed in bright reflective shade. The pots make it easier to move plants indoors in winter.

watering

Plants tell you when they are in need of more water by turning crispy or dry, or by leaves curling on the edges. Overwatering can cause them to die back. Holding back on watering causes some plants to be more aromatic. Brian Lawrence, PhD, author of a series of research volumes titled "Essential Oils," notes that chamomile, clary sage, coriander, and lavender are among plants from relatively dry climates that produce more essential oil when stressed by a lack of water. For my Mediterranean-climate plants, I follow the guidelines from the American University of Beirut in Lebanon for oregano and deep water them every other week during dry spells, or every week when daytime temperatures soar into the 90s. Israeli and Italian research found that some drought-resistant plants—such as lemon balm, marjoram, sage, savory, and scented geraniums—are more fragrant when they receive at least an inch per week. On the other hand, Lawrence points out that plants originating in more moderate climates, such as basil, caraway, and dill, tend to produce less fragrance unless they are watered on a regular basis.

If your garden is dependent on rainfall rather than irrigation, the amount of water is difficult to control, but fragrant plants tend to be versatile even if they do not produce the maximum fragrance. Jim Duke, retired USDA botanist, says that annual rainfall can range from twelve to fifty-four inches per year for lavender cultivation. Basil adapts to anything from twenty-one to one hundred seventy inches of rain annually.

garden mulch

Mulch retains moisture in soil, so helps cut down on watering requirements. It has its pros and cons. It tends to increase a plant's root growth. Organic material, such as straw and chopped leaves, are popular and inexpensive, but can become a haven for slugs, snails, pill bugs, and earwigs—and in humid climates, they invite disease. Make sure that the mulch you use does not contain seed, or you may be inviting a weeding nightmare. Sawdust and wood chip mulches work in some situations, but they can make the soil more acidic and invite harmful insects, including termites.

Mulching also offers roots some frost protection. Clear plastic mulch warms soil six to ten degrees Fahrenheit down to about six inches. Organic mulch keeps soil temperature slightly cooler, which honeysuckle loves, but culinary sage hates. Leaf mulch can cool the ground as much as twenty degrees, according to Allen Barker, soil scientist at the University of Massachusetts. I help some plants survive winter by mulching around their bases and placing a large pot or trashcan over them that has been lined inside with leaves. The container needs to be removed before plants leaf out in spring.

Many agricultural research stations recommend one to two inches of white sand, oyster shell, or pea gravel mulch to heat the

▼ Reflective sand mulch in a newly planted gray moon bed.

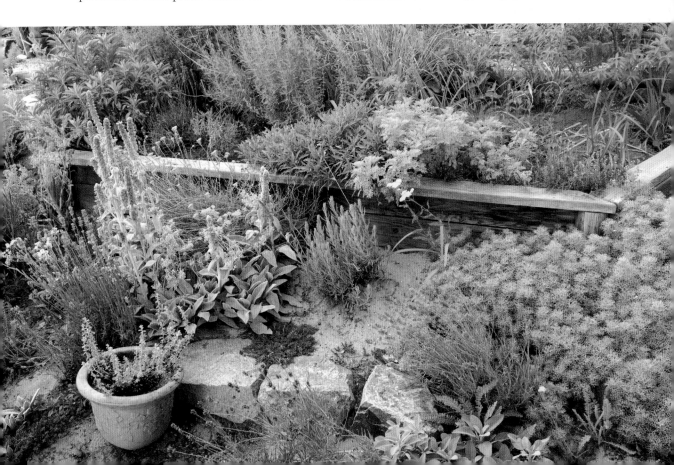

soil for Mediterranean plants. Plant researcher Dr. Arthur Tucker of Delaware State University found lavandin mulched with white sand grew larger, had more scent and a higher yield, and also had fewer fungal infections. Lavandin with fabric mulch also grew better, but did not winter over as well. The heating and cooling caused by the fabric might have been a factor. Plastic mulch increases growth of sun-loving basil and rosemary, though not parsley. Green or yellow mulch made basil more aromatic, while red mulch produced larger leaves. Plant scientists at Brazil's Universidade Federal de Sergipe and the Central Institute of Medicinal and Aromatic Plants in Lucknow, India, found that scented geranium yields more fragrance when mulched with white or black plastic or straw mulch. One reason may be because it increased the plant's ability to pull in nitrogen.

garden temperatures

Good soil drainage is important to get temperature-sensitive plants through a cold winter. Plants with roots sitting in water from winter rain or melting snow are more likely to freeze. The larger the plant and the deeper the roots, the better the plant handles cold weather. Plant early enough for roots to be well established before a freeze. A two-gallon-sized plant stands a far better chance than one in a four-inch pot. Kelp foliar spray applied to leaves in the fall helps perennials survive temperature extremes. It is well known that lavender is more fragrant when

grown at higher elevations than sea level in France. Some plant researchers say that has more to do with the cooler temperatures than with elevation.

Greenhouses and cold frames

Greenhouses and cold frames extend the growing season and may allow you to grow tropical plants. Just imagine entering your greenhouse to be greeted by the warm aromas of trumpet flower, scented geranium, patchouli, lemon grass, and orchid! It is a payoff, since these contained environments do create their own problems and demand diligence. The constant humidity and warmth encourages fungal diseases, white flies, aphids, and mealy bugs. Since plants are usually tightly packed in a greenhouse, disease and bug infestation can spread rapidly. In addition, running greenhouse lights, fans, and a heater can tax both your electric bill and patience. Plants are dependent upon being watered and having the temperature controlled, and even automatic systems are not foolproof.

An unheated greenhouse is easier to maintain, although it is more limiting since the plants inside are still subjected to cold temperatures. The advantage is that plants are never directly exposed to wind chill, hail, and snow. You can often winter over plants that are in the next highest gardening zone, but success depends on your location and the number of sunny days. The temperature inside tends to be a significant ten to fifteen degrees higher than the outside air. Having a sixty-watt, incandescent light bulb turned on inside adds a few more degrees. Cement

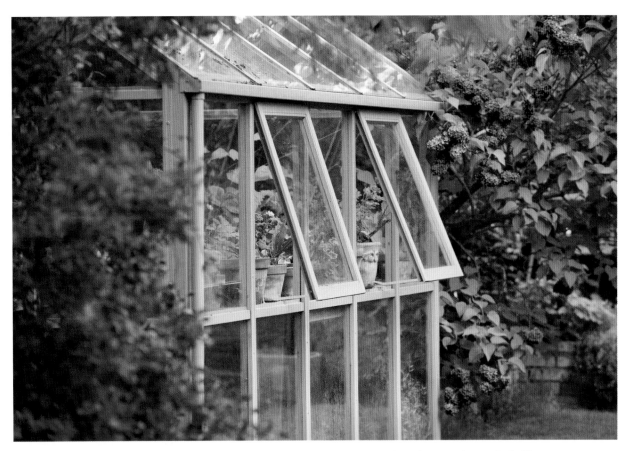

▲ A greenhouse demands attention but pays back with climate-impervious beauty and fragrance.

blocks, water or oil containers, double-pane windows, and clear plastic bubble wrap as insulation all help retain heat.

transplanting

If you have a garden, you will need to dig in plants from the nursery or from other parts of your garden. Only transplant healthy plants that are able to withstand some stress; the process should go as smoothly as possible to avoid overtaxing the plant. Annuals are generally transplanted in spring, once they have developed a root system. Perennials transplant best when they are dormant during winter or early spring. Transplant biennials before their second spring.

Most nursery plants have spent their lives in a protected environment, so even the healthiest ones benefit from a transition time before being planted in the garden. Nursery customers often select the largest plants with the most attractive and fragrant blooms, but plants that are in flower can have a difficult time reestablishing their roots. Go for the smaller, non-flowering options if there are any. If you must transplant while plants are in bloom, at least snip off the flowers. Transplant from a pot before roots grow into a mat and become root-bound. Dig a hole to accommodate the size of the plant when it reaches maturity. Add compost and any necessary amendments and wet the hole. The soil needs to stay consistently moist but not be displaced by heavy rains.

Even if a plant begins to droop, wait three weeks after transplanting to apply liquid fertilizer or it may burn any root endings damaged during transplanting. Sun and hot weather are stressors to new transplants. Sunlight stimulates the plant's chlorophyll and metabolic processes, but plants can use a break for a few days while they restore their root system. Transplant on an overcast day or cover the new transplant with nursery transplant cloth or with an upside-down, light-colored pot or cardboard box.

Annuals such as coriander, dill, and German chamomile have delicate root structures that are easily disturbed when transplanted. They are often planted directly into the garden or a container that will be their permanent home, to reduce root impact.

▶ The author tending her fragrance garden nursery, under the supervision of a friend.

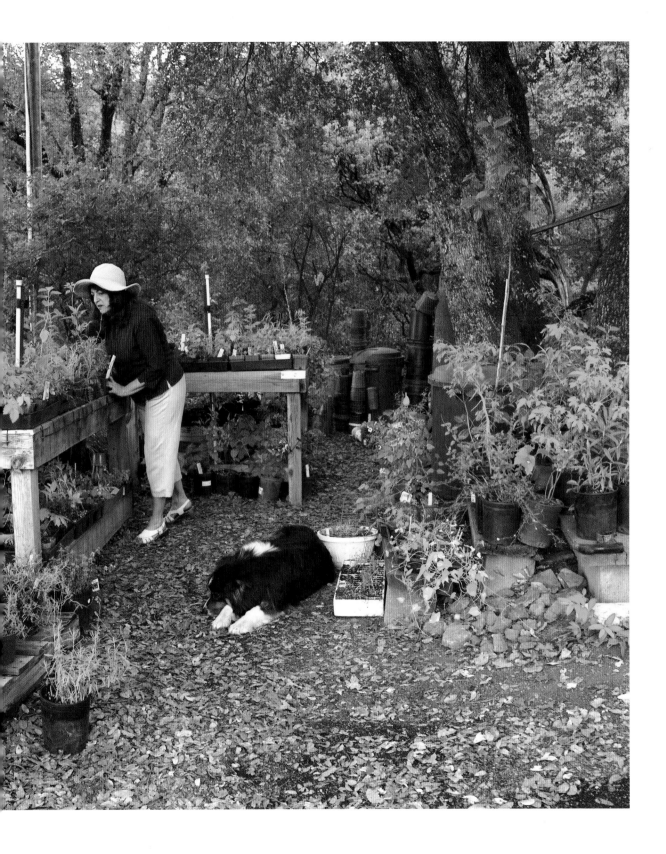

propagating plants

Propagation techniques help you expand your garden and keep your stock going when plants become old or fail. Add a bank of daphne, a hedge of lavender, a sage garden, or share plants with others. Sometimes, the only way to obtain the most aromatic varieties is to order seeds from specialty catalogs. The many cultivars of lavender, rosemary, thyme, and oregano should be propagated from cuttings or by layering since they may not come true from seed; this is the case with most named perennials. Peppermint and French tarragon offer little choice since they rarely produce seed. Cuttings also keep plants going when they are not winter hardy in your area. Robin Parer of Geraniaceae nursery in California (which specializes in geraniums) says that taking cuttings in the fall is the only way to maintain a collection of scented geraniums, unless you live in a climate that duplicates their South African homeland.

Propagating plants requires time, dedication, and diligence, but it is rewarding. A sense of wonder is evoked with every new seedling that emerges from the soil. Tending the baby plants in my nursery is one of my favorite garden activities.

Potting soil

You can purchase potting soil or make your own. A standard recipe is equal parts garden soil, homemade compost, and vermiculite. The ingredients can be altered for different plants. I keep soil additives on hand, such as mushroom compost, ashes from a wood stove, and peat moss (which makes soil more acidic and holds onto water and lime). Sand and large stones added to soil increase drainage; vermiculite, diatomite rock, clay beads, pumice, and clay soil slow drainage.

The gardener's dilemma: plants or seeds?

I am one of those people who would rather go to the nursery than the mall, but I also love witnessing the transformation of seeds into plants. The decision whether to purchase plants or seeds needs to be made for each addition to your fragrance garden. Many gardeners readily plant annual seeds since they sprout and grow quickly. Perennial seeds, on the other hand, demand time, dedication, and patience.

An advantage of starting with plants instead of seeds is that it saves the work and responsibility of growing seeds and the need to have a propagation area. Plants also offer a head start toward a mature garden. Perennials that are plants instead of seeds in the spring are larger when winter arrives and better equipped to survive. Some seeds can be difficult to germinate: rosemary, myrtle, orris root, santolina, sweet flag, and wintergreen are good examples. The same is true for many shrubs, vines, trees, bulbs, and tropical plants. Angelica seeds sprout readily, but they need to be planted within a few months of ripening—a fact that is the basis of a European folktale.

I have found gardeners to be a creative and frugal group. It seems to be in their nature to take on the challenge of growing plants from seed. They also know that a seed packet containing many potential plants is less than the price of one plant. One consideration is that seeds are often the only way to obtain a certain species or variety. This is especially true when seeking particularly fragrant plants, since nurseries favor hybridized plants for their color and improved durability. However, many of them sadly lose much or all of their scent when they are developed.

Hybrid seeds present their own problem: they often do not grow true to their parent plants. This means they may look different and can easily be less fragrant. Do not be surprised to find some plants and seeds labeled incorrectly. One way to deal with mislabeling is to see and sniff plants at a nursery, although the selection is more limited than on the internet. Even then, you can be fooled. I was once excited to find the very fragrant Cuthbertson sweet pea plants—only to watch them mature into ordinary, edible peas without scent.

Planting seeds

Seed viability is affected by quality. If seeds do not germinate, the fault may be old seed rather than your gardening skill. It is best to plant annual seeds when they are no more than a year old and perennial seeds within a couple of years.

Many commercial growers prefer planting their seeds in open flats because they take up less room in the greenhouse. I find seedling trays with individual compartments are easier since the roots of different plants do not become intertwined.

A sterile potting mix is recommended to eliminate weeds and prevent confusion over which seedlings you planted. It also discourages damping off disease, a nasty problem caused by microorganisms in soil that weaken the stems and cause seedlings to fall over. Plant the seeds by sprinkling them on top of dampened potting mix that has been lightly packed down to eliminate air pockets. Try to space seeds half an inch apart. Place a thin layer of soil (about twice the width of the seed) over the top. Gently tamp down the soil to hold the seeds in place and water with a light spray. Be sure that the spray does not displace the soil and expose seeds.

The soil mix must remain moist for seeds to germinate, but not be water-logged. The warmth of the soil and the amount of light determines how quickly seeds germinate. Overhead light is best for seedlings to grow straight. The preferred germination temperature for many seeds is around 70 degrees F. Tropical plants, such as cardamom, patchouli, and trumpet flower, like the soil a little warmer. To speed growth, use a horticulture heating pad under the flat and suspend grow lights six inches over the top of the seedlings. The lights should be on for sixteen straight hours a day. A liquid fertilizer can also be applied every few days once the seedlings are up. Annuals like dill and coriander are ready to plant just a couple weeks after they germinate. Basil needs only a few more days. Roman chamomile, lemon balm, catnip, and culinary sage are ready in about three weeks, while it takes thyme and oregano at least a month.

When seedlings emerge, the first seed leaves, called cotyledons, look different than the plant's typical leaf, so do not be fooled. Snip off extra seedlings with your fingernails or trimmers while plants are still small, so that they are spaced about an inch apart for good air circulation and to give the roots room to grow. This is always a difficult task for new gardeners, but plants grow stronger when they are not competing for nutrients, space, and air circulation. Do not let the soil dry. The tiny seedlings are ready for transplanting when they are just a few inches tall. Carefully remove each one with a small garden tool or a kitchen knife. Keep as much soil as possible around the root systems, which should be substantial enough to hold the soil around them. When seedlings are growing very close together, transplant them in a clump and snip them off later rather than disturbing the roots. Place plants into pots filled with nutritious potting soil. It is okay to bury the first cotyledon seed leaves. Push the soil down firmly around the plant and water it right away to eliminate air pockets in the soil.

Once seedlings have put on growth, gradually increase the amount of light they receive, until they are hardy enough to be moved into the garden or a pot. This process is called "hardening off."

Seedlings are vulnerable to insects, disease, sunstroke, and to being knocked over. As a result, gardeners often repot slow-growing perennials rather than placing them directly in the garden. Planting perennial seeds directly into the garden, or in open flats in the fall when their seeds ripen, often makes them stronger and hardier. This allows nature to take its course, and the seeds come up when the timing is right.

Making cuttings

Cuttings can be made from most perennial plants with woody stems. The best time is when the plant is in a growth cycle, but not

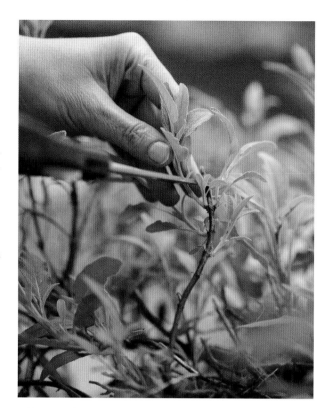

▲ Most sage plants are easy to start from cuttings.

in bud, flower, or seed. This is usually spring or fall. That catches the plant's hormones when they are oriented toward root growth rather than seed production. You should have easy success propagating scented geraniums, wormwood, lemon verbena, myrtle, curry plant, and most of the mint family, such as sage, from cuttings. Taking cuttings of shrubs and trees, such as bay laurel, can be done in early fall. Winter them over someplace where it does not freeze and they should be sufficiently rooted by early spring for transplanting.

Fill containers that do not have drainage holes with a rooting mix that contains few or no nutrients. This encourages the roots to grow as they reach out in search of nutrition. Coarse sandbox sand (not salty, ocean sand) used to be the favored choice, but many gardeners now prefer a mixture of the more absorbent perlite, vermiculite, and peat moss.

Use a clean knife to cut a four-inch spring growth sprig from a tip of the parent plant. Snip off all but the six or so leaves on the tip of the sprig. That leaves an odd-looking barren sprig with only a cluster of leaves at the top. Do this because there are not enough roots to support extra leaves, which will drop off anyway. Make more cuttings than you need since only the strongest survive. Using a rooting hormone powder is not necessary, but it may improve your success rate. Dip the lower third of the stalk into the rooting powder immediately after cutting it. Watering the rooting medium with a strong tea made from willow stems (which contain a growth stimulant) also encourages growth. You can make this tea by simply covering willow stems with water in a pail and letting the tea sit for a week.

Stand the cuttings in a wet rooting medium in a well-lit area that has at least ten hours of light a day, but not direct sunlight. The rooting medium needs to stay wet but not soaked, and the air humid. You can achieve both conditions by covering the pot with a clean plastic bag, opening the bag daily for fresh air. Some gardeners feed the cuttings with a liquid fertilizer.

After about ten days, carefully lift out a cutting with a thin blade to look for roots. If there are none, keep looking once a week. Be patient. It takes oregano, sage, and other members of the mint family about two weeks to develop roots, but it can take up to six weeks for some plants. The cuttings are ready for potting into nutritious potting soil when their roots are a few inches long. Pinching off the very tip of the cutting encourages growth rather than flowering. Keep the fledging plants in moist soil out of direct sun for a couple weeks while they establish a better root system. In a month or two, the roots will fill a four-inch pot and be ready for transplanting into the garden or another pot.

Layering stems

Layering is a useful propagation technique once you have an established garden. It works well with perennials that produce roots off their stems just under the soil's surface. Examples of plants to layer are anise hyssop, curry plant, santolina, wormwood, and tansy. This technique is especially easy with plants that have runners, such as peppermint, sage and other members of the mint family. It also works with shrubs such as lilac, rockrose, and Mexican marigold, and large vines such as honeysuckle, clematis, and jasmine.

Gently push an outer stem from the plant's base, leaves and all, to the ground. To speed root development, a tiny portion of the stem's outer layer can be scraped off and rooting hormone dabbed on that spot before burying the stem. Mound a pile of potting soil on top of the stem and pack it down, leaving at least five inches of the stem's end uncovered. Keep the area well watered for several weeks. If the potting soil is too loose to stay clumped around the stem, add a little garden clay or natural kitty litter to make it hold together better.

Be patient; it can take weeks for roots to develop, or "strike." The mints may do so in a couple weeks and rosemary and thyme take about three weeks. When a small root ball has formed, cut it from the mother plant with a shovel and transplant it into a pot to give it a couple months to develop before it goes into the garden.

To layer strong stems that do not bend, cover and pack the entire lower section of the stem with soil to create a mound. If it needs more stability, remove the bottom of a small plastic pot and slip it over one of the plant's stems, then fill it with potting soil and keep it moist.

Root division

Propagation by division can be done with perennials that form a crown, such as lemon grass, palmarosa, and valerian. This cluster of stems emerges close to the ground's surface from several places on the root. Plants need to be about three years old before their crowns are large enough to divide. Vetiver also has a crown, although its roots grow so tightly, it is not easy to divide them. Cleanly slice off a section of crown with a shovel and replant it or dig up the root ball and divide it. The root suffers the least injury when this is done in late fall.

Low-growing, fragrant plants that spread by their roots into mats can simply have a section dug and replanted. Examples of fragrant plants that expand into ground covers are creeping thymes, Roman chamomile, yarrow, violet, tansy, wintergreen, and sweet woodruff. Peppermint, spearmint, and pennyroyal easily spread by runners so they are especially simple to divide. Since they spread

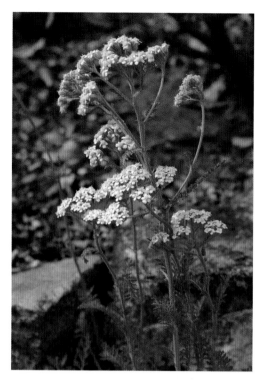

▲ Yarrow spreads via runners and is easy to divide by its roots.

so well, these plants can become invasive. Only grow them together if you want to have them freely intermingle, which can be a nice display.

Hyacinth, lily-of-the-valley, lily, and daffodil bulbs separate at the end of their growing season. Replant with the root side facing downward. Bury them about the same distance under the soil as the size of the bulb. Small bulbs can take up to two years before they flower after being replanted.

Orris root and sweet flag are treated in a way that is similar to bulbs. To divide them, dig the plant up and pull or cut apart the rhizomes. The portions are then replanted. They do better if the rhizomes are broken just enough to divide them.

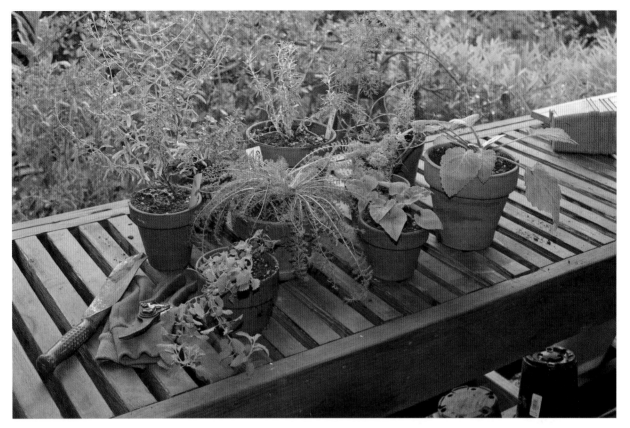

▲ Potted aromatic plants can be moved around the garden to fill gaps and suit changing conditions.

pots, planters, and window boxes

I love seeing pots in the fragrance garden. They are both attractive and useful. Potted plants can be placed along pathways, next to a bench, under house windows, or wherever their fragrance will be most enjoyed. They can highlight an especially attractive lemon verbena or scented geranium. Tuck pots of freesia, hyacinth, lily-of-the-valley, narcissus and other bulbs into spots in the garden or place them on a patio while they are in full bloom, then move them out of view once they die back. Culinary herbs in pots are convenient near the kitchen door, poised to grace your meals with their fresh flavor. Thyme, sage, and basil will grow in a south-facing window box. Perhaps window boxes filled with wallflowers, stocks, and violets should come back into fashion. They become aromatherapy air fresheners with every breeze, as the scent wafts into open windows. Star jasmine hangs off trellises around my windows to scent the house in early summer.

Planters solve many gardening dilemmas. Pots can be placed on driveways, rock walls, buildings, and all sorts of places you

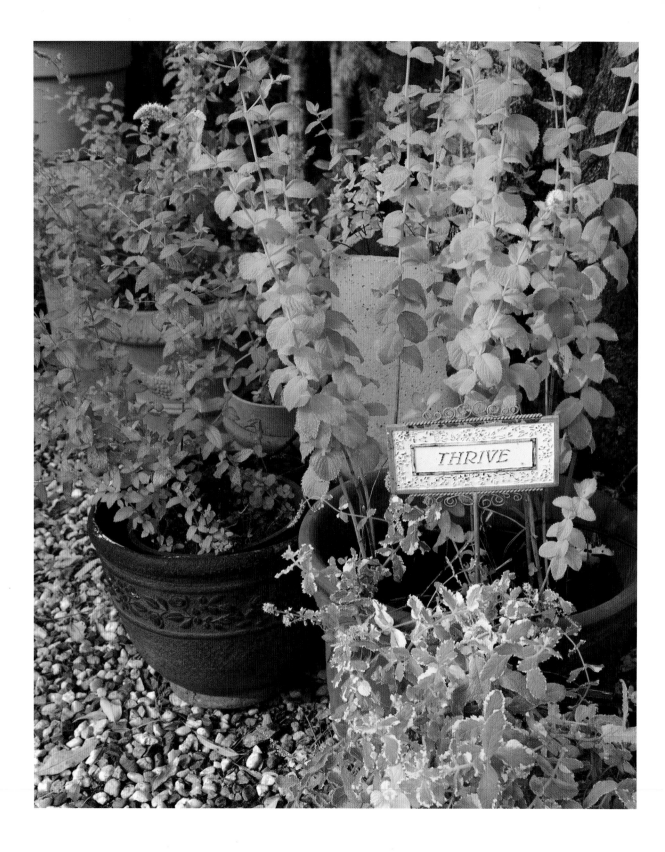

cannot or do not want to dig a bed. They are very handy to fill in empty garden spots. They keep rampant growers such as sweet woodruff, tansy, and mints from overtaking the garden. Angelica and valerian can be potted to stop gophers from eating their roots. Growing trees and shrubs in containers keeps them small and manageable in the garden by restricting their growth; potting bay and camphor trees helps them fit into the fragrance garden. Potting also allows convenient access for picking leaves and covering the plant during cold snaps, as well as simplifying transport to the indoors or a greenhouse—or planting in the ground to survive winter's cold temperatures. Bringing them out in the spring results in an instant garden. Some botanical gardens have entire sections of potted plants buried in mulch. This trick can quickly fill gaps in the landscaping before hosting a garden tour.

For all their advantages, potted plants demand more attention than plants growing in the ground. Containers restrict growth and plants in them dry out and freeze more easily. Plants in pots also run out of nutrition, especially if the container is small. From a size standpoint, choose at least two-gallon pots. Feed potted plants several times during their growing season so that they receive sufficient nutrition. Make sure containers have drainage holes in the bottom to prevent stagnant water from inviting disease.

Growing plants in pots makes it especially challenging to keep them sufficiently watered. Despite being attractive, unglazed clay pots are particularly difficult because they dry out quickly, pulling nutrients from the soil in the process. Experiments show that they lose half their water during one hot, summer day. Even in the winter, plants grow better and faster in plastic pots. To have the best of both worlds, slip plastic pots inside clay pots and conceal the lip of the inner pot with mulch or potting soil. This makes transplanting and moving plants easier. A clay pot is less likely to crack if it is not filled with soil that expands and contracts with temperature extremes.

Customize soil for potted plants, seedlings, and nursery plants. This will provide better drainage for sage and lavender, and keep the soil moist for lily-of-the-valley, sweet pea, sweet flag, and wallflower. In wet climates, Mediterranean plants stay drier when their pots are under a roof or overhang. In dry regions, pots can receive extra water with drip lines and emitters that are different sizes to regulate the amount of water each plant gets. Large rocks in the bottom of a container increase drainage; small rocks compress and can hinder it.

◀ A potted mint garden.

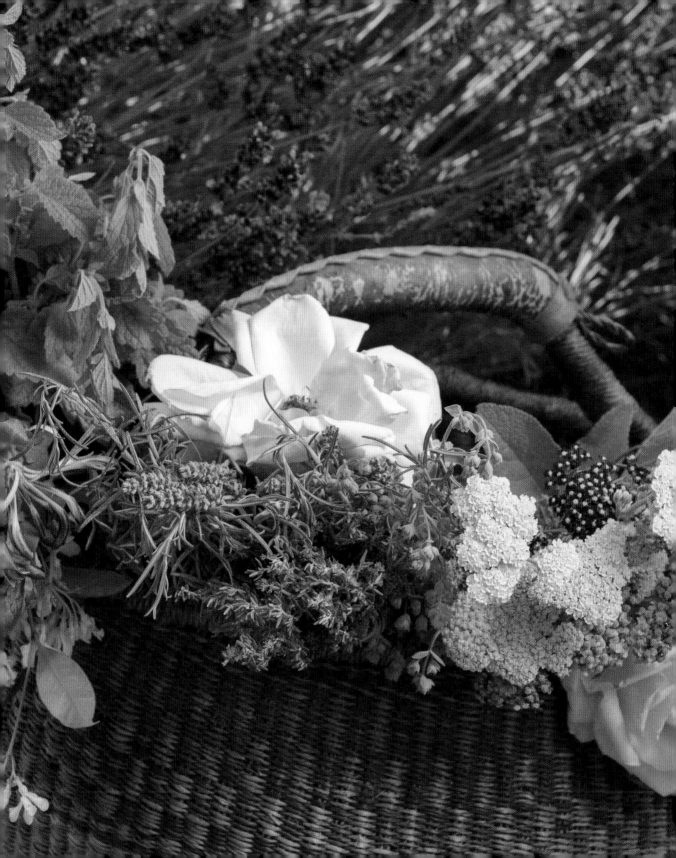

a harvest of scents and flavors

One of the joys of a fragrance garden is the ongoing bounty it produces. Aromatic plants from your garden enhance your life with scent and color throughout the year. Make a habit of strolling through the garden, basket in hand, happily clipping and snipping. Bring gorgeous, fresh flowers into your house for most of the year and have dried bouquets that last all winter. Fill your kitchen spice cabinet with savory, aromatic herbs from your garden, such as rosemary, mint, oregano, thyme, sage, and dill—after all, researchers say that about 80 percent of what we taste comes from what we smell.

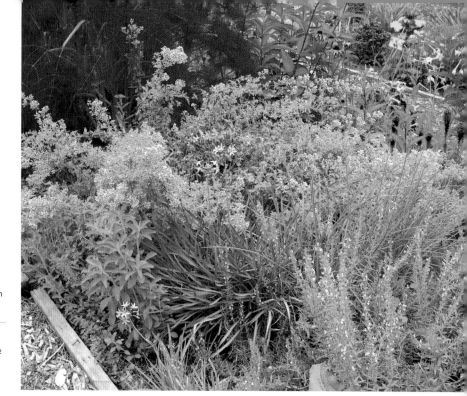

▶ Culinary bed with herbs in bloom.

▼ During the growing season, you can expect multiple cuttings of fragrant flowers and herbs. Garden at the Herb Pharm, Williams, OR.

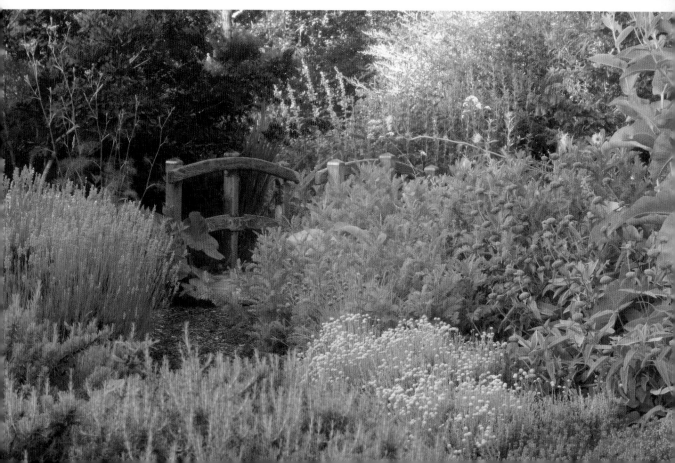

Use your harvest to create aromatherapy personal care products like body and massage oil, culinary treats such as herbal vinegars, and potpourri for yourself or as gifts for others. You can even make your own bug repellents from your garden.

the gathering

Harvest plants when they reach their peak fragrance. There is no need to refer to charts. Simply watch and smell your garden as it grows. As plants with fragrant foliage get close to blooming, their aroma becomes stronger and concentrates in the upper leaves. The lowest leaves on the stems not only have less scent, they also begin to die back. This is why herb books say to harvest the topmost leaves of aromatic plants as they go into flower. Rather than depending upon this rule, give plants a sniff test to determine for yourself the most aromatic parts to harvest. Choose only strongly fragrant and vibrant-looking plants and avoid yellow, dry, or bug-eaten leaves and flowers.

Collect leaves, flowers, and seeds when their scent is strongest, in the early morning. After that, the aroma dissipates into the air throughout the day. The hotter and drier the weather, the more quickly scent is lost. Moisture on plants also encourages fragrance to evaporate. Plants that are dusty or dirty should be rinsed off before they are cut, but make sure they are thoroughly dry before collecting them. The same goes for plants that are wet from rain, morning dew, or watering.

Use a sharp knife, clippers, or scissors to cleanly cut stems. Tearing plants or making jagged cuts injures them. For flowers on long stalks, such as lavender, curry plant, sage, daffodil, freesia, lilies, and orris root, cut them off at the base of each stem, just above the leaves. This not only looks better, but the plant does not waste unneeded energy trying to feed those empty stalks. Take rose and gardenia flowers down to at least the second set of leaves on the stem. It may be more practical to pinch individual leaves off shrubs that have thick stems, rather than cut off a branch, especially if you only need a few bay leaves for soup.

Make sure to leave enough on the plant so that it remains healthy and continues growing. This varies with each plant, but take a quarter or less of the plant mass. Chances are that you can have more than one harvest in the growing season. Cutting back the budding tops of lemon verbena, scented geranium, and most species of the mint family encourages fresh growth and branching. Basil is a good example. Keep pinching off budding tops down to the next set of leaves and it will branch out, increasing its yield three-fold. If you intended to harvest basil, marjoram, or oregano, but it is already in bloom, the flowering top is potent enough to use for a culinary herb.

Flowers are so beautiful in the garden; it's often a conflict whether to cut or leave them! You can compromise by taking only some of the flowers, and remember that the more flowers are picked, the more the plant continues to bloom. Most flowers are harvested while in full bloom. Lavender is an exception. The stalks are cut just before the buds open and release their fragrance. Thankfully, it flowers again in another month or so. The long lasting bloom of yarrow and tansy flowers can be enjoyed in the garden for a couple weeks as long as you catch them before they begin to brown around the edges.

Spring or fall is the most aromatic time to dig angelica and vetiver roots and the rhizomes of orris root, spikenard, and sweet flag. These underground portions of the plants are most potent then, since that is where they store nutrients to get through winter. Wash roots and rhizomes right after harvesting them. They can be soaked in water, but only long enough to loosen dirt, since water pulls out their scent. If the water becomes fragrant, they soaked too long. Thick roots and rhizomes like these dry more easily if they are sliced into thin strips or cut into quarter-inch pieces with garden clippers.

Keep all parts of the plant out of direct sun and high heat right after they are cut. The light and heat increase oxidation, which darkens them and causes their aroma to more quickly evaporate into the air.

DRYING AROMATIC PLANTS

Dry fragrant plants carefully, so that they retain as much scent and color as possible. Even then, they will typically lose as much as thirty to forty percent of their fragrant essential oils. Plants dry quickly in a warm, dry place that has good air circulation to move out the moisture. Too much heat pulls the aromas into the air. If your dried plants are headed for the kitchen for spices or tea, be sure to dry them in a clean environment that is free of bugs and dirt. Drying time depends on the climate. It can be only a couple days if the air is warm and dry, but humidity and cold slow down the process, often to as much as a week. Drying time also depends on the plant. Yarrow and lavender contain little moisture, so they dry quickly, while fleshy leaves of basil, lemon balm, and peppermint take longer.

Hanging plants to dry

Tying plants into bunches and hanging them upside down from their stems is a classic drying method. Depending on the plant, climate, and weather, tie together three to twenty stems. You may need to experiment in your area to make sure there is sufficient airflow and to prevent molding. Fortunately, many of the same essential oils that make plants smell so good are also mold inhibiters.

Hanging plants are fragrant and picturesque, but this drying method is also a practical way to keep stems straight. It makes it easier to run your fingers along the stem to strip off dried leaves of lemon balm, lemon verbena, or peppermint for tea; and basil, marjoram, rosemary, sage, and thyme leaves for the spice jars. Straight stems also mean that lavender, roses, tansy, yarrow, and the various sages stand upright in dried flower arrangements.

Drying bouquets are beautiful wherever they hang, but not every house has rafters. Be creative. If you have a ceiling or wall rack

---

▶ Lavender harvest for potpourri, tea, and lavender cookies.

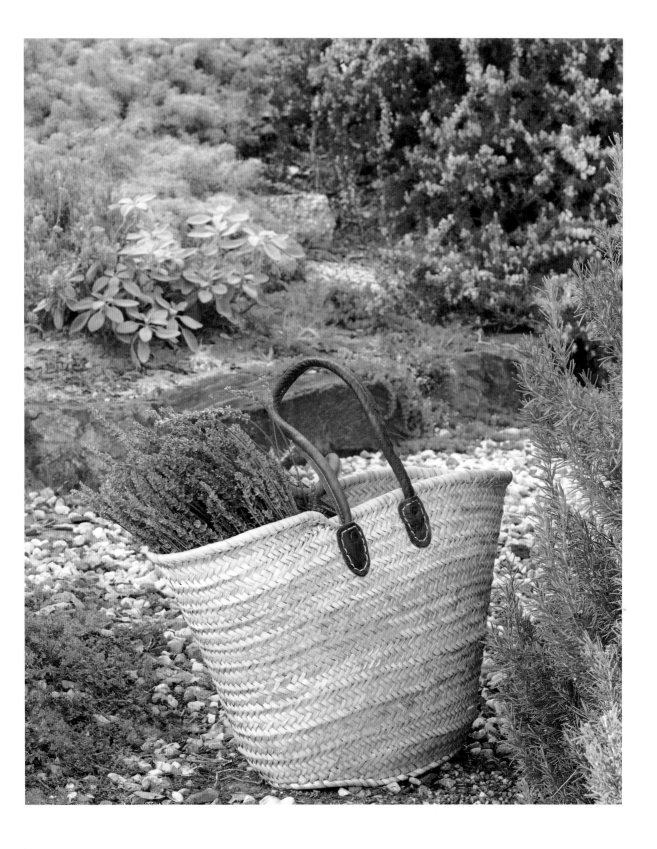

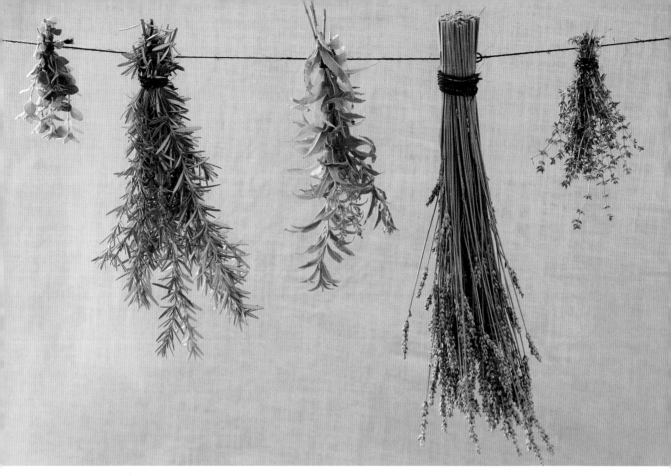

▲ An easy and efficient way to dry herbs is to hang them.

in your kitchen for hanging pans or baskets, perhaps part of that can be appropriated during the harvest season. Wall racks that fan out to dry dish towels work equally well for plants, and those racks fold flat against a wall when not in use. Coat pegs or hooks can be pressed into service. A folding clothes-drying rack with a series of parallel dowels holds about fifty small bundles of drying plants. It is also portable, so it can be set up almost anywhere, then folded to store. If nothing else is available, string a clothesline in a shady outdoor area or even inside the house. Be forewarned that when crispy plants are removed from their drying area, small pieces may crumble or break.

Other drying methods

I am always seeking easy solutions to harvest my large garden. Paper bags and porous cloth bags make handy, portable dryers. They keep dust and sunlight off the drying plants but still allow them to dry. To increase air circulation and drying, cut little "u" shapes into paper bags and open the resulting flaps. Place a bunch of plants on the stem into the bag with the stems protruding from the top. Tie a string firmly around the top of the bag with the ends of the stalks sticking out. Use the strings to hang the bag or catch them on a hook. A flat-bottomed paper bag can also be used for individual flowers, leaves, and seeds. Place a thin layer on the bottom of the bag. Shake it at least once a day to redistribute the plant material so that it dries evenly. Hang drying bags almost anywhere. Even tree branches will do, although your neighbors may think you invented a new way to keep away crows! These bags can be easily moved from one place to another.

Bags are also very helpful to harvest and dry seeds. Collecting and drying angelica, coriander, dill, and fennel seeds can be tricky because they fall off the plant as soon as they are ripe. Just before seeds ripen, slide a bag made of paper or porous cloth over the seed head. Tightly tie the bag's opening to the stalk. One bag can hold several stalks of plants that are growing very close to each other. When the seeds begin to ripen and fall inside the bag, cut off the stalk, and put it on a shelf—or hang it, bag and all. Once the seeds finish falling into the bag, they are ready to pour into storage jars.

A screen is also an excellent way to dry plants. It works especially well for leaves that are not dried on the stalk, and for flowers, seeds, and root slices. Use a clean window screen or make your own by stretching and adhering flexible hardware screening over a wood frame, such as a heavy-duty picture frame. Screens can hang from the ceiling or be stacked about eight inches apart using clean bricks or wood blocks. When I was drying plants for commercial tea blends, I had custom-made racks that held a series of six-by-four-foot screens. Place drying screens where there is good airflow. Keep plants in a thin layer so that they dry rapidly and evenly. Limp plants, such as basil, need to be stirred at least once a day so they do not overlap too much.

Plants quickly dry in a forced-air food dehydrator. An oven set on warm also works as a dryer, although it is not very energy efficient. Open the door to allow moisture and excess heat to escape. In a microwave oven, place individual leaves, seeds, or petals between two paper plates or paper towels and set the oven on low. Check every two minutes to see if the plants are dry and do another round, if needed. Remove the plants just before they are completely dry, and finish by air-drying or they will become too crisp.

PRESERVING AND STORING

Plants are ready to store when they are dry enough to break or crumble. Clean, dry, airtight glass containers retain the most fragrance, but airtight plastic jars or bags also work. If moisture begins to form on the inside of the storage container, the plants were not dry enough. Act quickly to rescue them. Once mold sets in, it ruins the plant's color and fragrance.

It is best to store dried plants fairly whole, but without too much air in the container. Lightly crumble leaves, and store seeds and petals whole. Store tea herbs in canning jars with wide lids for easy access, and culinary herbs in six-ounce jars. For the best flavor, hand grind culinary herbs just before they go into a dish you're cooking. A coffee grinder can be used to pre-grind small amounts; keep those herbs close at hand, perhaps in a spice rack on your kitchen wall.

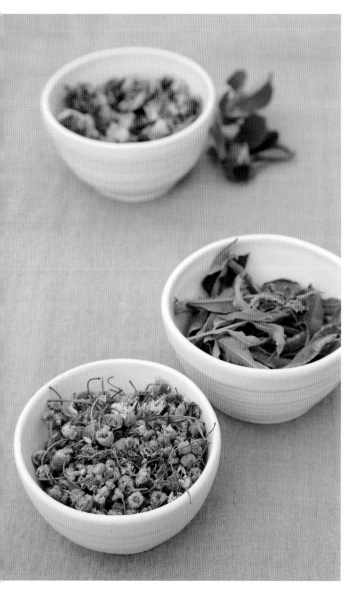

The aroma of dried plants slowly dissipates over time. There is no clear cutoff, but they last about two to three years if kept in sealed containers in a cool, dark place. They keep much longer refrigerated. If they still smell good, they have maintained enough potency to use.

The same mealy moths and grain weevils that eat grain also go after dried plants. The telltale signs are webs forming in the container. Fortunately, many fragrant plants are bug repellent. The more potent a plant smells, the less likely it is to become infested. A few bay laurel leaves in a container of grain has long been used to protect it from bugs. Freezing plants kills the bugs. My refrigerator freezer is already packed with herbal concoctions, but I put jars of vulnerable dried plants, such as rose petals, outside overnight when temperatures drop near freezing. Freezing tea and culinary herbs retains their scent and flavor. Fleshy culinary herbs, such as basil, lemon balm, and peppermint, can be chopped or blended with dried herbs into tasty combinations. Pack them into containers to freeze. A small ice-cube tray creates individual portions that melt quickly when you need to spice up a meal. Concentrated teas can also be frozen. Fresh, whole petals of roses, leaves of peppermint or scented geranium, and slices of lemon peel can be frozen in ice cubes to make fun additions to cold drinks.

▲ Aromatic herbs and flowers provide a wide selection of tasty teas.

in the kitchen: aroma and flavor

Your fragrance garden is filled with many herbs that are just waiting for experimentation. The flavor and scent of any aromatic plant come from the plant's essential oils. When you have one, you have the other. One way to judge the quality of the culinary herbs in your garden is simply to smell them. When you dry aromatic herbs, retain as much of the scent as possible to make sure they maintain a deep, rich flavor.

GARDEN HERB BLENDS

The fragrance garden is also the chef's garden. You can have all the basic flavorings necessary for many recipes. Grow your own basil, coriander, dill, fennel, marjoram, rosemary, sage, and thyme, and maybe even your own bay leaves from your own bay laurel tree. Culinary herbs can spice up your cooking, and your life. They are all aromatic, because the same essential oils are responsible for both taste and scent. You can even judge the quality of their flavor by smelling them.

Chefs say the secret to fine dining is to use herbs fresh from the garden, because they have the most flavor. I used to ship just-picked herbs from my farm on cold packs overnight from California to exclusive New York restaurants, so they could have the superior taste of fresh herbs. You can have the same quality in your home cooking. Store-bought spices are no comparison to the sensory superiority and deep satisfaction of cooking with your own homegrown herbs. Grind your garden herbs in a coffee

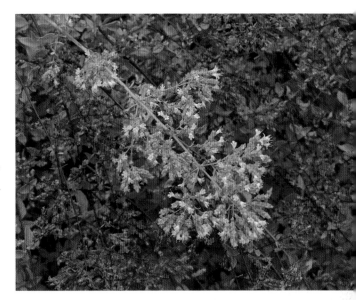

▲ Oregano's white flowers contrast with all types of marjoram blooms.

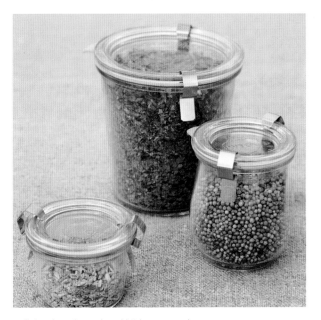

▲ Spices from the garden add rich aromas and tastes to a variety of dishes.

grinder, blender, flourmill, or by hand with a mortar and pestle. Then fill your spice jars.

Make spice blends by combining powdered herbs. You can even make theme blends. An Italian mix of basil, marjoram, and oregano can be sprinkled on pasta, pizza, and just about any tomato dish. For a French flavor, combine marjoram, rosemary, sage, and thyme. Instead of grinding these herbs, you can tie them into little bundles for your own French-style bouquet garni to flavor soups and stews. If you do not already have your favorite blend, keep it simple and use equal parts of each herb. To make herbal salts, mix an herb blend with an equal amount of coarsely ground salt.

If you like to think outside the box, try rose petal sorbet. Mexican marigold can substitute for tarragon, which is not always easier to grow. Peppermint goes into Mexican mole. Rose geranium gives cakes an amazing flavor. Curry plant leaves are not the perfect substitute for curry, but they're not bad with rice. For Thai cuisine, mix lemon grass leaves, curry plant, and cilantro with chili peppers.

Herbal vinegar

Aromatic plants can turn an ordinary bottle of vinegar into a gourmet delight. You can even make vinegars to replace toxic commercial house cleaners. Vinegar infused with aromatic plants is one of the most versatile culinary products you can make from your garden. The most popular blends are the herbal ones, such as basil, dill, marjoram, oregano, rosemary, sage, and thyme—but don't stop there. Put your imagination to work and try bay laurel, coriander, fennel, lemon, lemon grass, lemon verbena, and peppermint. Or how about curry plant or lavender? The different flavors of basil are also tasty. Any type of vinegar can be used. White vinegar brings out the colors of the plants, such as the rich hues of purple basil. Apple cider vinegar is sometimes preferred for its flavor and health properties. Other types, such as wine, barley, and rice vinegars also work well.

To make herbal vinegar, you need about a cup of chopped fresh or dried herbs from your garden. Place the herbs in a clean, wide-mouthed jar and cover with about one pint of your choice of vinegar, so that the herbs are completely submerged. Stir to eliminate any trapped air pockets and put a lid on the jar. Keep it at room temperature for two weeks, then strain out the herbs. This is a concentrate, so dilute it with an equal amount of pure vinegar before using it in salad dressing, mustard, pickled foods, or any recipe calling for vinegar. The final touch can be to submerge a few sprigs of a fresh or dried plant in the infused vinegar.

Infused vinegar can also be used for hair rinse, by diluting it with an equal amount of water instead of vinegar. Use lavender, rosemary, and sage for the infusion. The vinegar scent dissipates quickly, leaving hair bright and shiny.

▶ Herbal vinegars bring the garden to your table throughout the year.

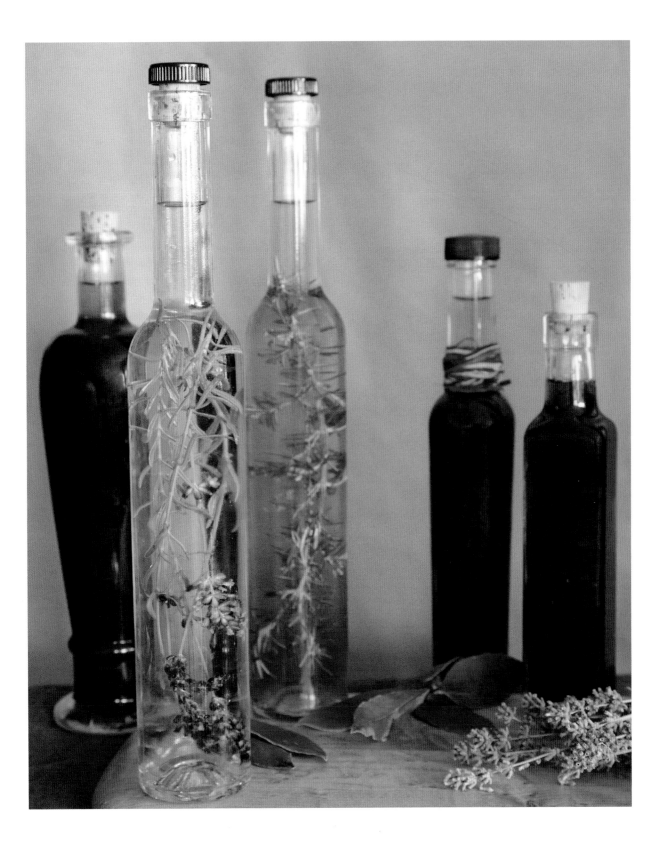

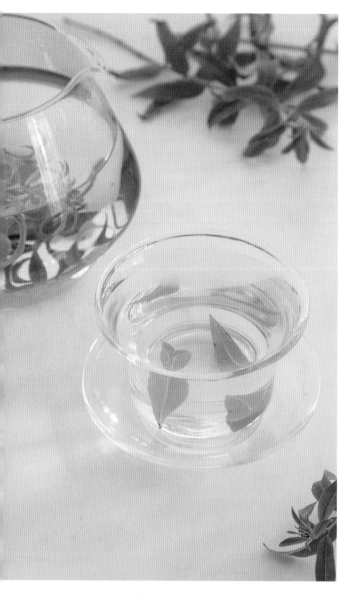

▲ A cup of cool tea is always welcome on a hot summer day.

A perfect cup of tea

After working in your garden, nothing is more rewarding than taking a tea break with an herb tea—from your own garden, of course. Garden visitors are always delighted to be served a cup of tea from the garden. Sitting down to a hot cup while poring over seed catalogs is a popular winter pastime of gardeners. There is nothing like the aroma of summer to bring back memories of a garden filled with color and fragrance. And cool tea on a warm day refreshes and restores the spirit.

To make a good cup of hot tea, choose either fresh or dried herbs. Use about one teaspoon per cup (more dried herbs fit into a teaspoon, so they will make a stronger tea than fresh herbs). Steep flowers, leaves, and seeds in a teapot, pan, or cup by covering the herbs with boiling water. Place a cover on the container and let it sit at least five minutes. Roots, rhizomes, and barks need to be simmered for about fifteen minutes. Often, a second batch can be made from them. Keep the heat low and cover the container to reduce the escape of steam and retain the aroma and taste.

Herbs such as German chamomile, lemon balm, lemon verbena, lemon grass, peppermint, and wintergreen make tasty tea when used alone or in combinations. The first three are relaxing, while peppermint and wintergreen provide a pick-me-up. Fennel seed or anise hyssop add their licorice-like taste. Few people drink lavender or rose petal tea any more. Lavender is strong, so use a half-teaspoon per cup for a lighter taste. Scented geranium comes in many scents, each with a corresponding flavor. Other unique flavors to try are rosemary, sage, basil, and holy basil or tulsi. It only takes a couple of fresh or dried jasmine flowers to flavor an entire pot of green, black, or herb tea. Lemon peel goes well with almost any herb tea.

creating aromatic products

Bringing the garden's aromatherapy into your house can be as simple as having a vase of flowers on a table or sideboard, or incorporating homegrown herbs into your cooking. You can scent the air by gently simmering a handful of aromatic plants in a pan of water. But taking the time to create your own fragrant home accessories and personal care items can be especially satisfying. Body care creams, lotions, tonics, and hair rinses not only improve your complexion and hair, the fragrance also has healing potential. Herbal vinegars can be used either for body care or in the kitchen.

FRESH AND DRIED BOUQUETS

Nothing is as uplifting as having fresh, fragrant flowers throughout the house. More than a third of the people surveyed by the Flowers and Plants Association said scent influenced their choice when they are selecting cut flowers. To help bouquets last longer, put them in water immediately after they are cut. Another trick is to slice stems diagonally—increasing the surface area of the cut allows the stem to draw in more

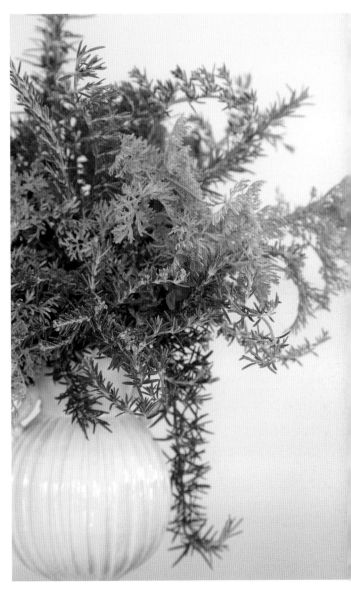

▲ Rosemary and wormwood for memory, reminding you to bring garden herbs inside.

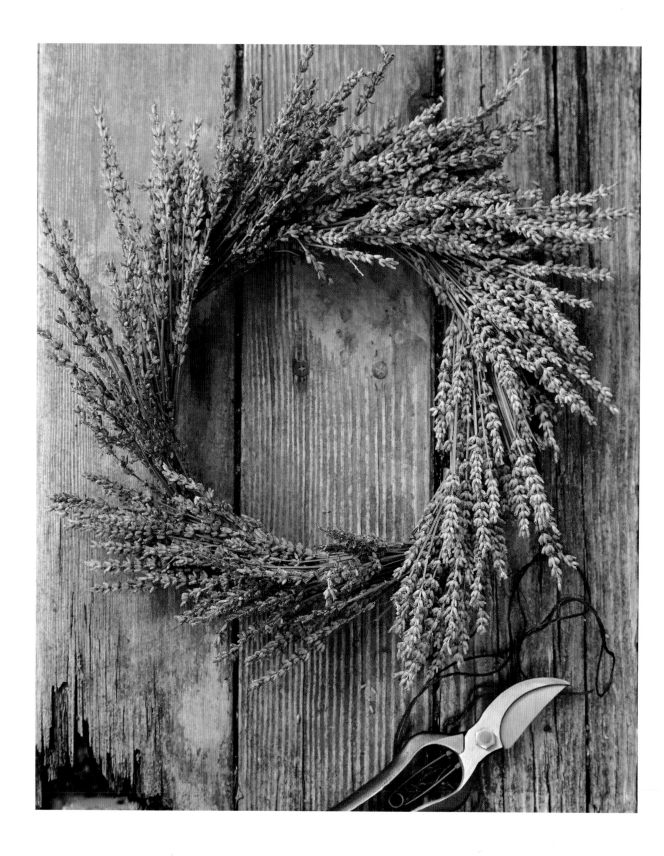

water. Many flowers last longer if the leaves are snipped off the stem before putting them in water. For example, lilacs do not last very long as a cut flower, but remove their leaves and they will look vibrant for an extra day.

Do not overlook violets, pansies, hyacinths, and English primroses as cut flowers. They may have rather flimsy, short stems, but they make beautiful, early spring bouquets when they are placed in a short vase. Combine them in one vase and their textures and colors will play off each other. The stems of gardenia and daphne flowers are too crooked for vases, but the flowers look stunning floating in a shallow bowl of water. Just a few flowers will fill the immediate area with fragrance. Jasmine vines are not long lasting, but they can still be twined into a bouquet of other flowers. Lavender, rosemary, tansy, and yarrow are summer blooms with tough stems that dry nicely in the vase. Pull them out of spent bouquets, cut off the wet portion of the stems, and they are ready for dried arrangements.

When winter sets in and the garden no longer offers fresh flowers, turn to dried bouquets. Roses, tansy, and yarrow flowers can be accented with the leaves of bay laurel, juniper, myrtle, oregano, rosemary, and thick-leaved sages. The shorter stems of santolina, southernwood, and wormwood also dry nicely for accents, although they dry quite brittle.

Dried plants keep their color and fragrance best when stored out of direct sunlight. Most dried leaves last about a year, while dried flowers keep for several years. Take dried arrangements outside occasionally to shake off any dust that has accumulated. When the plants look spent or brittle, toss them out and rearrange the bouquet with new additions. Beautiful wreaths and wall swags can also be created from dried plants.

SHARING THE SCENT

Close your eyes and the fragrance of dried flora can transport you to the middle of your garden, no matter where you are or the time of year. Gardeners used to concentrate on growing the most aromatic plants and then preserving them, to keep enjoying the garden's fragrance throughout the winter and to share with others. What better way to show off your garden all year long?

Potpourri

Potpourri is composed of sweet-smelling, dried petals, leaves and spices that release their perfume over time. They are mixed together mostly for fragrance, but also for the visual appeal of contrasting colors and textures. The word "potpourri" is translated from French, meaning a "combination of diverse elements." As with good perfume, the individual scents become slightly elusive when they blend into unique fragrances.

Potpourri was the original air freshener. The natural scent is much purer and more appealing than modern so-called potpourri plug-ins that contain overly sweet, synthetic scents. Some potpourris need the addition of essential oils to enhance their scent, but not

◀ Lavender wired on a ring becomes a decorative, fragrant wreath.

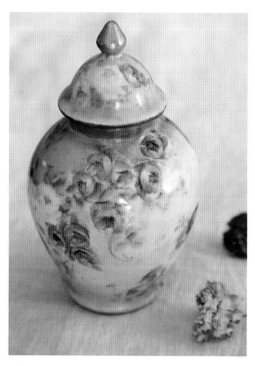

▲ The author's grandmother Irene's potpourri jar.

southernwood, wormwood, and the various sages can also be added. Other possible ingredients that add visual appeal as well as scent are coriander seeds and lemon peel.

Plants that become more fragrant as they age also make potpourri last longer. They are called "fixatives" because they fix the scent. Finely chopped orris root is the most popular fixative due to its light, violet-like aroma, although some people have an allergy or sensitivity to it. Alternative fixatives from the garden are patchouli, sandalwood, vetiver, and Cleveland sage, each of which contributes its own scent to the mix.

Stovetop or simmering potpourri is a variation on the theme. When a handful of potpourri is very lightly simmered in a quart of water, the steam that is produced scents an entire room. Try this on a cold winter's day, to bring back the aroma of a summer garden. The stovetop potpourri's scent only lingers as long as it is simmering, though, so keep a large jar of potpourri on hand.

Sachets

Grind potpourri into coarse powder in a coffee grinder and it becomes a sachet. The powder is used to fill a paper envelope or a bag. A common method of holding sachet is to bring the ends of a small, square cloth together and tie them in a bow. Sachets of roses or lavender have long been tucked into dresser drawers to make clothes smell sweet. I first encountered the heavenly smell of lavender when I opened my grandmother Irene's lingerie drawer. I was just tall enough to hang my nose over the edge of the drawer, which I did at every opportunity when no one was looking.

those made from the garden. As a child, I remember opening a jar of rose petals to inhale the wonderful fragrance every time I visited my grandmother, Irene Keville. She left me that jar, which still retains a strong scent after seven decades.

Many different potpourris can be created from your fragrance garden. You cannot go wrong with any combination. The flowers of chamomile, gardenia, lavender, rose, and yarrow dry nicely for potpourri. There are a number of dried leaves that work well, such as bay laurel, juniper, lemon verbena, patchouli, marjoram, myrtle, and scented geranium. Small amounts of the sharp-smelling leaves of rosemary, santolina,

Moth-repellent sachets in your woolens make eco-friendly replacements for toxic, smelly mothballs. Fill them with southernwood, camphor leaves, or patchouli to deter clothes moths. They work as well as the renowned smell of cedar. Other moth repellents are bay laurel, camphor, lavender, and culinary sage. Your cat will appreciate a catnip sachet on a string to bat around, although the ball may not stay on the string for long! My cats like to play their version of soccer with them.

Dream pillows

Dream pillows contain potpourri herbs thought to enhance dreams. Ask anyone who has slept on a mugwort pillow and they should confirm that they dreamed through the night. Mugwort can be mixed with other herbs. Plant lore associated with dreams says that thyme prevents nightmares, lavender makes dreams more pleasant, while roses instill love. Rosemary is said to improve dream recall, while everlasting flowers such as curry plant help dreams make a lasting impression. You may want to combine all these—except maybe the curry plant, which smells like curry and makes me hungry rather than dreamy.

If you prefer to sleep rather than tossing and turning with dreams, stuff a pillow with hops and lavender. "Dilly" pillows filled with soothing herbs (such as dill seeds and chamomile) have long been used to put babies to sleep and settle fussiness. Many of my aromatherapy students who learned to make dilly pillows in class say how well the sleep aids have lulled their own children and grandchildren to sleep. When I travel to

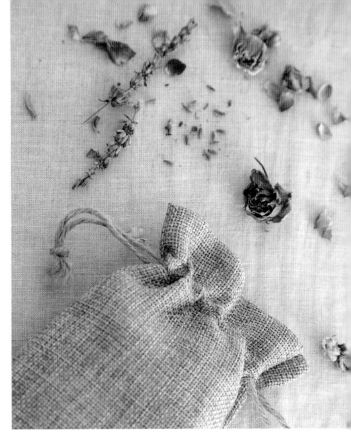

▲ Roses and lavender make for sweet dreams.

teach seminars, I always carry an herbal sleep pillow. It really does work, and it is far simpler to roll over while groggy and grab the pillow than to wake up and make tea.

Mugwort and hops were once used to stuff large bed pillows, but modern dream and sleep pillows are typically about six inches wide. This makes them small enough to tuck inside a pillowcase next to the pillow. They can be made from simple cotton fabric or fancy satin or velvet with laces and ribbon edgings. Potpourri pillows last for quite a few years, especially if they are kept away from heat. When the scent begins to wane, squish the pillow and the herbs inside will release more fragrance.

aromatherapy body oils from the garden

Long before there were essential oils to purchase, people made aromatic body, hair, and anointing oils from their gardens, using favorite fragrant plants such as sweet basil, gardenia, jasmine, and spikenard. To create soothing and fragrant body oils today, simply soak aromatic plant materials in a warm carrier oil. A carrier oil is a vegetable oil such as coconut or grapeseed oil that serves to "carry" the essential oil. Carrier oils are readily infused with the tiny essential oils, and thus the scent. I suggest that you try small batches when you start out to master the technique. In addition, some delicate flowers that are difficult to steam-distill into essential oils, such as jasmine, are sensitive to any heat used in processing. The result is an infused oil that smells good, but never smells as beautiful as the pure essential oil.

To make your own aromatherapy oil, finely chop dried or fresh garden plant material. Fresh plants are trickier to process since they mold more easily. Either way, the plants generally represent about half the amount by weight of the carrier oil. So if you have eight ounces of plant material, use about sixteen ounces of oil. However, it is difficult to give exact measurements for each herb, because they have varying weights, volumes, and rates of oil absorption. The plant material should be completely submerged in the carrier oil, with the oil barely covering it. Place it on very low heat—no boiling or even pre-boiling—for at least five hours. The ideal temperature is between 80 and 90 degrees F. To maintain this state, you may want to use a double boiler or a rice cooker, or a crock pot if it has a very low setting. If the room fills with a lovely aroma, the temperature is too hot and you are losing the plant's scent into the room.

An alternate method uses solar heat. Place chopped, dried plant material in a clean, wide-mouthed glass jar. Pour the carrier oil over the top, then stir it to release any air bubbles, and affix a lid. If the air is humid, cover the top of the jar with several layers of cheesecloth instead of a lid, and secure the cloth with string or a rubber band to allow moisture to escape and to prevent molding. Check the mixture in a few hours; you may need to add more oil if the plant materials are very absorbent. Let the jar sit in the sun for three or four days. This technique works best on hot days since the temperature inside the jar will be about five degrees cooler than the outside air. Fluctuations in temperature from day to night will not harm the process, but if daytime temperatures temporarily cool down, leave the jar in the sun for a few extra days. You can also keep the jar in another warm place, such as next to a heater, wood stove, or fireplace.

With either the stovetop or the solar method, when the plants are ready, strain the oil through a fine kitchen strainer, cheesecloth, or muslin. Before you strain out the plant material, however, make sure that the oil has taken on the color and aroma of the plant. Stick a clean knife into the oil. Pull it out and smell the oil residue on the knife to make sure it smells like the plant(s) you used. If it doesn't, try processing the oil a little longer. If you used fresh plants instead of dried, you may end up with a few drops of

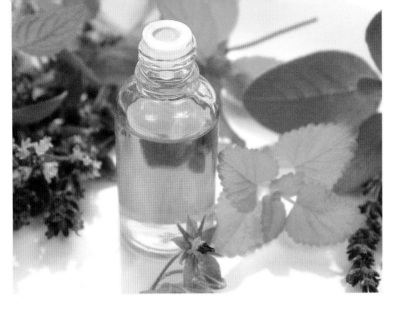

◀ Nothing smells or feels as good on the skin as body oil made from plants you've grown yourself.

water at the bottom after the oil is strained. Discard it with the last little bit of oil, or save it for your next bath. Once the oil is strained, you have your own body or massage oil or hair treatment from your garden.

Following are some simple formulas. You do not have to follow them exactly. Feel free to stick to the plants you have in your garden. Simply use equal parts of whatever plants you choose, put them in a jar and cover them with a carrier oil.

Gardener's heating liniment When a long day in the garden has your muscles aching, you can turn your garden plants into a pain relief liniment with basil, bay laurel, eucalyptus, and juniper leaves. To create a liniment-like sensation of heat, also add camphor or peppermint leaves.

Lavender-rose anti-inflammation oil This formula can ease muscle cramps or pain from arthritis, and the same plants also reduce inflammation from bruises and sprains—injuries that gardeners know all too well. Use the flowers of lavender, German chamomile, and curry plant; and leaves of marjoram, rose, and rose geranium.

Sleep and de-stressing massage oil Try gentle aromatherapy by making a massage oil with the flowers of German or Roman chamomile, clove pink, lavender, orange blossom, and rose; and the leaves of bee balm, lemon balm, and marjoram. This oil may also be rubbed on the temples.

Antidepressant massage oil One of the main features of aromatherapy is how fragrances act on the mind. Take advantage of this by creating oils with aromatic plants that are used to increase a sense of happiness, such as bee balm, clary sage, lavender, lemon balm, lemon verbena, jasmine, orange blossom, and rose geranium. This oil may also be rubbed on the temples.

Sensual massage oil A number of plants have age-old reputations as aphrodisiacs, such as clove pinks, jasmine, orange blossom, rose flowers, and patchouli leaves. Coriander can be added to this list, but it, as well as the others, are obviously not good additions if the object of your affection does not find the scent pleasing.

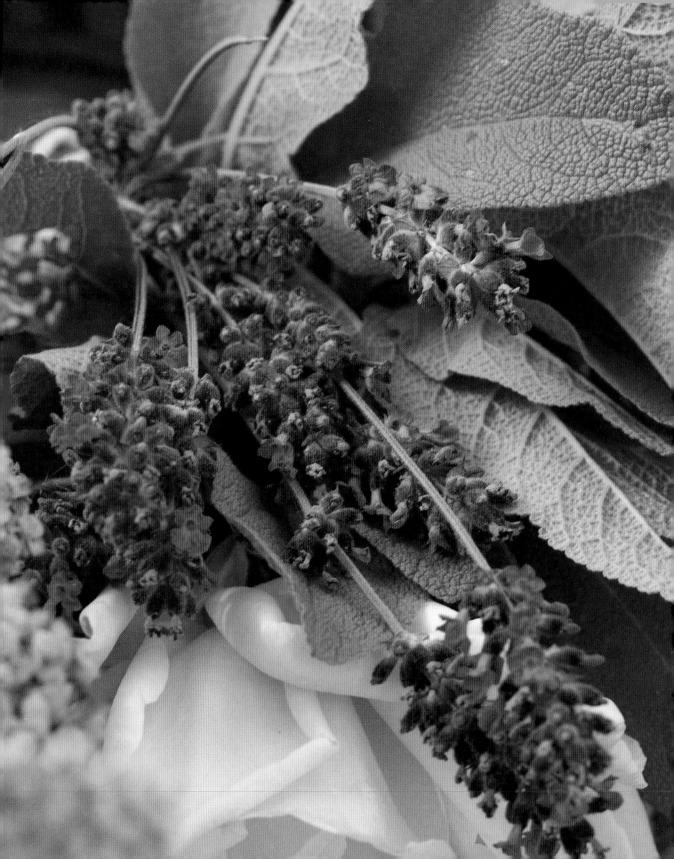

profiles of
aromatic plants

Most gardeners agree it is a joy to be surrounded by aromatic plants. No wonder we love gardening! Yet, it is easy to see in today's nurseries and garden catalogs that color and form have won out over fragrance. In the quest to develop good-looking plants, hybridization sadly left scent behind. Take the rose and sweet pea. Both were originally highly aromatic, but modern varieties with perfectly formed, more-abundant flowers generate little scent. Even lilacs, once famed for their fragrance, are now available in practically scentless varieties.

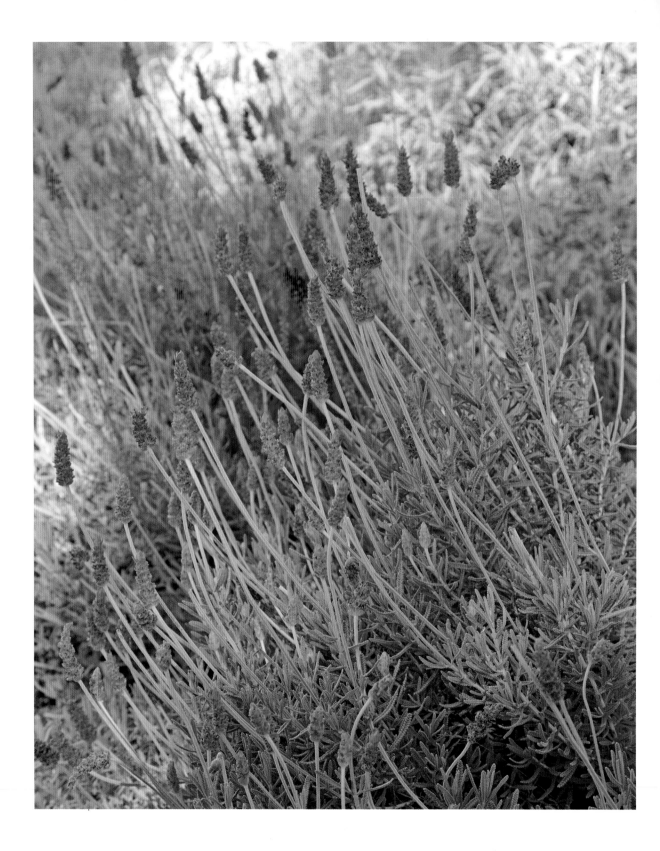

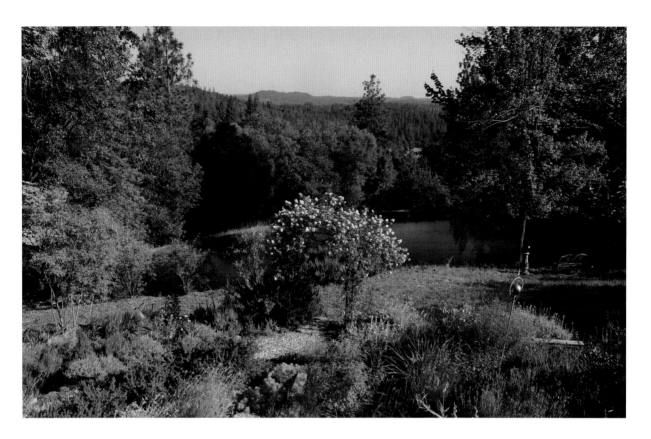

Gone, too, are the plant catalogs that wove elaborate descriptions of each plant's scent, and gardening books that lusciously described fragrances of honeysuckle, daffodil, pansy, and primrose.

Despite the modern lean away from fragrance, nurseries say customers are often looking for aromatic species. There may be an innate desire within us for our plants to be endowed with scent. Imagine opening your door or window to be greeted by the fragrance of your garden. A selection of aromatic plants from around the world is available to the modern gardener.

I carefully chose my favorite fragrant plants, along with their scent-laden relatives. Each is distinctive for its abundant, interesting, or beautiful aroma. These old friends have graced my fragrance gardens for decades, and they are more than pretty smells. Their aromatherapy properties are a constant source of emotional uplifting and healing for me.

▲ The fragrance garden offers a place to contemplate the world.

◄ One of the delightful smaller lavenders preferred for tight landscaping.

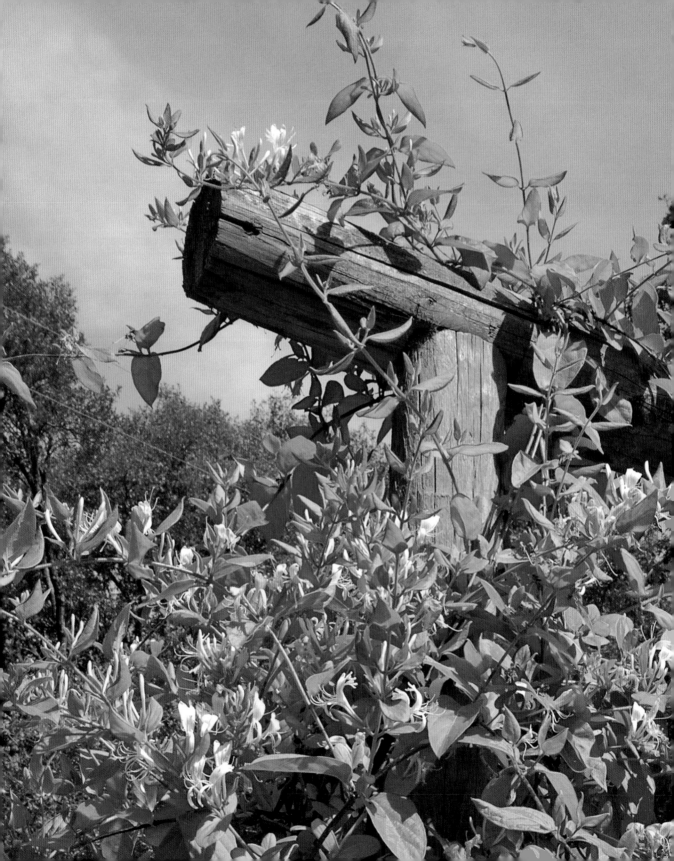

plants to breathe life and joy into your garden

Here I offer classic aromatherapy choices, as well as describing the healing potential of other fragrant garden plants, based on their history. Suggestions highlight a range of species and varieties, indicating which are most fragrant, as well as profiling different aromas. Guidelines are provided on cultivation and harvest, including plant care requirements, to help you choose aromatics that will best suit your garden and home. Wherever possible, I offer a glimpse into the colorful folklore of aromas.

Botanical names and hardiness zones

Botanical names can help you keep track of which plants are related. First the genus, then the species name is listed. For example, in the case of *Lavandula angustifolia*, *Lavandula* is the genus from which lavender is produced, and *angustifolia* is the species. This plant is a member of the large, highly aromatic mint family, the Lamiaceae. If slight differences occur in a species, they are designated as varieties. Botany is organized by visual similarities and differences in plants. Plants do not always fit perfectly into botanical groupings, so there is some pushing and shoving, as well as changes in nomenclature. But botanical names are still helpful in organizing and remembering plants and their relationships to each other.

Latin and some Greek words designate plant names. A plant is typically named to honor an individual or to describe its characteristics or use. It is not difficult to guess why a species of daphne is named "odora," both violet and mignonette have "odorata" species, and a particularly heady species of honeysuckle is called "fragrantissima."

The USDA Hardiness Zone Map is a valuable tool that indicates a plant's hardiness to freezing temperatures, and can help you determine what plants will survive in your area. The map divides North America into eleven zones that differ by about ten degrees Fahrenheit for each number. Zone hardiness is based on an average weather year; obviously there are weather events that happen that are not typical of a zone, but it is good for general determination. This map can be found at planthardiness.ars.usda.gov/PHZMWeb.

◀ Fragrant honeysuckle loves to climb, spreading its sweet aroma.

Angelica

Angelica archangelica

Carrot family: Apiaceae
Biennial (may live three years before flowering)
Zones 4–9

Both angelica root and seed have a deep, herby aroma with a spicy high note that leaves a lingering sweet and bitter scent. It is musty, quite sharp, and a little like celery with a touch of alcohol, yet hauntingly attractive. It could be a designer drink that combines celery and gin. The musty spiciness reminds me of walking through an East Indian bazaar rich with spices incense. Pinching either the leaf or stem releases a lighter version of the same unique aroma.

Angelica gigas, with its attractive red stems and seed heads, has the same aroma and is a favorite among gardeners. Daegu Haany University in South Korea found in 2005 studies that *Angelica gigas* regulates mood changes by moderating dopamine, a brain neurotransmitter. Simply inhaling the aroma seems to help smokers quit their habit, by preventing the addictive high that usually results when tobacco spikes dopamine levels.

Both the Europeans and the Chinese burned the aromatic root as incense for its calming effect and to protect them from disease. The aroma is said to relieve depression and frayed nerves, and to generate creativity.

The plant grows abundantly in Iceland and Finnish Lapland, where angelica garlands are presented to poets in the hope that its perfume will provide inspiration. Benedictine monks in the Middle Ages added the aromatic root to wines and elixirs for its uplifting and medicinal properties. It still flavors Cointreau and Chartreuse liqueurs, as well as some vermouths and gins. The hollow stems are candied for a crunchy, bittersweet treat to ease a sore throat. All that sugar brings out angelica's sweeter side. In Norway, the powdered seeds flavor bread. An essential oil is produced from both the root and seed, but it needs to be well diluted, as its strength can cause a temporary skin reaction.

The species name *archangelica* is appropriate, considering how this six-foot-tall plant dramatically hovers over the garden with wide, spreading leaves. Its strikingly large white umbels flower in its second or third year. Position individual plants separately throughout the garden, or showcase them as a focal point in the center of a bed. The flowers attract many beneficial insects. Ultraviolet nectar guides that we cannot see on the angelica blooms lead honeybees to their target. Keep angelica away from the door since flies flock to its aromatic blooms, including the beneficial tachinid flies that attack harmful insects.

Garden lore says angelica's fragrance increases when stinging nettles are planted nearby. The plant prefers a rich, moist, slightly acidic loam in a cool climate. It can adapt to full sun provided it receives sufficient water. If potted, it needs a five-gallon container or larger to accommodate its taproot. Angelica will not grow from cuttings or easily reseed, and unless refrigerated, the seeds are only viable for six months. The roots are harvested for tea in the first fall or second spring.

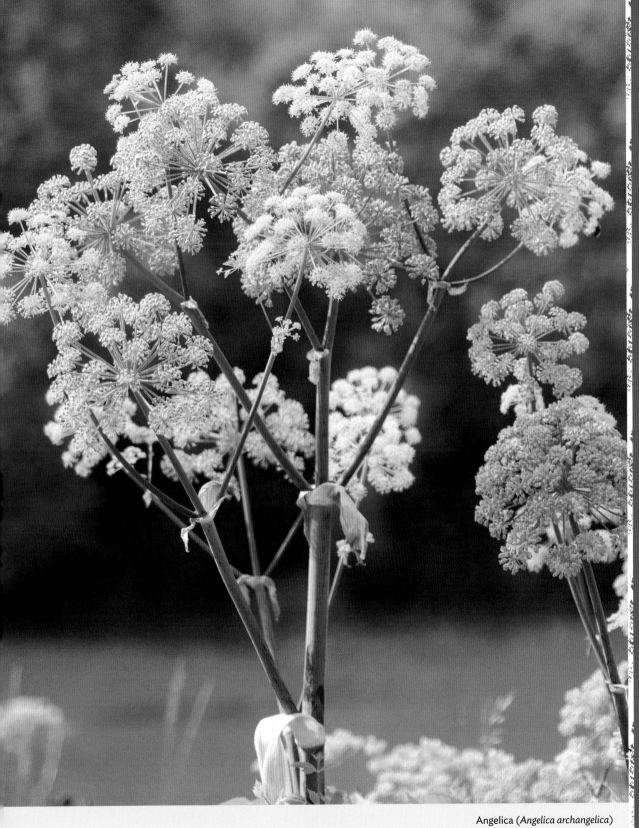

Angelica (*Angelica archangelica*)

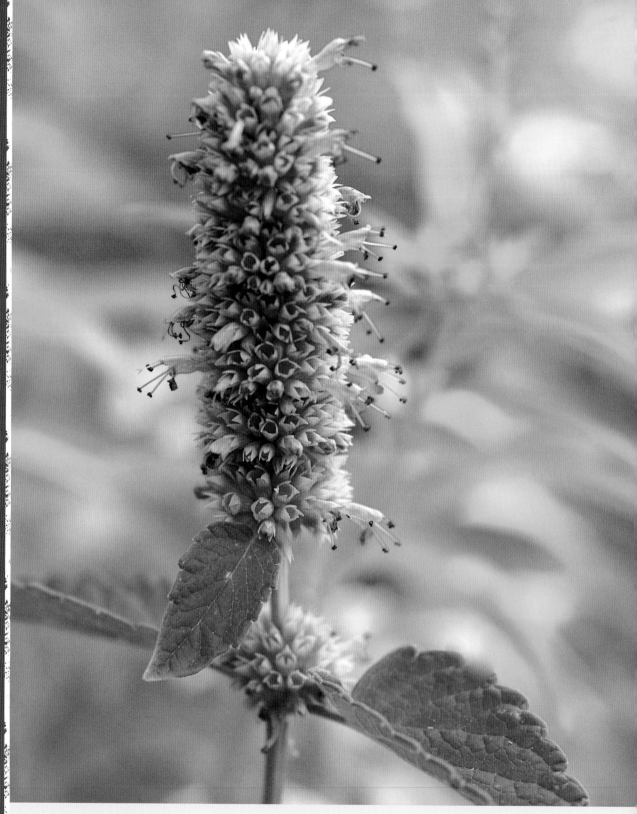

Anise hyssop (*Agastache foeniculum*)

Anise hyssop

Agastache foeniculum

Mint family: Lamiaceae
Perennial
Zones 4–10

As its name implies, the aroma of anise hyssop leaves and flowers is similar to anise, though more precisely, tarragon. Imagine licorice candy combined with an herb-like scent, backed by mint and a faint hint of pineapple, and you get an idea of the fragrance's complexity. Another comparison might be sweet licorice mints combined with chamomile herb tea.

A fragrance garden cannot have too many of the dozen *Agastache* species. They provide a variety of scents with anise or licorice as their theme. Purple giant hyssop (A. 'Fragrant Delight') is a cultivar that is often sold as anise hyssop, although its scent sways more toward pennyroyal. One of my favorites is the showy A. 'Tutti Frutti', with its lemon-mint scent and flavor. The raspberry-purple flowers are a favorite with hummingbirds. It grows to zone 6. Licorice mint hyssop (*A. rupestris*) has bronze-colored flowers surrounded by lavender calyxes and a lovely mint-licorice smell and taste. Native to southwestern North America, *A. aurantiaca* comes in several sweetly anise- scented varieties that have orange flowers. Mexican giant hyssop (*A. mexicana*) is also minty, with beautiful pink to crimson flowers. Korean mint (*A. rugosa*), a Chinese medicinal species, comes in two distinctly different versions, or chemotypes; one is clove-scented and the other smells more like patchouli.

Like anise, the aroma of anise hyssop is a pick-me-up. Its sweet scent and flavor have been well appreciated by Native Americans. The Plains tribes sweetened their food with it. The Cheyenne used it as aromatherapy for those who felt disheartened. They scented medicine bundles with the flowers and burned the leaves as incense during healing ceremonies, as well as placing the bundles on hot rocks in the sweat lodge to scent the air.

The licorice aroma is mirrored in the taste, so anise hyssop is used as a tarragon substitute. It also makes delicious herbal tea; mix it with peppermint or spearmint to bring out its minty side. Serve your guests a cup and they will think it is a tea blend. Sweeten tea with anise hyssop honey, which has a subtle mint flavor. The flower yields so much nectar that anise hyssop has been called the "wonder honey plant." It actually attracts more wild bumblebees than honeybees, as well as other pollinators such as hummingbirds, moths, and butterflies.

The bushy anise hyssop grows three feet tall, producing striking blue-purple, flowering spires beginning in midsummer. Use it as a background for shorter plants with vivid flowers such as calendula. Grow it with other *Agastache* species to contrast their colors and scents. It can be grown into a small hedge to showcase other plants. It is also perfect for a bee and butterfly garden among other plants that attract pollinators, such as blue- and red-flowering salvias.

Provide a well-drained, sandy, rich loam. Anise hyssop is not as drought tolerant as Mediterranean plants, so requires more watering. Give it full sun or, in hot climates, filtered light to prevent the thin leaves from drying out. The clumps look good for a couple years before beginning to die out. The seed-nutlets germinate easily, and having new seedlings every year maintains a succession of vibrant plants. The stalks can be hung to dry.

Balsam fir

Abies balsamea 'Nana'

Pine family: Pinaceae
Evergreen
Zones 2-8

The fragrance of fir is that of the forest on a hot day when the wind blows its sharp yet balsam-like fragrance your way. Since it is the aroma of the traditional Christmas tree, many people associate it with the spirit of that season. Fir is used more often in aromatherapy than the much sharper-smelling pine. An essential oil is distilled from the twigs and needles of balsam fir and also its less-sweet cousin, Siberian fir (*Abies sibirica*). The scent is used by aromatherapists to inspire goodwill, make one feel more grounded, and for those who feel emotionally blocked.

This species is a dwarf evergreen fir that is good for gardens since it only grows one to three feet tall, but the use for fir is the same no matter the size. The dense, rounded silhouette with a flattened top makes it a favorite in Japanese rock gardens. Grow it in slightly acidic, well-drained but moist soil without too much sun, to keep the needles looking good. It prefers hot, dry climates at low elevations. Unlike many plants in the fragrance garden, this bush tolerates windy areas.

Basil

Ocimum basilicum

Mint family: Lamiaceae
Annual

Basil's spicy clove scent, with its hint of mint and pepper, makes it delightfully sweet, hot, and sharp all at the same time. It is often referred to as sweet basil. The aroma definitely smells good enough to eat, like a slightly sweet and spicy herb blend designed for a Middle Eastern meal. The genus name *Ocimum* fittingly comes from the ancient Greek word that meant "to smell."

Crossbreeding among the basils has resulted in many varieties. There are also numerous aromatic types, or chemotypes. Lemon-scented basil (*Ocimum ×citriodorum*) from Thailand adds a citrus scent. Cinnamon basil (*O. basilicum* 'Cinnamon') is an extra spicy plant with purple flower spikes. The other approximately sixty basil species are so diverse that some botanists would prefer to reclassify them according to fragrance. Camphor basil (*O. kilmandscharicum*) from Kenya has an intense sharpness. Holy or sacred basil (*O. tenuiflorum*), known as *tulsi* in its native India, comes in three scents that are more herby than spicy.

Basil's uplifting fragrance improves mental work and decision making, but also reduces stress. Japanese researchers have found that the aroma stimulates the brain's beta waves, which increase alertness. Aromatherapists also suggest basil for those who tend to be tense and hold in anger. In Greece, it has a reputation of helping those who are in mourning. Sixteenth-century herbalist John Gerard said it "taketh away sorrowfulness." A popular basil-scented hand and face wash from that era doubled as a mood-enhancing cologne.

For the Italians, the scent of sweet basil signifies love. Even today, a suitor can proclaim his

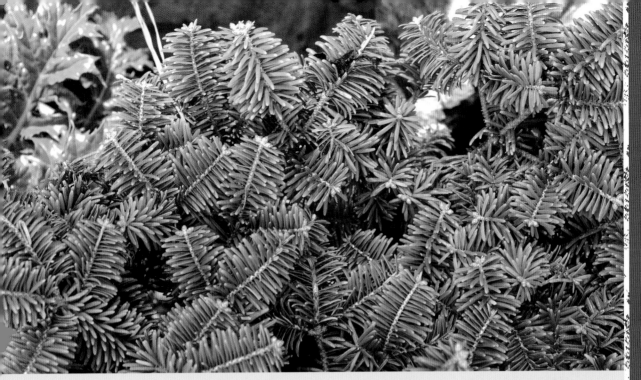

Balsam fir (*Abies balsamea* 'Nana')

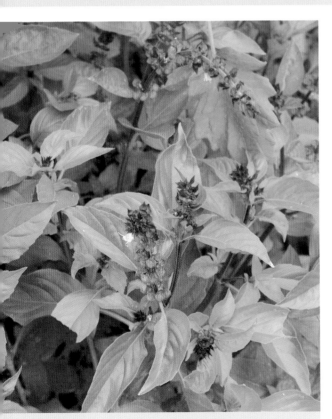

Basil (*Ocimum basilicum*)

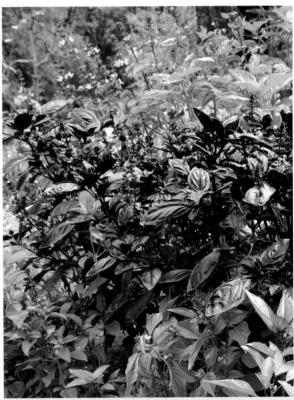

Purple basil (*Ocimum basilicum* var. *purpurascens*)

intentions by wearing a basil sprig. Apparently, a pot of basil on the porch also puts out an invitation to one's lover. A mainstay in Mediterranean and Middle Eastern cooking, sweet basil often sits on the porch close to the kitchen.

Basil's essential oil scents soap and other body care products. In perfumes, it serves as an inexpensive substitute for mignonette. Aromatherapists suggest rubbing sweet basil massage oil into overworked muscles to ease tightness, mental tension, and headaches. Ancient Egyptians burned it with myrrh as headache-relieving incense. A popular sixteenth-century snuff, powdered basil treated headaches and colds. It was a favored remedy for restoring the sense of smell after sinus problems.

Take advantage of the plant's speedy growth to temporarily fill empty garden spots. Wherever you place basil, its shiny leaves add contrast. Growing different basil species alongside each other not only showcases the varied leaf shapes and colors, but makes them convenient to harvest. Both honeybees and butterflies pollinate sweet basil. It discourages mosquitoes and flies.

A native of the tropics, basil grows like crazy when daytime temperatures reach the 80s and nights do not drop below 60 degrees F. The soil should be rich, but do not overdo it or basil's scent and taste can suffer. Basil likes full sun and regular watering. Overhead watering followed by direct sun produces unsightly water spots. Researchers found green mulch under basil plants makes them more aromatic and red mulch makes the leaves larger. This perennial also winters over as a houseplant potted in a two-gallon container.

Basil makes a delicious pesto filled with health benefits. You can harvest several pounds of leaves from just one plant by cutting back the uppermost leaves weekly. I do this to make small, perfect-sized portions of pesto throughout the summer. Hang the stalks or spread the leaves on screens to dry.

Bay laurel
Laurus nobilis

Bay family: Lauraceae
Perennial
Zones 8-10

Break a bay laurel leaf and you'll smell a sharp, pungent aroma spicy enough to create a tingling sensation in your nose. The aroma invites you in with its intriguing warmth and sweetness, yet literally holds you at bay because it is so intense. I compare it to walking into a woodworking shop where the smells of cedar, pine, and other scented woods combine with wood varnish. The best way to experience bay laurel is to crack a leaf and hold it away from your nose to appreciate its underlying aromas. Bay laurel varieties offer scents ranging from lemon to almost no aroma at all.

Bay laurel's sharp fragrance is mentally stimulating and improves memory. Wreaths of bay laurel adorned Greek scholars and poets and European doctors during the Renaissance, as a symbol of intelligence. Symphony conductors are still crowned with them. We also continue to honor graduates with bay, although in name only—bay laurel is the source of the Latin word baccalaureate. The antiseptic smoke from burning bay laurel leaves was used in ancient Rome to purify air. One old headache remedy was to hold a bay laurel leaf on the forehead. It works, except that smelling bay laurel can produce a headache as easily as cure one! Some historians think that smoke from burning bay laurel leaves was inhaled by the ancient Greek priestesses at Delphi to enhance their prophetic visions.

Scientists at the Second University of Naples showed that bay laurel's potent antioxidants can protect the brain and nervous system. The aroma may help treat neurodegenerative diseases that

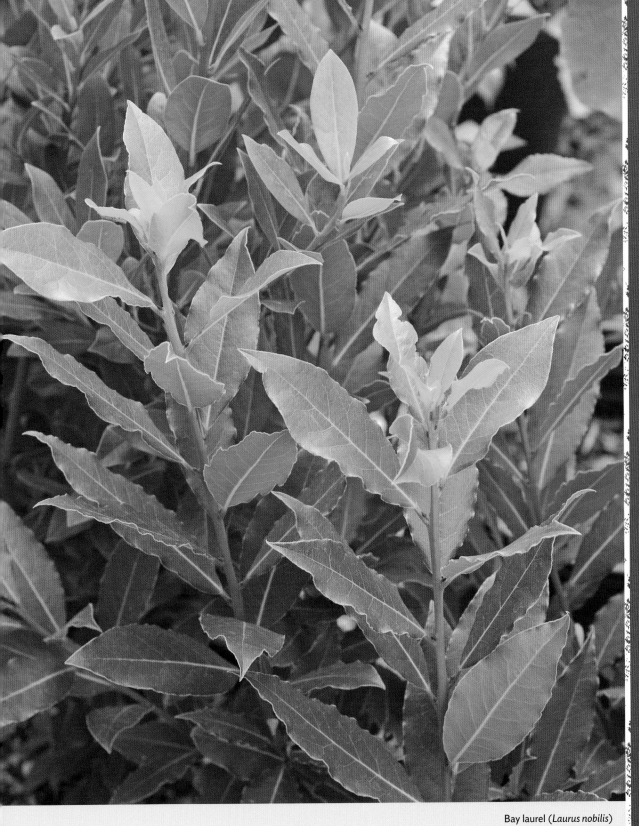

Bay laurel (*Laurus nobilis*)

affect memory, such as Alzheimer's disease. A Russian convalescent hospital has used it to sharpen their elderly patients' minds.

Bay laurel's shiny, deep green leaves and black berries make it stand out in the garden. Its tiny, white flowers attract honey and bumblebees and the western tiger swallowtail butterfly. On the other hand, the smell of its leaves sends cockroaches running.

You may need to give it a sheltered location in zone 8, or cover it with protective cloth during cold snaps. The plant typically handles temperatures down to 28 degrees F, although an extended freeze can kill it. Bay laurel only requires a little water and well-drained soil. Full sun in hot, cloudless climates can burn the uppermost leaves. It has thick enough growth to be pruned into a standard or a hedge. Botanical gardens often have bay laurel trees in pots that can be rolled into a protective shelter for the winter. An attractive way to display potted bay laurel is to grow shorter plants around the base. To propagate by cuttings, use first-year growth that is still green but stif. Bay cuttings are aided by use of a rooting compound. Growing it from seed can produce variations. The scent and flavor reach their peak just before the tree flowers, but the leaf aroma is strong enough that leaves can be harvested throughout the year. Harvest them individually and dry on a rack or in a paper bag.

Bee balm
Monarda didyma

Mint family: Lamiaceae
Perennial
Zones 4–10

Blend orange with mint and sugar and a little basil, and you'll come close to bee balm's unique, fresh fragrance. You'll know the scent if you have ever sipped an orange mint julep, the citrus version of that famous cocktail from the American South served with sprigs of fresh spearmint.

Scarlet bee balm (*Monarda didyma* 'Cambridge Scarlet') is an old, showy, popular variety. *Monarda didyma* 'Earl Grey' leans toward the scent of the citrus bergamot used to flavor that tea. Lemon bee balm (*M. citriodora*) has citrus-scented leaves and attractive, blue flowers. Its subspecies, *M. citriodora* subsp. *austromontana*, is an oregano substitute with a thyme-like flavor and scent. *Monarda fistulosa*, *M. clinopodia*, and *M. pectinata* are other strongly scented species that are cultivated for the perfume industry. Bee balm combines the aromatherapy actions of orange and peppermint to encourage relaxation and reduce anxiety, while at the same time increasing awareness. It is likely one of the plants

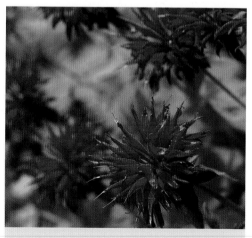

Bee balm (*Monarda didyma*)

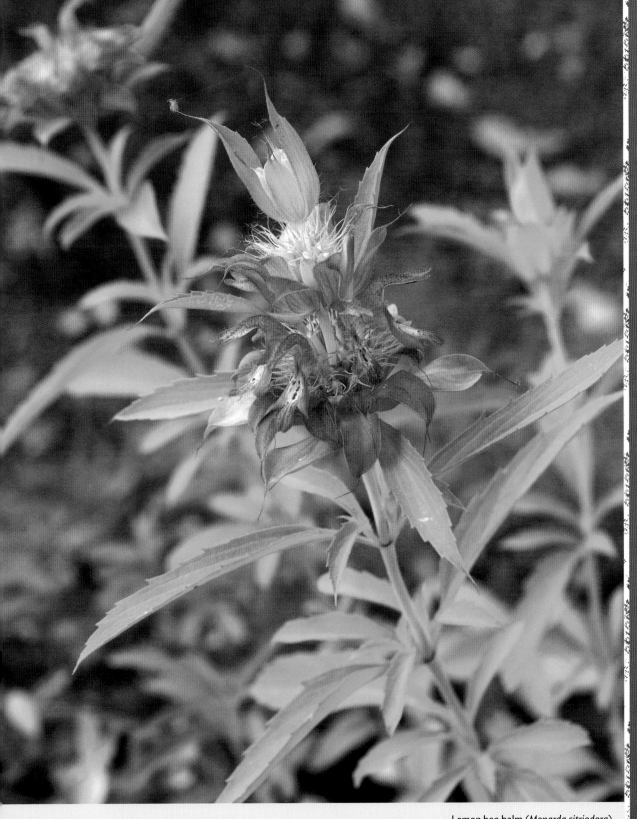

Lemon bee balm (*Monarda citriodora*)

that lessens the adrenal gland's negative response to stress. Do not confuse it with lemon balm, also sometimes nicknamed bee balm or orange bergamot (*Citrus bergamia*), two other plants that also have aromatherapy applications.

The showy, bright red-orange flowers on two- to three-foot-tall bee balm highlight the back of a bed, but look beautiful placed anywhere in the garden. This North American native does well naturalized along a stream or pond or in informal gardens. Combining different species results in a blast of color. Deadhead old flowers to keep them blooming. Bee balm is a favorite for a bee and butterfly garden. True to its name, honeybees flock to bee balm, as do butterflies, the ruby-throated hummingbird, and the evening sphinx moth.

This native of the Northeast is not fussy, but prefers rich, moist, cool soil in full or partial sun, and wilts if under-watered. Planting it in sun helps reduce the tendency for the leaves to develop mildew. It spreads easily through the garden via runners—perhaps a little too easily—but forms an attractive, thick patch. The center of the clump eventually dies out, but pinching back the tops and transplanting it every few years keeps it lush. Harvest the stems and hang them to dry.

Bitter orange

Citrus ×aurantium

Citrus family: Rutaceae
Tender perennial
Zones 9–11

Flowers of the bitter orange tree have a heavenly, sweet aroma that is perfume all by itself. It is obviously citrus, but with exotic accents of jasmine and rose rolled into one fragrance. Bitter orange trees in Sicily, Israel, Spain, and the United States produce slightly different scents.

Bitter orange blossom's antidepressant fragrance treats nervous strain, confusion, shock, fatigue, and insomnia. International Flavors and Fragrance Inc. has been investigating aromatherapy for years. They patented a blend of neroli, valerian, and nutmeg after studies showed all three scents help reduce stress, anxiety, fear, and blood pressure. Similar to oranges, the flowers may affect the brain's neurotransmitters and balance stress levels of cortisol. I experience an almost disorienting relaxation when walking through orange orchards in full bloom. Flowers from the edible, sweet orange tree (*Citrus sinensis*) are not as deeply scented, but an essential oil is produced from its peel. The trees are commercially grown in Brazil, where the Universidade Federal de Sergipe found their tranquilizing scent helps relieve anxiety.

Bitter orange essential oil is known as neroli, probably named after Anna Maria de la Trémoille (1670–1722), the princess of the Roman province Nerola, and the first person to have it distilled. The essential oil has been the base of Eau de Cologne since then. The classic formula also contains bergamot, lavender, and rosemary. The fragrance gained preference over the highly popular apple blossom scent to become the rage during the Italian Renaissance. Victorian-era

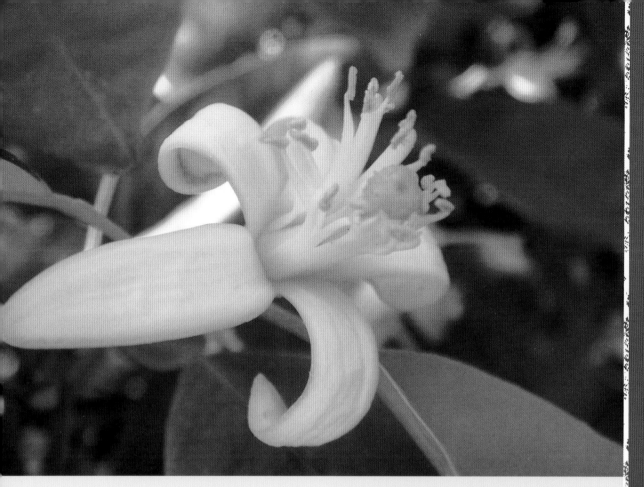

Neroli comes from bitter orange (*Citrus ×aurantium*)

brides attached circlets of the blossoms to their bridal veils to scent the air around them. The flowers were in such high demand that the flowers were shipped fresh from Florida throughout the United States. The aroma represents purity, although it is considered a potent aphrodisiac. In Iran, fresh flowers go into the sweet-smelling but bitter orange-blossom jam called *moraba-ye bahar-narenj*. Oranges are featured in Botticelli's famous fifteenth-century painting representing spring, *La Primavera*. The plant actually blooms several times a year, attracting bees that produce a refreshing honey smelling lightly of citrus. The flowers gradually lose their scent, even when

they are carefully dried, making it nice to have your own tree.

This twenty-five-foot tree obviously needs room and a warm climate or greenhouse to grow. You can keep it trimmed to make it easier to contain and also to reach the fruit, since most of it is produced on the bottom branches. Only prune deadwood or overlapping branches. It requires full sun and very well-drained soil that is amended with compost three times a year. Water established trees about once a week and those growing in pots at least twice a week; more often in hot weather. Let the surface of clay soil dry out between waterings.

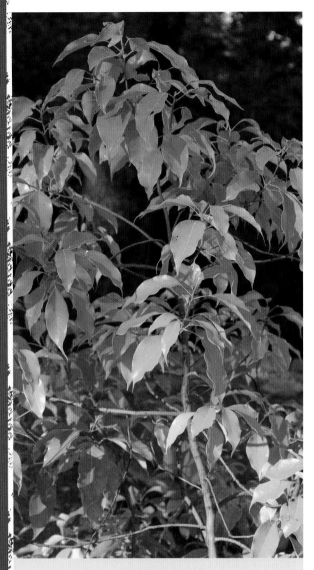

Camphor (*Cinnamomum camphora*)

Camphor
Cinnamomum camphora

Laurel family: Lauraceae
Evergreen
Zones 8–11

The shiny leaves and wood of the camphor tree give off a strong smell when crushed. Many fragrant plants are described as camphorous, but this is the full-force, nasal-crushing scent from camphor itself. It has often been compared to mothballs, but true camphor is much warmer and sweeter, borrowing a faint amount of scent from its cinnamon tree relative. The aroma varies depending upon the country of origin, but it is generally very stimulating. It was the aroma in Victorian-era smelling salts that pulled a person out of a fainting spell or from a deep sleep.

This slow-growing tree is used in its native China and Japan to make incense and fragrant statues of the Buddha. Cloth bags filled with mashed camphor leaves are heated and placed on sore muscles during Thai massage. The scent is a potent moth repellent. I have an intricately carved Chinese chest made from camphor wood to keep moths out.

Small, fragrant yellow flowers are followed by blackish fruit in warmer climates. Foliage can turn a variety of attractive bronze shades in early spring. Camphor grows in sun or partial sun and is drought resistant. Plant it in a large pot if you wish to keep it to a reasonable size.

Cardamom

Elettaria cardamomum

Ginger family: Zingiberaceae
Tender perennial
Zones 10–13

The spicy fragrance of cardamom seed smells of freshly baked gingerbread cookies, although it is sweeter, smoother, and not as spicy. It also carries a surprisingly nice touch of eucalyptus. You know the aroma if you have hovered over a steamy chai tea or Turkish coffee, both of which it flavors. The best-quality seeds are sweet, while inferior ones smell harsh and too strongly of eucalyptus. The base of the crushed leaves has the same fragrance but is much lighter.

Cardamom's fragrance eases nervous tension, but it is also invigorating. This combination is used to improve mental concentration, making chai tea a good substitute for your morning coffee. The plant originates from India, where ayurvedic medicine recommends it to increase focus and attention and to prevent light-headedness resulting from nervous indigestion. Sniffing a combination of cardamom, ginger, and mint decreased nausea after surgery at the Carolinas Medical Center–University, in North Carolina. It may lower blood pressure, which is an indication of relaxation.

Throughout India, Egypt, and the Middle East, cardamom is best known as an aphrodisiac. Called the "queen of spices," the seed has been an important commodity since the early spice trade transported precious aromatics to markets in Babylon, Carthage, Alexandria, and Rome. It was valued as a spice and perfume ingredient. The ancient, cardamom-scented Egyptian *kyphi* perfume was recreated for Denver's King Tut museum exhibit.

Still an international best seller for the perfume industry, cardamom scents the modern

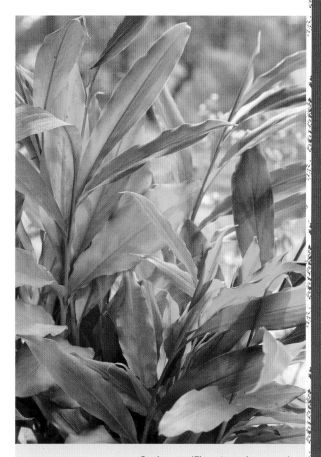

Cardamom (*Elettaria cardamomum*)

perfumes Devotion and Gujarat. Cardamom lends its spiciness to the strongly aromatic Chartreuse and Cordial Medoc liqueurs, and Angostura bitters.

This is not your typical garden plant, unless you live in the tropics. Chances are that it will never flower or produce seed. I still enjoy its attractive, aromatic leaves. A well-mulched plant winters over for me in zone 9, but is slow to put on spring growth. Keep it potted for a garden accent during summer, and a houseplant during winter. Cardamom likes rich soil and thrives in partial shade, provided it is well watered.

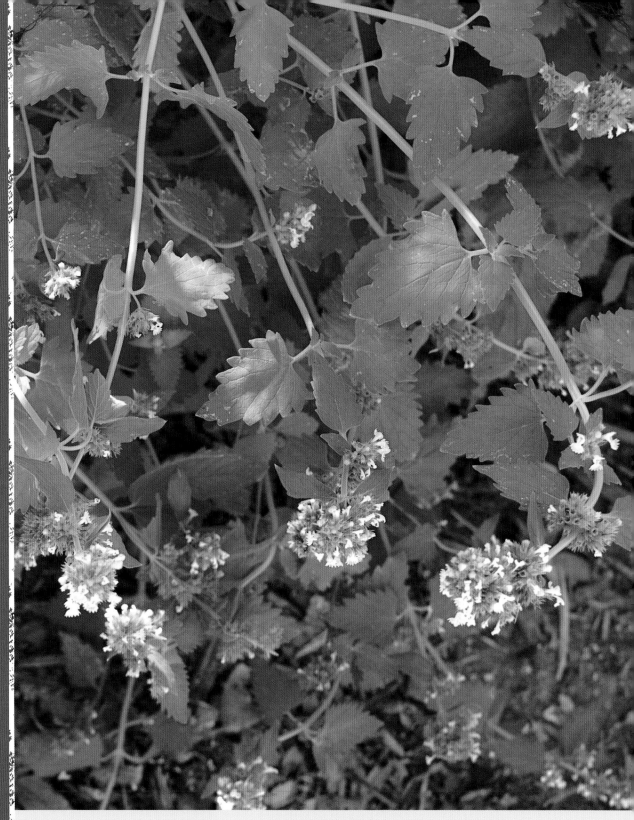

Catnip (*Nepeta cataria*)

Catnip

Nepeta cataria

Mint Family: Lamiaceae
Perennial
Zones 3–9

Catnip leaves have a musty, pungent, mint aroma with something that is almost some dull floral scent in the background. This soft and sharp combination of scents is appealing, except that it is a little too sharp. It smells a lot like a bouquet of wormwood, tansy, and peppermint.

Lemon catnip (*Nepeta cataria* 'Citriodora') adds a lemon scent to catnip's aroma. *Nepeta ×faassenii* has a lighter version of catnip's scent, although it still attracts cats. The dainty leaves and deep blue flowers look beautiful cascading down a hanging pot that is far out of a cat's reach.

The French once considered catnip a culinary seasoning, but its pungency eventually restricted it to medicinal tea. The aroma is relaxing for humans but is the opposite for many cats. At least half of adult domestic cats react to an aromatic compound called nepetalactone that converts in their nerve receptors to mimic a cat pheromone. This hereditary reaction is stronger in male cats and in breeds with European ancestry. Just a couple hours after smelling catnip, a cat will react again. However, if exposed to catnip more than a few times a week, some cats eventually become immune. The opposite reaction occurs when felines eat catnip—ingested, it acts as a mild sedative. Some zoos give it to their big cats for entertainment.

Interestingly, the nepetalactone compound that attracts cats has been found more effective as a mosquito repellent than DEET. Iowa State University Research Foundation applied for a patent to develop it into insect repellent.

The blue-gray leaves blend nicely with blue-flowering plants and contrast with dark green leaves. Catnip forms a tall border that can be somewhat shaped by pruning back new growth, but it refuses to completely lose its wild look and becomes straggly when going to seed. The tiny flowers attract the equally tiny skipper butterflies.

Catnip prefers dry, well-drained, fairly rich soils, but it will grow in clay soil. It also handles partial shade, but is less fragrant than when in full sun. It grows easily from seed. An old saying recommends sowing the seed for propagation because cats will roll over cuttings: "If you set it, the cats will eat it. If you sow it, the cats won't know it." Harvest catnip by hanging the tall stems.

Chamomile

Matricaria recutita

Aster family: Asteraceae
Annual

The fruity scent of chamomile (also called German chamomile) smells so much like apples, Greeks call it *kamaimelon* or "ground apple." The Spanish name *manzanilla* also means "little apple." Besides apple, the complex fragrance carries a hint of pineapple and bitter butterscotch that makes it smell good enough to eat—like hot oatmeal covered with maple syrup, topped with butterscotch chips, and very lightly sprinkled with marjoram and rose petals. If you have ever enjoyed chamomile tea, you know the aroma very well.

Roman chamomile (*Chamaemelum nobile*) makes a perennial ground cover that emits a sweet aroma when walked upon. Although it is in another genera and contains a few different aromatic compounds, it shares chamomile's fruity fragrance, but with slightly more bitterness. It makes a fragrant lawn, pathway, or a seat. I have it planted as the seat of a medieval-style stone bench, similar to ones that "comforted" the mind in times past when someone sat upon them and released the fragrance.

Chamomile is an antidepressant that aromatherapists recommend for emotional and physical oversensitivity. Studies show that it helps with anxiety, stress, and insomnia. Marie Curie Cancer Care in London found that patients felt less anxious when massaged with oil containing Roman chamomile than with unscented oil. In a Chiba University study, Japanese women's studious alpha brain waves relaxed when they sniffed German chamomile. The women said they were more "comfortable" and relaxed. The tea calms both new mothers and hyperactive children. Fussy babies cry less when they smell chamomile.

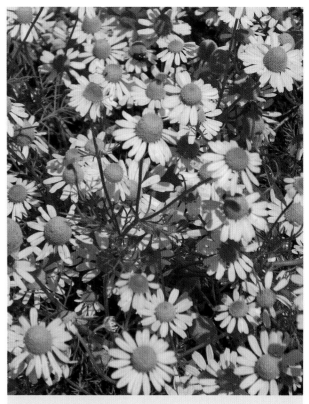

Chamomile (*Matricaria recutita*)

The pretty little daisy-like chamomile flowers look picture perfect among other plants. Chamomile is said to help ailing plants, so grow it near plants you find difficult to cultivate.

The two-foot-tall annual needs to be seeded every year and dislikes transplanting. It prefers fairly nitrogen-rich soil. Give it full sun where there is some cloud cover, otherwise, partial shade. Harvesting the small flowers individually is time consuming, so commercial harvesters use a fine rake that pops the heads off the thin stems. Dry the flowers in a thin layer on a screen or in the bottom of a paper bag.

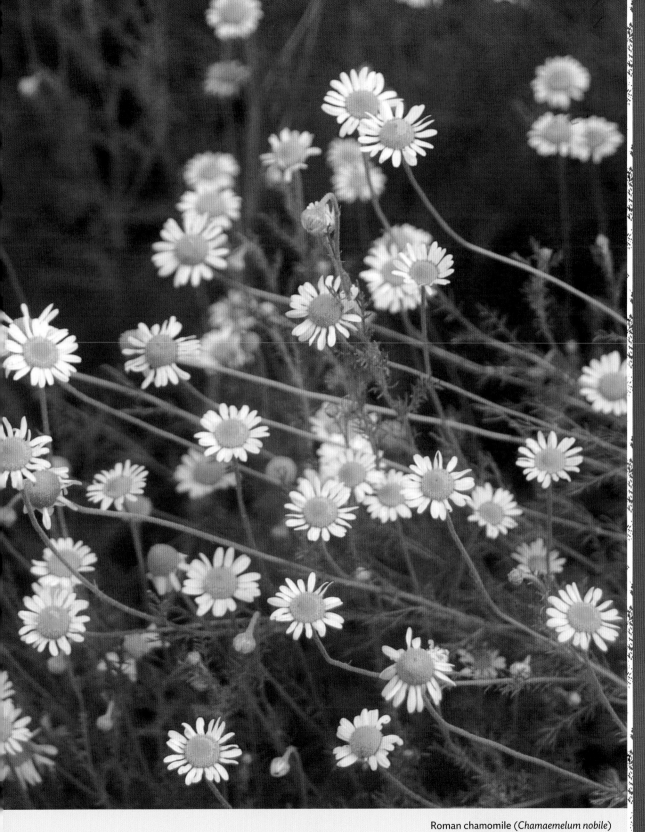

Roman chamomile (*Chamaemelum nobile*)

Chinese wisteria

Wisteria sinensis

Pea family: Fabaceae
Perennial
Zones 5–9

Chinese wisteria's fragrance is floral and much like lilac, but a little sweeter with a touch of creamy honey vanilla and wispy note of jasmine in the background. There is also something else that might be equated with burnt toast. It is certainly a scent that keeps you coming back for more to try to grasp it. The complexity makes it difficult to describe. It is perfume and dessert at the same time.

White-flowering wisteria (*Wisteria sinensis* 'Alba') has a slightly different aroma that is more pungent and spicy enough to almost be cinnamon. It tends to be sweeter, and many gardeners say more fragrant, but that depends upon the plant and growing conditions. The fragrance of Japanese wisteria (*W. floribunda*) is also pungent, but more sugary. It tolerates lower temperatures. If you cannot tell from the fragrance, Chinese wisteria twines in a clockwise direction, while Japanese wisteria grows the opposite way. Silky wisteria (*W. brachybotrys* 'Shiro-kapitan') is a fragrant wisteria with less rampant growth, making it more easily contained. The North American natives are less aggressive, but have little scent.

Chinese wisteria is a large vine that sends out long branches that twine around a support or anything they can find. Like many members of the pea family, it is an aggressive grower that will probably need to be cut back or trained. Prune it into the framework you want from an early age, and cut off any of the long, aimless streamers every summer. I have been in an amazing, two-story tree house taken over by a live wisteria. Both Chinese and Japanese wisterias become invasive in many locations, and both are

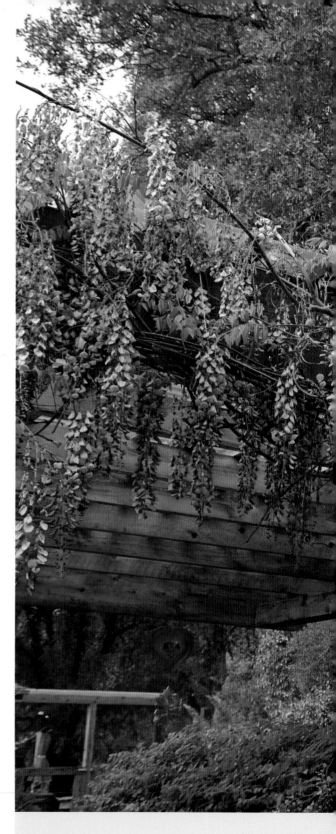

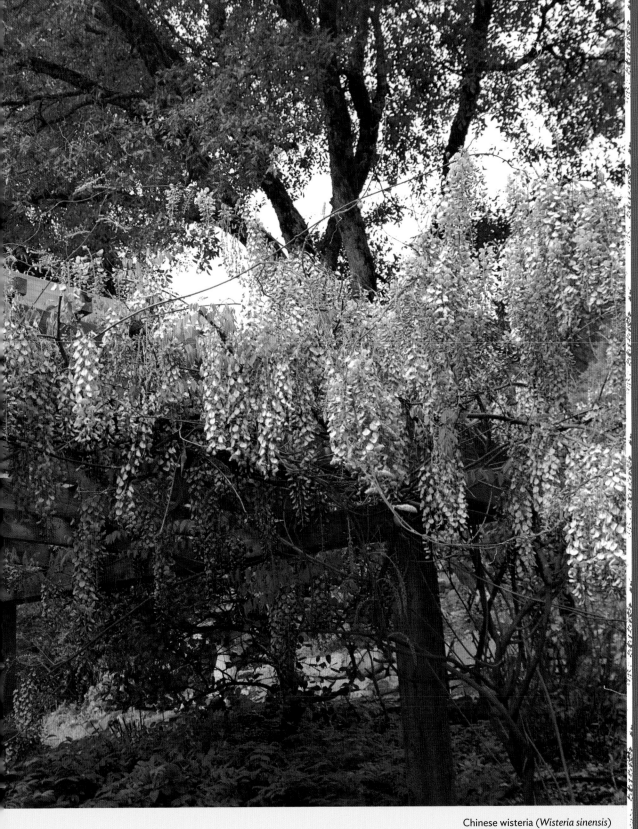

Chinese wisteria (*Wisteria sinensis*)

restricted in private gardens in some states. You may want to cut off the seedpods before they mature to avoid having dozens of seedlings. Keep the seeds out of the garden compost!

The plant requires drainage and prefers slightly acidic, rich soil. Preparing the soil well before planting pays off, since this is a long-living plant. Feeding it in the fall or winter assures masses of fragrant blooms permeating the air for yards away. It needs full sun and a balanced diet. Too much nitrogen versus phosphorus will keep it from flowering, as will too much pruning, although that is difficult to do with wisteria! It is pollinated by hummingbirds, as well as honeybees and bumblebees.

Clary sage

Salvia sclarea

Mint family: Lamiaceae
Biennial
Zones 5–9

The potent aroma of clary sage is pungent and musky, yet also sweet and sour. It has an odd, underlying scent similar to sweat—almost like culinary sage doused in clingy, sweet perfume. This cloying, intense fragrance is not for everyone, although those who appreciate it seem to love it. The secret is to enjoy it from a few feet away rather than up close.

The fragrance is thought to produce joyfulness to counter depression. Even working in the garden around clary sage makes me a little giddy. Classes always break out in laughter when I pass it around. Aromatherapists also use the scent to treat hormonal imbalances, such as postpartum depression and menopause. A clary sage spray works well for menopausal hot flashes. Studies show that it does affect the mind in a way that is similar to hypnotic pharmaceutical drugs. Researchers at the Korea University College of Nursing in Seoul suggested clary sage could be developed into a treatment for depression after the aroma proved more successful as an antidepressant than either lavender or chamomile. Clary sage seems to work by affecting brain receptors. It also has a rare compound called sclareol in its essential oil that influences estrogen hormones and is likely responsible for some of its actions.

Perfumers and aromatherapists have learned to blend small amounts of clary sage with much lighter fragrances. It scents several perfumes, as well as muscatel wine. It is one of the few aromatic crops in the United States, where it is primarily grown and distilled into essential oil to scent and flavor tobacco.

The towering four- to six-foot-tall clary sage is a showstopper even when placed in the back of a bed. It can span three feet by its second year, so give it room or the lower leaves will cover smaller plants. It is good in the background, so that garden visitors do not touch the leaves before being warned that the strong scent will linger on their hands. This also keeps all of the honeybees and bumblebees it attracts off the pathway. Even though it produces a large taproot, it will grow in a pot or in poor soil, though either method stunts it. Although it is a biennial, wait until spring to pull out seemingly dead plants, since new growth can emerge from the base. It reseeds so abundantly that you may want to keep the seedling stalks out of the compost pile, to avoid clary sage taking over your garden the next year. Instead, throw them into fall bonfires to release their pungent scent.

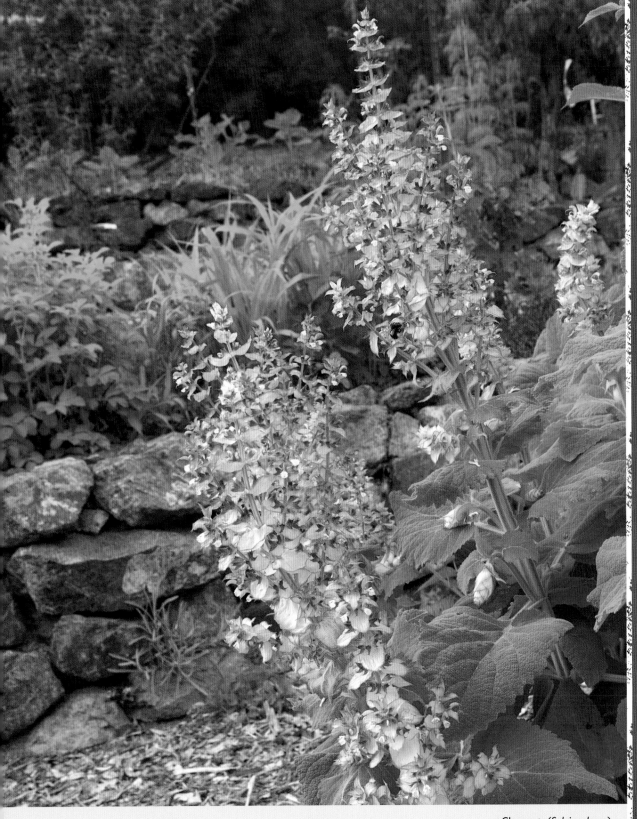

Clary sage (*Salvia sclarea*)

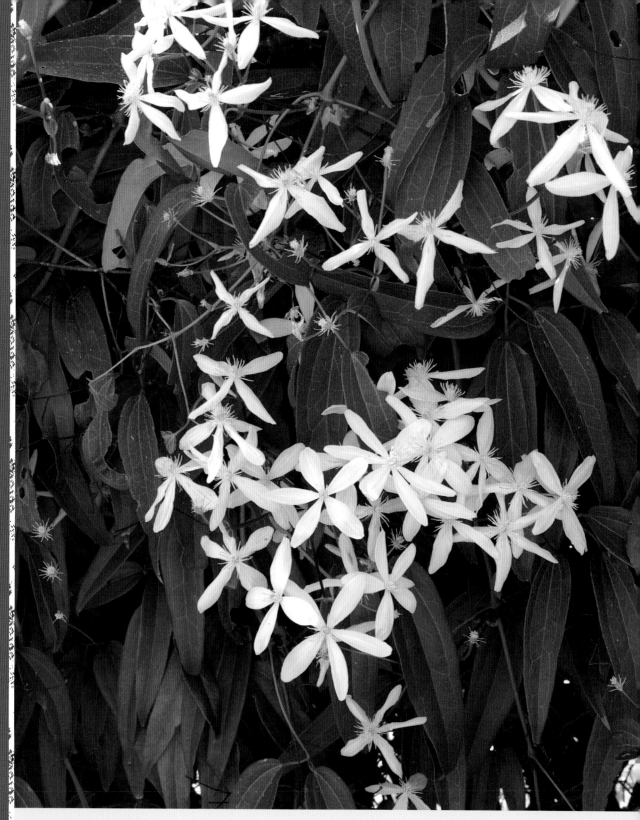

Clematis (*Clematis armandii*)

Clematis

Clematis armandii

Buttercup family: Ranunculaceae
Perennial
Zones 7–9

The flowers of *Clematis armandii*, often called evergreen clematis, fill the air with a delicious scent of bitter almonds, vanilla, and a sweet touch of honey. Imagine honey-vanilla ice cream topped with toasted almonds. This has to be the closest scent to dessert that the garden offers. The fragrance of clematis reaches across a garden bed.

Clematis armandii 'Apple Blossom', with cream-colored flowers, is probably the most fragrant cultivar. Himalayan clematis (*C. montana*) is the first to bloom in spring, when its eye-catching, large white flowers smell like a chocolate milkshake. The varieties of this species can be disappointingly less fragrant. Blue jasmine (*C. crispa*), with compact growth and blue flowers, has an orange-vanilla scent similar to the Orange Julius drink. Virgin's bower (*C. flammula*) puts out a strong, vanilla-almond scent from a profusion of dainty white flowers in late summer. Sweet autumn clematis (*C. terniflora*) handles hot summers and blooms heavily in autumn with a softer, but delightful, vanilla fragrance. Gardeners take advantage of the rampant growth of *C. terniflora* to cover structures, although it can become invasive, and is restricted in private gardens in some states.

Plants such as evergreen clematis that have a vanilla aroma are calming and emotionally comforting, easing frayed nerves. Western, Chinese, and India's ayurvedic medicines treat nervous system problems with the dried plant. Clematis has such an appealing aroma that a clematis craze developed in the nineteenth century, when stylish women wore fragrant flowers instead of perfume. It was one of the most sought-after cut flowers in Parisian markets, drenching flower stalls with fragrance. The scent is captured when clematis flowers are dried for potpourri.

The glistening white flowers of *Clematis armandii* are spring bloomers that are over two inches wide. Curious beard-like seed tufts keep clematis attractive long after it flowers, and give it the name old man's beard. Support this twining plant on a trellis or let it intertwine with other fragrant climbers, such as honeysuckle—a duo that creates striking combinations of color and scent. For a change of pace, plant evergreen clematis during its winter dormancy in rich soil in a hanging basket. Hang it in filtered light, give it plenty of water, and the flowers will cascade over the edge. Since the stems break easily, plant it away from garden foot traffic.

This native of China grows fast and can be trained, but requires a lot of pruning to cut off dead parts of the vine. Be careful when pruning it after the plant is dormant, because the live wood looks dead. Clematis requires sunlight and rich, loose, very well-drained soil, plus monthly boosts of compost in the growing season. It prefers moist shade on its roots from mulch or a ground cover. It does well in filtered light in hot climates. The leaf tips burn if there is salt in the soil or water.

Clove pink

Dianthus caryophyllus

Carnation family: Caryophllaceae
Perennial
Zones 6-8

The aroma of clove pink is predominantly that of cloves, delightfully softened with sweet floral and honey fragrances. Imagine being in a room filled with bouquets of fragrant roses and steaming, clove-flavored mulled cider sweetened with honey. One old gardening book suggests duplicating the scent by cooking cloves with Damask roses.

Dianthus 'Can Can Scarlet' is among the most fragrant varieties. 'Bookham Perfume', with its deep crimson flowers, is especially clove-like. 'Gloriosa' is an old hybrid with pale pink flowers that emit a rich, clove scent. 'Pheasant's Ear' is a lesser-known cultivar from the seventeenth century. Its semi-double white flowers are centered and fringed with burgundy. Sweet william (*D. barbatus*) is the more common species that also smells fairly strongly of cloves, especially in the evening.

Much like cloves, the scent of clove pink flowers is both energizing and relaxing, helping to overcome mental fatigue, nervousness, and poor memory. It encourages joyfulness and represents love, graciousness, and gratitude. These qualities led to it becoming the official flower for first wedding anniversaries and Mother's Day. Egyptians chew the small seeds to make the breath smell sweet. Perfume the house with a vase of the cut flowers.

Clove pinks are distinctively clove-like because they contain eugenol, the same fragrant compound in cloves. Smelling them produces a response of happiness in the brain. Studies, such as those from the Kagawa Prefectural College of Health Sciences in Takamatsu, Japan, indicate that eugenol reduces stress by moderating neurotransmitters and GABA receptors in the brain and reducing adrenal cortisol levels that typically increase during stress. Most people rate clove's scent as very pleasant, although it appeals to women more than men. It is no wonder that it is a component of so many men's colognes! A small amount of carnation essential oil is produced by chemical extraction, but it is expensive, so most carnation-scented colognes use clove instead.

The white, pink, red, and striped flowers dress any garden with color, as well as fragrance. Accent these short plants by planting them toward the foreground or in raised beds that bring the flowers closer to nose level. They are especially wonderful combined with Persian catnip to edge a bed of lavender. Clove pinks prefer cool temperatures, and dislike humid weather. Plant them in good soil and do not overwater.

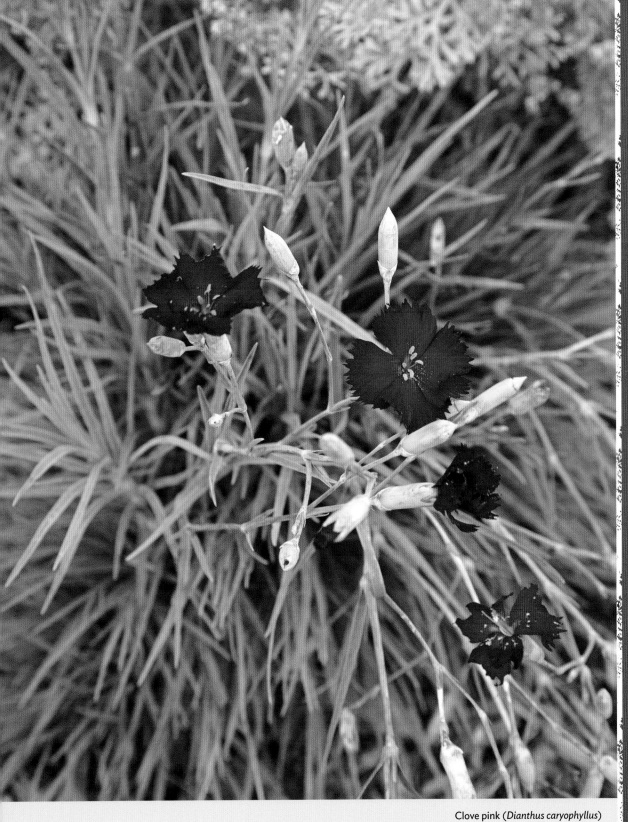

Clove pink (*Dianthus caryophyllus*)

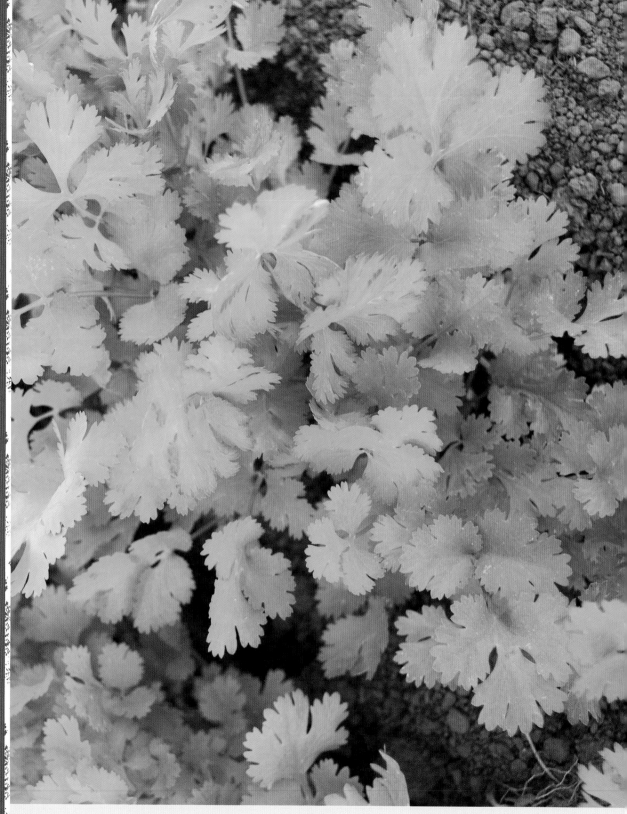

Coriander (*Coriandrum sativum*)

Coriander

Coriandrum sativum

Carrot family: Apiaceae
Annual

Coriander, also known as cilantro, is two plants in one. The seed is spicy and almost fruity, combined with some sharp pepper, a dash of floral scent, and a nutty aroma. This makes a unique, all-in-one kitchen herb. Think of an unsweetened apple turnover filled with nuts and flavored with rose water. The leaves have a similar aroma, but one that is fuller and not so sharp. It is very appealing unless you are one of the few people who carry a gene that makes coriander smell and taste like soap.

Aromatherapists consider coriander seed an uplifting scent. They use it to help individuals overcome stress, insomnia, and lack of motivation. Medieval texts said that the aroma calms nervousness. Head wreaths of the flowers are worn for special celebrations in Europe. The Egyptians called it the "secret of happiness" and made an aromatic concoction that mixed coriander with wine. The herb is currently being studied for its ability to help relieve anxiety, depression, and the oxidative stress that occurs with Alzheimer's disease.

It may seem surprising, but according to Scheherazade's story from *The Arabian Nights,* coriander was used as a powerful love potion. The seed does scent perfumes, such as the spicy Coriandre perfume by Jean Couturier for Women. The secret is in the blending. Small amounts mixed with more floral oils makes coriander less overpowering. The fourteenth-century nuns of St. Just included the seed in their popular Carmelite complexion water that was splashed on the face. It served as an early form of cologne called Eau de Carmes for four centuries. Coriander continues to scent soap and deodorant. The seed flavors tobacco and liqueurs, such as Cordial-Medoc and Danziger Goldwasser, as well as gin, vermouth, and Belgian wheat beer. An essential oil is produced from both seed and leaf for the food industry.

The plant is too small, wispy, and short-lasting to do much for garden design It matures in a month and bolts as soon as the weather turns hot. It is best grown in a patch where it can be replaced by other plants once it is harvested. The flowers are visited by honeybees.

Sow coriander seeds directly in the ground, because its small taproot dislikes being transplanted. Thin out the seedlings to about six inches. Harvest the young leaves as needed for the kitchen and the seeds when they mature. Cut plants when the ripe seeds are still on them and put them into paper bags, so that the seeds conveniently fall off into the bag.

Curry plant

Helichrysum italicum

Aster family: Asteraceae
Perennial
Zones 8, 9

The fragrance of curry plant is spicy, sweet, and warm, with an underlying fruitiness. When I ask my garden tours to guess the scent, anyone with a good nose picks out cumin, coriander, turmeric, or fenugreek—curry's basic ingredients. It is that pungent, sweet, and spicy combination of aromas that greets you when you walk into an Indian restaurant.

Helichrysum italicum, often called *H. angustifolium*, has at least three subspecies. *Helichrysum italicum* subsp. *italicum* is either nearly two feet tall or a much more compact shrub, and comes in at least three chemotypes with different scents. *Helichrysum italicum* subsp. *microphyllum*, from the island of Sardinia, grows under twelve inches. It produces at least two chemotypes with an especially sweet curry aroma.

French helichrysum (*Helichrysum stoechas*) is highly aromatic with long-lasting flowers that give it the name immortelle. *Helichrysum orientale* has a similar aroma. Both plants are used by the perfume and flavor industries.

The scent of curry plant is gently stimulating and uplifting. It helps alleviate nervous exhaustion and lethargy, and associated stress and depression. *The Journal of Alternative and Complementary Medicine* reported less burnout both at work and at home when participants used a personal inhaler containing curry plant, peppermint, and basil essential oils throughout the day. University of KwaZulu-Natal in South Africa found that four helichrysums out of the forty-six wide-ranging plants tested were among the strongest to enhance relaxation by affecting the brain's GABA receptors.

The plant has been called poor man's curry because it was used in place of curry in Europe when imported spices from India were very expensive. It lends a bitter but interesting flavor to rice and other dishes, but does not have curry spice's heavy, sweet spiciness. Curry plant is closer to curry powder in aroma than in taste. An expensive helichrysum essential oil is used to make skin care products. You can distill the flowers yourself to make a fragrant hydrosol water, and also infuse almond oil. The shrub has been stuffed into pillows, added to dried potpourri, placed in linens, and used as a fragrant broom.

In the garden, curry plant is an attractive, gray or gray-green shrub that stands out, especially during the few weeks in summer when it is covered with bright yellow flowers. Curry plant has a similar growth pattern to lavender and is attractive placed with *Lavandula angustifolia*, next to dark green leaves, or interspersed with yellow and pink yarrow. Consider shaping curry plants into rounded forms every fall so they do not become too gangly. However, cutting back a well-established plant for the first time results in unsightly gaps.

This plant likes a dry, well-drained soil and plenty of sun. It grows in partial sun, but will sprawl toward the light. I have seen it growing wild in France in rocky, forlorn places. Cuttings are more reliable than seeds, but it self-seeds in my gravel pathways, which must remind it of its home on rocky Mediterranean hillsides. Harvest the flowers before they turn into pale fluff as they go to seed. There is usually a second, sparse flowering.

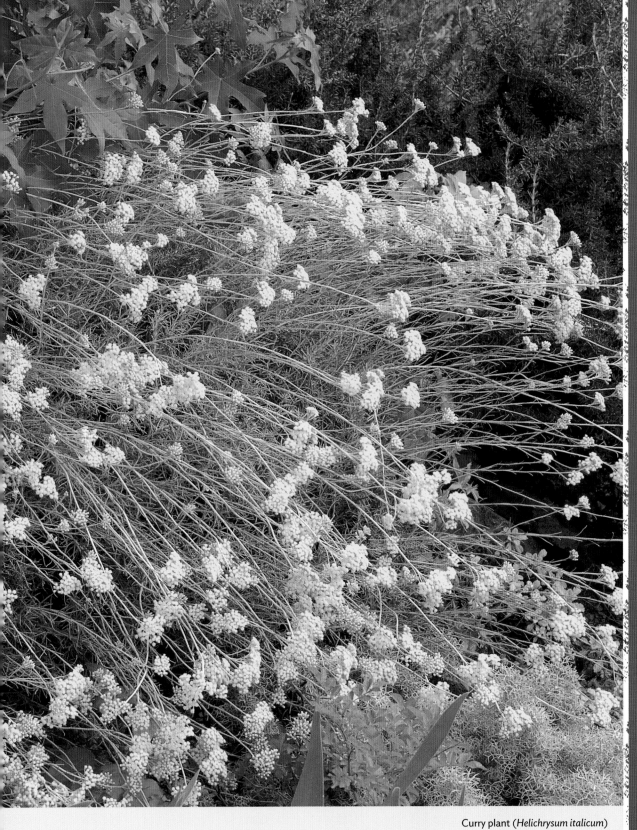

Curry plant (*Helichrysum italicum*)

Damask rose

Rosa ×damascena

Rose family: Rosaceae
Perennial
Zones 3-10

Damask rose has layers of fragrance reminiscent of floral balsams, butter, and sweet honey. Trying to describe it sends your nose swimming among dozens of aromatic compounds that create the scent. It is one of those perfect fragrances that changes with each inhale. Damask is one of the three most fragrant roses in the world, according to modern fragrance technology. Old-fashioned roses like this were developed before 1867, when tea rose hybridization began. Many hybrids with perfectly formed flowers bloom throughout summer, but alas, often have no fragrance.

The two other most fragrant roses are also old-fashioned. Musk rose (*Rosa moschata*) has ivory-white, single-petaled flowers that bloom in the summer with a sweet, honey-like scent. Its dense, flat-green foliage covers arching canes. Cabbage rose (*R. centifolia*) has arching, prickly stems that are heavy with intensely fragrant, white or pink flowers. Its common name comes from the densely packed inner petals that are clutched by larger, outer petals to resemble the packed look of cabbage leaves. All three of these rose forms—damask, musk, and cabbage—are distilled into essential oils for the perfume industry. There are many fragrant cultivars. Musk roses are varieties of damask and cabbage roses that have balsam-scented glands covering unopened buds and sometimes leaflets. The flowers are white to red. Musk roses derived from *R. ×damascena* are soft to the touch, while *R. centifolia* musk roses are prickly.

Over twenty-five distinct rose scents have connoisseurs comparing the different aromas much like fine wines. Red and pink blooms generally have a sweeter scent, while yellow and white flowers tend toward scents that resemble violet, lemon, or nasturtium. Orange shades can also go toward violets and nasturtiums, plus fruit and clover scents, although a hot day makes clover smell more like bay. Other rose scents are more like clove or citrus. They may also have hints of pepper, anise, bay, or raspberry—or fern, moss, or quince.

As with all fragrant roses, the therapeutic use of damask rose revolves around the heart. Called the "queen of flowers," rose is an almost universal expression of love. It has inspired poets and lovers in Europe, China, India, and the Middle East. In all of those regions, it is also considered an aphrodisiac. The fragrance eases sadness, grief, heartache, loss, depression, and lack of confidence. It encourages receptiveness to people, places, and new ideas. It also instills heart-felt spirituality. Mohammed said the scent of rose was the closest thing to God's heart. A generations-old tradition creates rosary beads from rose petals. The warmth of the fingers praying with them releases the aroma.

Tottori University Faculty of Medicine in Japan and other research centers studying aromatherapy found rose's fragrance relaxes muscles, emotional tension, pain, and the sympathetic nervous system. Rose helps the body deal with long-term tension, diminishing the adrenaline stress response by about a third. It seems to do so by working through the brain's hypothalamus and pituitary glands, as well as affecting GABA activity, which has a calming effect on the body. Studies sponsored by the Shiseido fragrance company showed how inhaling rose scent increases relaxation as much as forty percent. Rose has also reduced the need for pharmaceutical drugs. According to research from the Islamic Azad University, there is a chance that the essential oil lessens mor-

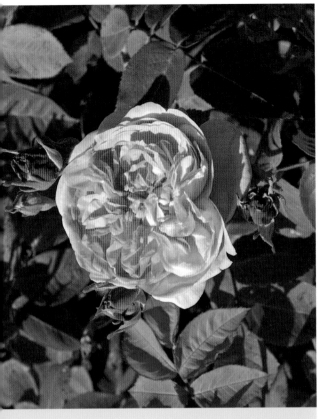

Cabbage rose (*Rosa centifolia*)

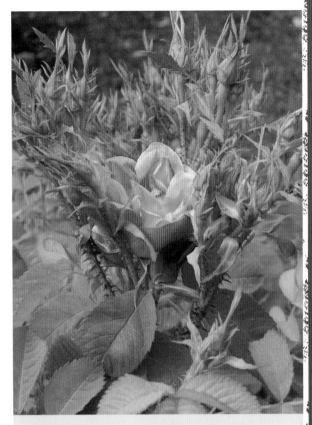

Damask rose (*Rosa* ×*damascena*)

phine withdrawal symptoms, by affecting the brain's neurotransmitters.

Rose helps rejuvenate skin and is used in body care products, especially for complexion. It is expensive, so is usually reserved for high-end perfume. It takes about sixty roses to make just one drop of the costly essential oil. It is also expensive because the shrubs need a lot of care and the roses are handpicked.

Plant rose shrubs together in a rose garden or place them individually to highlight different areas. The pink and white damask flowers are borne on long canes, so need room in the garden. Most damask varieties flower in spring. Autumn damask rose (*Rosa* ×*damascena* var.

semperflorens) blooms in the fall. Grow a variety to have cut flowers throughout spring and summer.

As much as I love roses, I am trying to maintain my collection at thirty shrubs—that is, until another rapturous scent entices me. They are high maintenance, with all of the pruning, deadheading, spraying, and regular feedings. Deeply water them, but not from overhead, which spots the leaves and encourages fungal growth. It is important to clear away fallen diseased leaves from around plant bases, because infected leaves carry black spot and other diseases.

Daphne

Daphne odora

Daphne family: Thymelaeaceae
Perennial
Zones 7–9

Hidden under daphne's cloying, heady perfume is a hint of citrus and the sharp scent of the bay laurel tree. Said to be the most fragrant of all garden flowers, daphne is famous for a pervasive, sugar-citrus scent that can extend across the landscape for twenty feet or more. It smells as if someone ground up lemon peel, bay laurel leaves, rosebuds, and brown sugar, then blended them with orange blossoms into a mix—a mix that is too strong to eat, but with an aroma perfect for a hot bath. I find it intoxicating, although perhaps this is because daphne blooms in winter when few other plants care to flower. Nineteenth-century novelist Henry Kingsley, in *Silcote of Silcotes*, elaborately describes daphne as having "the most rich, glorious, overpowering scent in the world, to which that of the magnolia seems like a grocer's spice. How do the storms and frosts of a bitter northern winter develop such a pure sweet scent?" Daphne's intense scent is relaxing to the point of being sedative. It alleviates stress, helping one forget one's problems. In China, it was originally called *shuixian*, or sleeping scent.

Daphne has small, pink flowers. *Daphne odora* 'Aureomarginata', with deeper pink flowers and yellow-edged leaves, is extra hardy and is perhaps the easiest daphne to cultivate. It has the Royal Horticultural Society's Award of Garden Merit. Nepalese paper plant (*D. bholua*) is not a great beauty until it bursts into intensely fragrant, lilac-colored flowers in late summer. February daphne (*D. mezereum*) bears aromatic, striking red flowers.

The shrub looks good throughout the year, even when not flowering. It is poisonous to ingest and its flowers do not last once picked, making daphne best enjoyed in the garden. I have 'Aureomarginata' next to my hot tub. Need I say more? Surround it with shade-loving ground covers such as sweet woodruff. Daphne dies easily so it pays to carefully prepare a spot with rich, alkaline humus and diffused light. Try to not move it once established.

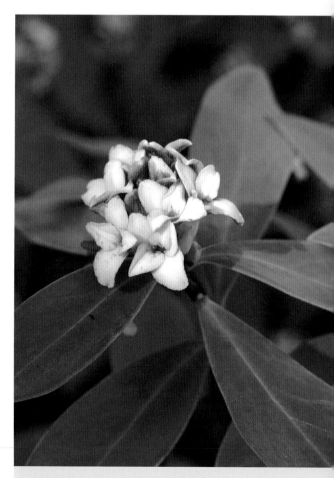

Daphne odora blooms in small clusters known for big fragrance.

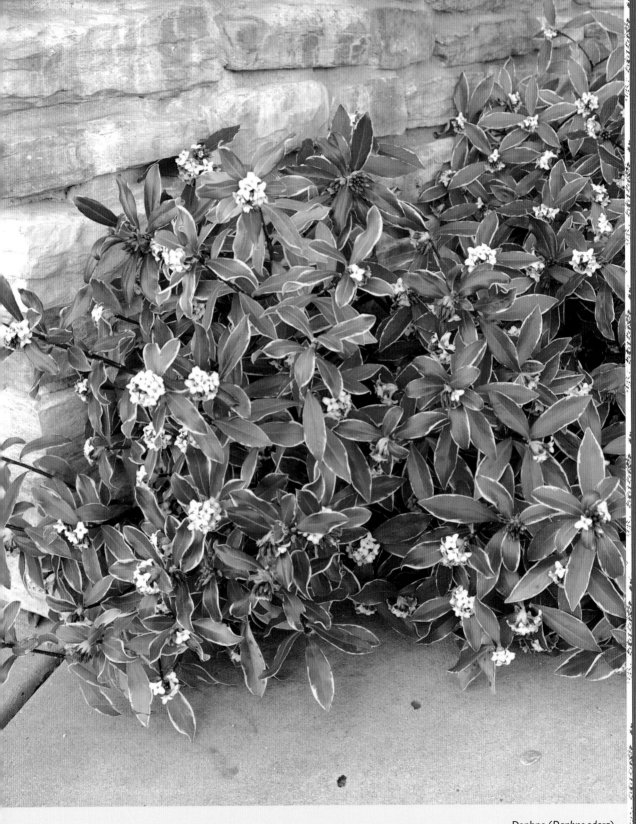

Daphne (*Daphne odora*)

Dill

Anethum graveolens

Carrot family: Apiaceae
Annual

Dill is a familiar aroma. Open a jar of dill pickles to be instantly struck by its distinctly herby and sharp features, with slightly grassy overtones. It smells similar to but less bitter than caraway. The two share many aromatic compounds. Both dill leaves and seed have a similar smell and taste, with the seed a little sharper.

Dill is said to strengthen the brain and improve one's mood. It once symbolized good luck, fortune, courage, and protection from harm. As a result, dill sprigs have been tucked into head wreaths that were placed on scholars, war heroes, and brides, and hung over baby's beds. The name dill comes from the Scandinavian word that means "to lull," probably because it calms babies. In Europe, babies were put to sleep with "dilly" pillows filled with dill seeds and lavender. I have encouraged my students to bring back this tradition for so long, that now, young women who had dilly pillows in their cribs are making them for their babies. A dill remedy with the descriptive name "gripe water" was also given to colicky babies.

The ancient world considered *dille* so important that it was exchanged as money. Greeks who could afford it burned the oil in lamps as an ancient house freshener. It is a surprisingly pleasant house scent, but it can make one hungry. Puritans tucked dill "meetin' seeds" into their Bibles to appease their appetite during long services. Dill perfumes soap and occasionally goes into perfume. The seeds make a good breath freshener. Ethiopians chew the seeds to banish headaches.

The short, feathery plants look best combined with fuller plants such as marjoram. They are tall enough to go in the middle of a narrow bed or wispy enough to be in front. If planted in the spring, dill seeds and dies back before summer is over. If it is planted as a solid bed, another plant can fill its place in late summer. Dill attracts the western tiger swallowtail butterfly.

Plant dill in moderately rich soil where there is full sun. This annual does not like to be transplanted so it is often planted directly into its permanent bed. If you do transplant it, do so when the weather is cool. Sow dill seed in full sun directly where it will grow and you will have dill seed in two months. Keep the area weed-free for a more productive dill crop.

Dill can be harvested several times during the summer. Use it as a fresh kitchen herb. Harvest the seed heads just before the seeds are completely dried and fall to the ground. I stick them in a paper bag to fully dry, then shake the bag to make the seeds fall to the bottom.

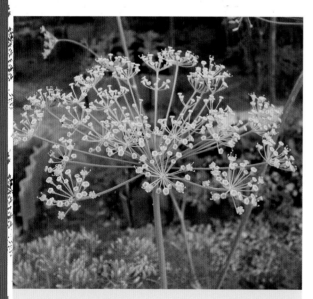

Dill (*Anethum graveolens*)

Fennel

Foeniculum vulgare

Carrot family: Apiaceae
Perennial
Zones 5–10

Fennel's aroma is very much like licorice or anise with the addition of an herby, sharp scent. It fills your senses with the thought of biting into a licorice candy that has ground dill seed in it. That may not sound very tasty, but fennel still manages to smell great.

Bronze fennel (*Foeniculum vulgare* 'Purpureum') has the same scent, with attractive bronze-colored leaves. Florence fennel or finocchio (*F. vulgare* var. *azoricum*) has a swollen, bulb-like, licorice-scented base that is eaten as a vegetable.

Twelfth-century abbess Hildegard von Bingen said sniffing fennel makes you happy. Stimulating and revitalizing, fennel is used to increase self-motivation and enliven the personality. Science credits "green odors" like fennel with protecting the body from stress. Shiseido fragrance company research determined that inhaling the aroma of fennel spikes nervous system activity. Fennel's stimulating aroma does appear to enhance activity of the pituitary, adrenal, and hypothalamus glands to reduce stress and the negative impact it has on the body. These areas of the brain work together to keep the body running smoothly. Maybe this is why fennel has represented strength and longevity since ancient times.

Fennel lends small amounts of its licorice scent to cologne, perfume, soap, and especially to cordials and liqueurs. It is used in body care products and facial steams for its reputation to slow the aging of skin and prevent wrinkles.

I place these six-foot-tall plants in the middle of a large bed so their feathery leaves and tiny,

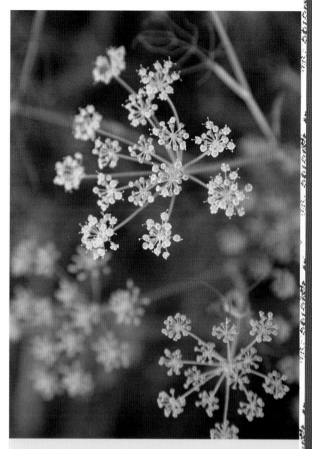

Bronze fennel (*Foeniculum vulgare* 'Purpureum')

yellow flowers can provide interesting contrasts in color and texture with shorter, denser herbs, such as lavender and sage. Fennel will grow into a green screen during the summer to hide a fence or structure. I grow extra plants for the anise swallowtail butterflies that are attracted to fennel.

This plant prefers nitrogen-rich soil in full sun, but manages to grow in the wild in all sorts of conditions. It easily self-seeds, maybe too easily, since fennel has naturalized in the West and is considered invasive in some areas. It is easy to pull until the taproot develops. That taproot makes it difficult to transplant, so think ahead when choosing a garden spot and seed it directly.

Flowering tobacco

Nicotiana alata

Tomato family: Solanaceae
Tender perennial
Zones 9–10

The warm aroma of flowering tobacco is sweetly exotic. It is reminiscent of jasmine and a complex scent. The fragrance seems magical, but that is probably because the tubular white flowers seem to glow at dusk, when they scent the air and draw in moths that flit about like fairies. The fragrance smells as if someone took several different high-quality jasmine perfumes, poured them together, then heavily misted it into the night air.

The old-fashioned, white-flowered tobaccos are the most fragrant, while most red flowers and hybrids in a variety of fun colors offer little scent. Some have been bred to stay open during the day, which must frustrate the night moths that pollinate them. *Nicotiana alata* cultivars 'Fragrant Cloud' and 'Grandiflora' are the most fragrant. *Nicotiana sylvestris* has a more exotic fragrance.

Flowering tobacco's aroma calms emotional agitation, nervous energy, and overactivity. It is hypnotic enough to dull the senses. Some programs to stop smoking claim success when participants just smell it. Since jasmine is an aphrodisiac, flowering tobacco must be as well. Perfumers use a solvent-extracted absolute of tobacco for the dry, masculine scent with a heavy base note. The dried leaves, with their own, mustier aroma, have long been smoked by Native Americans during pipe and healing ceremonies.

Flowering tobacco looks good as an edging for a border garden since the tall, narrow stalks do not hide plants behind them. Plant flowering tobacco near a window to enjoy its evening fragrance. Large gray hawk moths, attracted to the scent, descend on the flowers in the evening to pollinate them. Tomato worm moths sometimes choose tobacco over tomatoes, but aphids hate the smell. Gardeners use this to their advantage by making a tobacco leaf spray.

Flowering tobacco is a perennial, but usually it is grown as an annual. It needs moist soil in sun or shade. Plant the seeds in relatively rich, regular garden soil in full sun and give it regular watering.

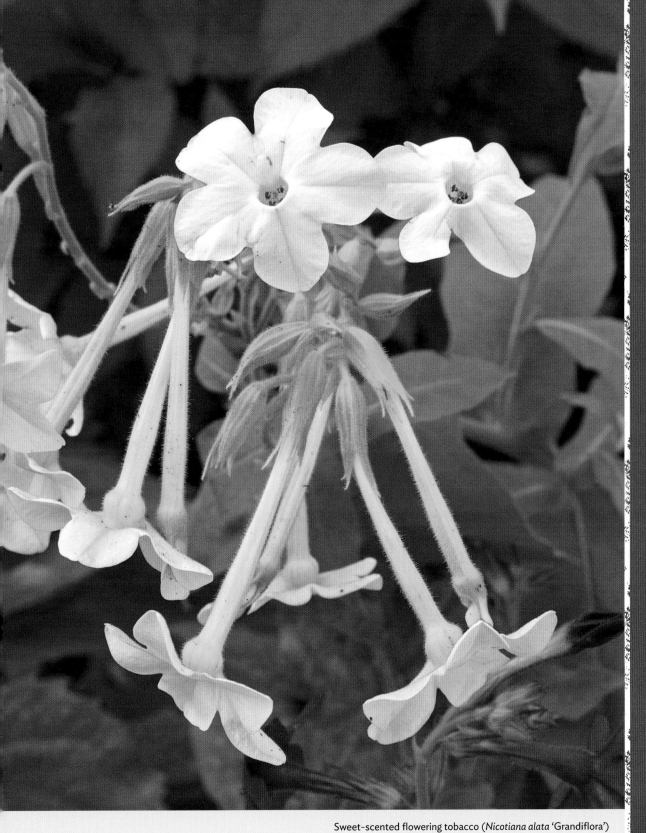

Sweet-scented flowering tobacco (*Nicotiana alata* 'Grandiflora')

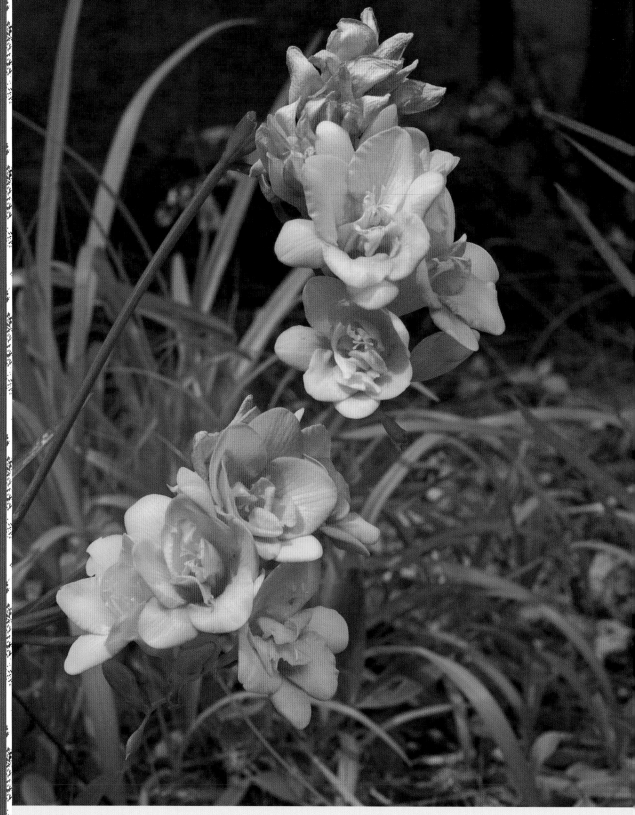

Freesia (*Freesia refracta*)

Freesia

Freesia refracta

Iris family: Iridacea
Perennial
Zones 9–10

Freesia presents a refreshing and sharp, peppery jolt of sweet, pervasive aroma. The complex scent carries the deep tones of jasmine, a touch of citrus, and coriander. There is also an elusive violet fragrance, although its presence is fleeting and disappears once the flowers are cut. A patch in bloom fills much of the garden and cut flowers perfume an entire room. One florist described it well by saying the scent "knocks your socks off, like trumpets in an orchestra; everyone sings backup, even the lilies."

Yellow flowers are the most fragrant, followed by white blooms that smell spicier. Next in line are the blues and purples. *Freesia refracta* 'Gold Flame' and 'Aladdin' are good examples of strongly scented yellow flowers. *Freesia refracta* 'White Swan' has a white flower that is nearly as fragrant. Brightly colored freesias are popular, but their greener, grassy aroma makes them the least fragrant.

Freesia creates a sense of happiness. It represents friendship and innocence, according to old European lore. A bouquet is presented on the seventh wedding anniversary. Synthetic freesia essential oil scents cream and bath oil, but it smells overly sweet compared to the real thing.

Freesia quickly became a hothouse favorite when it was introduced to Europe from South Africa. It continues to be one of the most popular cut flowers in the florist industry and certainly one of the most fragrant. The flowers attract beneficial butterflies, hummingbirds, and moths.

Grow freesias among other fragrant spring-flowering bulbs, such hyacinth, or as a houseplant. The bulbous corms need rich, porous, damp soil in full, but not too hot, sunlight. In zone 8 or colder, freesias can be potted in the fall and stored in a garage until spring.

Gardenia

Gardenia jasminoides

Coffee family: Rubieceae
Shrub
Zones 8–10

The scent of gardenia flowers in bloom is heady, heavy, exotic, very sweet—and a bit spicy. As with jasmine, a collection of light, sweet scents dance on heavier, exotic aromas that predominate. The fragrance brings to my mind a hot, sultry night at a garden party, women in their summer dresses wearing heavy, exotic perfumes and walking among the flowers. The mingling scents hang in the air.

The dwarf *Gardenia jasminoides* 'Prostrata' endures slightly cooler temperatures, and makes a good houseplant, but has a muted, less musky aroma. *Gardenia augusta* 'August Beauty' is another cultivar that has an especially strong, gardenia fragrance. The scent of the blooms of *G. florida* and *G. thunbergia* are so strong, they are grown for their essential oils, although neither of these two species handles frost.

Sniffing the aroma of fragrant gardenias can be so relaxing that it becomes difficult to concentrate. Studies back the traditional Chinese medicine use of gardenia as a muscle relaxant and to treat nervous system problems, pain, and emotional distress. German researchers at Ruhr University Bochum were granted a patent after gardenia proved to be the most relaxing of one hundred calming scents tested. It seems to act much like sleeping pills that increase GABA in the brain. Nanjing University of Chinese Medicine is studying the antidepressant properties of the fruit's oil.

Many cultures regard scented gardenia as an aphrodisiac associated with love and marriage. Polynesians wear heavily scented gardenia leis. They infuse coconut oil with the flowers, then use the oil, called *monoï* (scented oil), to improve skin and hair. *Monoï* is also used as massage oil to relax muscles. Perfumers consider gardenia the perfect scent since it combines top, middle, and low fragrance notes. At least fifty perfumes are based on gardenia, although many of these use the less expensive synthetic oil. Despite their short, twisted stems, gardenia flowers are popular cut flowers for their fragrance. They are the traditional French gentleman's formal *boutonnière*.

The scent of cape jasmine gardenias in bloom wafts throughout the garden from the minute the pure white flowers begin to unfurl like pinwheels. In warm climates, they flower all summer, the flowers contrasting beautifully against the shiny leaves. The best bloom is when night temperatures do not dip below 60 degrees F. Gardenia sometimes tolerates occasional temperatures below 20 degrees F, although it will die back. If it gets colder where you live, they grow well as houseplants if given a large pot and a sunny window. They like humidity and misting can prevent flowers from dropping off early when grown indoors or in a hot, dry climate. Plant the shrub in acid soil where it is out of direct sunlight. Fertilize these heavy feeders every other month while they are in flower.

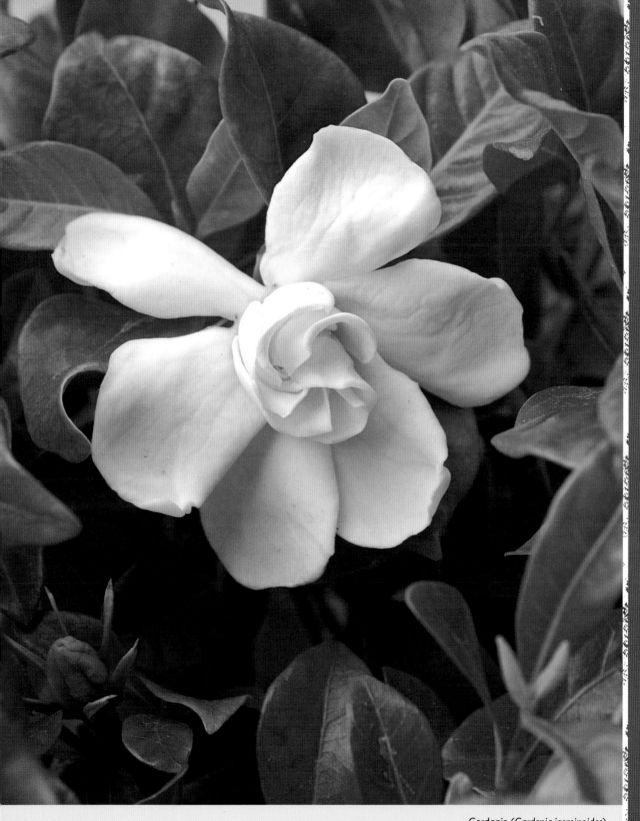

Gardenia (*Gardenia jasminoides*)

Harlequin glorybower

Clerodendrum trichotomum

Mint family: Lamiaceae
Shrub
Zones 7–10

Asian native *Clerodendrum trichotomum* is cultivated for its sweetly scented, late summer blossoms and metallic-blue fruit. The strong, nutty aroma of the heart-shaped leaves gives it the well-deserved nickname of "peanut butter tree." The flowers, on the other hand, have a sweet, honey fragrance. Depending on whom you ask, they also smell of rose, vanilla, banana, melon, lemon, cream punch, black currant, or nuts. Harlequin glorybower actually contains an aromatic mix of all of these. This makes its fragrance quite complex and difficult to describe, except as divine. It is exotic, but not cloying. Fortunately, it is the flower, not the leaves, that heavily perfumes the air around the bush.

Over five hundred *Clerodendrum* species are distributed throughout the world. While the aroma of some of these might make you hungry, others have been described as evil-smelling. *Clerodendrum trichotomum* 'Fargesii' received the Royal Horticultural Society's Award of Garden Merit. Glory flower (*C. bungei*) blooms famously smell just like Froot Loops® cereal. A Mexican native, it is a popular landscape plant in the southeastern United States. *Clerodendrum inerme* flowers are worn as fragrant head wreaths and leis in Polynesia and are also extracted into coconut oil to make a relaxing massage oil.

The individual aromas in harlequin glorybower flowers combine to create a relaxing effect. It is rarely used for aromatherapy, although a study did find anti-anxiety and sedative actions that appear to be mediated by GABA brain receptors in the roots of *Clerodendrum mandarinorum*. A number of species are burned and the incense-like smoke inhaled to treat asthma and headaches, as well as to deter mosquitoes.

The flowers of this tropical bush are used medicinally in China, India, Thailand, and Africa. The leaves are actually eaten, but are cooked first to remove their strong, aromatic flavor. A vase of the beautiful white and cream-colored flowers easily perfumes an entire room. Hummingbirds, moths, and masses of swallowtail butterflies are attracted to the blooms.

Harlequin glorybower gets its name from its strikingly colorful flowers. It grows ten to fifteen feet in height and width. It is deciduous and freezes to the ground, but will vigorously come back the next spring. It can get leggy, so many gardeners surround the base with low-growing plants. The bush can be shaped and the flowering stems pruned down to the ground every two to three years. Some gardeners report getting it through zone 6, and even zone 5 winters, as long as it is planted in a protected place and well mulched. Give it partial shade and well-drained soil with sufficient water.

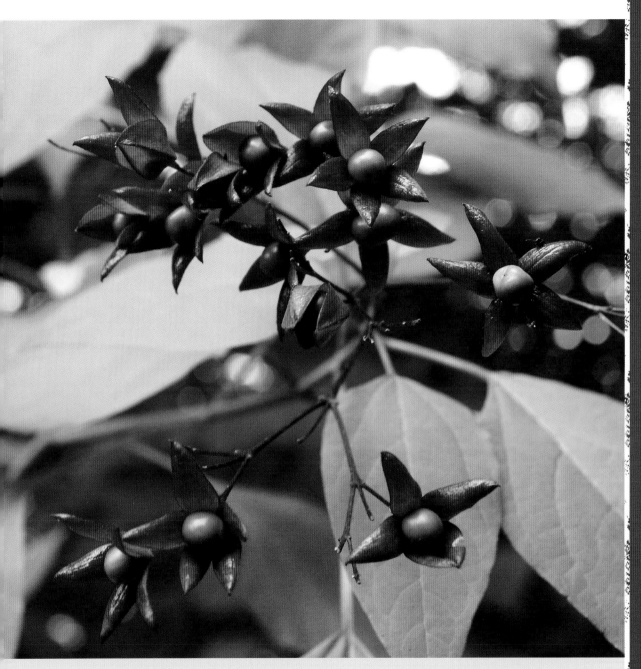

Harlequin glorybower (*Clerodendrum trichotomum*)

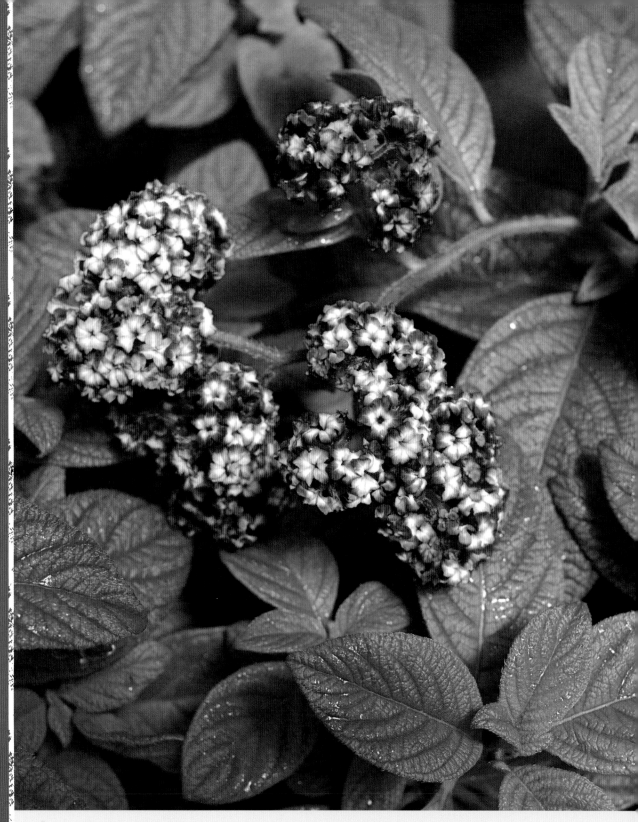

Heliotrope (*Heliotropium arborescens*)

Heliotrope

Heliotropium arborescens

Borage family: Boraginaceae
Tender perennial
Zones 9–11

Heliotrope's aroma is of almonds and cherries. The aroma resembles cherries so much that its nickname in England is cherry pie. Some say it is more vanilla and warm, caramel apples, or cherry vanilla crumb cake made with chopped, roasted almonds. Or have you ever smelled cherry amaretto? Thomas Jefferson called it a "delicious flower." He talked about the care needed to winter it over inside, but added "the smell rewards the care." Plants with pale mauve flowers often have the most scent.

When the French brought it from Peru in the mid-eighteenth century, it was an immediate hit. It was used in flower arranging and called the *herbe d'amour* (the herb of love). It is an easy flower to love with its rich aroma, but this more likely comes from Greek mythology, in which it represented unrequited love that is followed by forgiveness and acceptance. A flowering, potted plant was a common gift in Victorian times as a symbol of devotion.

The modest-looking heliotrope is grown more for its fragrance than beauty. Plant breeders have been striving to develop flowers with deeper blue hues. However, there is already a tendency for blue flowers to be less aromatic and the effort is causing heliotropes to lose some fragrance.

Heliotrope was a popular Victorian edging for rose beds. It works well along a pathway leading to the house, although it is more often grown in a container. It grows well potted for several years and can be trained into a standard by removing the lower leaves. To prevent it from becoming tall and leggy, pinch out the top and force it to branch. The flowers take a little longer to bloom, but the reward is many more blossoms.

As with many tropical plants, heliotrope appreciates very rich soil. With that wonderful perfume, you want as many blooms as possible in order to increase the intensity of the fragrance. For propagation, cuttings are easier than growing it from seed. Many gardeners treat it as an annual or grow it in a greenhouse. If conditions are right, they bloom in the winter in a cool greenhouse that is not above 50 degrees F at night.

Hyacinth

Hyacinthus orientalis

Lily family: Liliaceae
Perennial bulb
Zones 6–9

The fleeting sweetness of hyacinth fills the early spring air. The flowers are balsamic, rich, very sweet, and both floral and fruity. There is a definite musky scent that is almost starchy, making the aroma somewhat haunting. I've heard it described as the most ravishing perfume of the spring garden. Roman poet Ovid, from the first century BC, said that the fragrant breath of the flowers could "perfume the skies." The flowering stalks can be nicely displayed in bulb vases to fill a room with their fragrance.

Hyacinthus orientalis 'China Pink' has sweetly-perfumed, soft-pink flower spikes. *Hyacinthus orientalis* 'Hollyhock' is noted for double pink flowers with exceptional fragrance. *Hyacinthus orientalis* 'L'Innocence' is heavily perfumed and often grown in a pot indoors. Surprisingly, the other two species in this genus have no scent.

Hyacinth's aroma sends the mind into a dreamy state. The aroma is sedative, soothing, and emotionally uplifting. It helps treat nervous exhaustion and fatigue by lowering stress levels. This was one of most popular ancient Greek flowers to refresh and invigorate the mind and improve memory. Poet Oliver Wendall Holmes commented in the nineteenth century how the sweet smell bewitched him with memories. Try it yourself by placing a bouquet into a short vase to bring in the house, or by growing them indoors. The plants were introduced to England in the 1500s, when heavy scents were the rage. By the mid-eighteenth century, "hyacinthomania" was sweeping through the gardening world much like

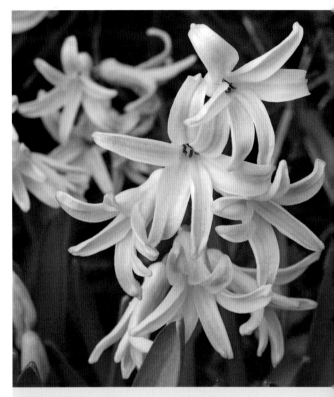

Hyacinth flowers open into a bundle of stars.

the previous tulipomania. Rare hyacinths were selling for two hundred pounds a bulb.

The fragrant, waxy blue flowers last only a couple of weeks in spring but each stalk can have up to sixty individual florets. The plants progressively become less showy in a few years, so many gardeners replace them every other year. They grow well in small pots either outside or inside. They can be forced into early bloom in bulb vases containing pebbles, marbles, or decorative crystals. Hyacinth loves sandy soil in the sun, but can handle some shade. Wear gloves when planting the bulbs, since touching them can irritate the skin.

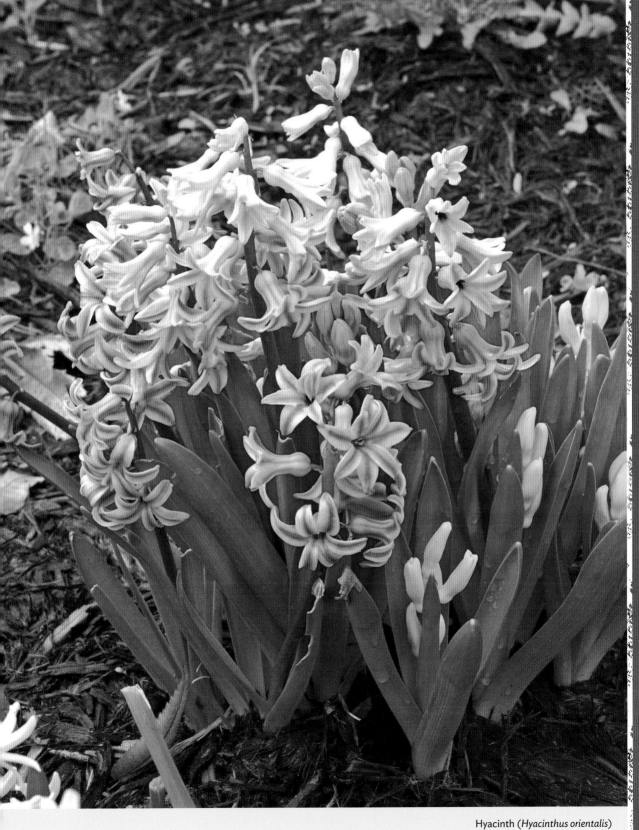

Hyacinth (*Hyacinthus orientalis*)

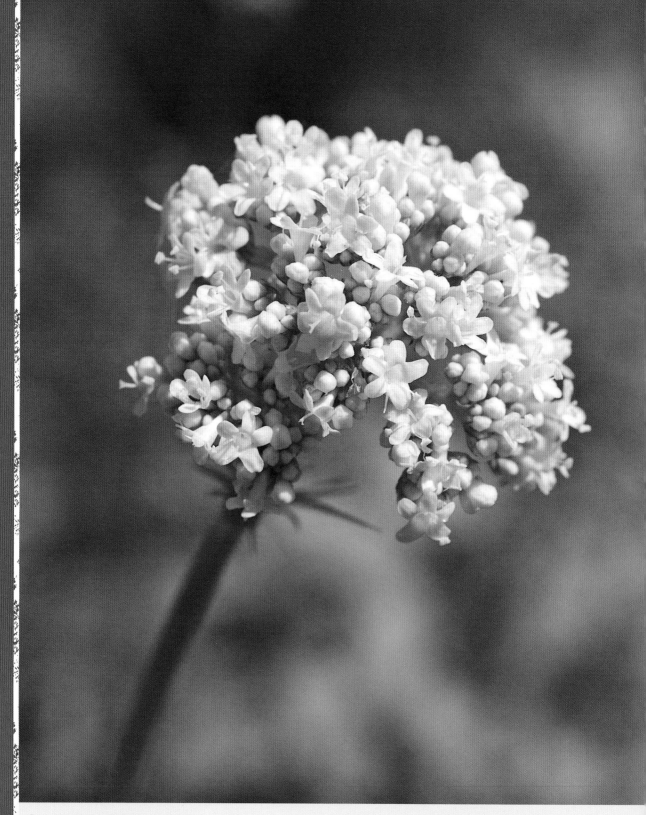

Common valerian (*Valeriana officinalis*)

Indian Valerian

Valeriana jatamansii, syn. *V. wallichii*

Honeysuckle family: Caprifoliaceae
Perennial
Zone 7

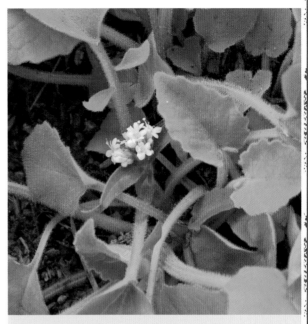

Indian valerian (*Valeriana jatamansii*, syn. *V. wallichii*)

Valerian from India has a rhizome with a deeply earthy and woodsy fragrance that is almost animal-like. It has the strong (and slightly objectionable) scent of European valerian root, or common valerian (*Valeriana officinalis*), which has been compared to dirty socks. Ancient Greeks called valerian *phu*, which described the typical reaction to it! Yet, the scent of valerian from India maintains a sweeter, more perfumey aroma, to earn a valued place in the fragrance garden. All valerian has a calming, sedative, and antidepressant effect. It helps resolve restlessness and irritability. Ayurvedic medicine uses it as a tonic for the nervous system and a way to treat headaches, tremors, hyperactivity, and anxiety. Traditional Chinese medicine prescribes it for mood disorders. A traditional ayurvedic massage oil can be created by infusing sesame oil with the roots. Just rubbing the aromatic massage oil on the soles of the feet sends most people to sleep.

Spikenard (*Nardostachys grandiflora*) has a similar, but even richer scent. It is wonderfully rich and sensual, leaning more toward perfume and patchouli's sweet muskiness. It smells old, even ancient, like a fragrance that could unfurl the history of exotic places, if only it could speak. How it affects the brain is very similar to its cousin, Indian valerian. Sometimes, the two are used interchangeably. Spikenard's fragrance increases the calming, meditative, theta brain waves, as well as deeply relaxing delta waves. In the Middle East, the tea treats heart and nervous conditions. It was an important ingredient in ancient perfumes, including the famous Roman *nardinum* and the ancient Egyptian temple incense-perfume, *kyphi*. It is perhaps best known as the expensive oil that Mary, often referred to as Mary Magdelene, poured over the feet of Jesus in the Bible. Very small amounts of this heavy fragrance still round off gentler scents in perfume.

Compounds in valerian, as well as spikenard, work together in an impressive, synergistic way to relax the brain, muscles, and nervous system. Several studies, reported in journals such as *Phytomedicine*, *Phytotherapy Research*, and the *Journal of Ethnopharmacology*, call them natural tranquilizers, antidepressants, and mood regulators. These herbs all seem to act as GABA inhibitors to regulate serotonin and dopamine neurotransmitters in the brain. They apparently temper stress by balancing the activity of the hypothalamus as well as the pituitary and adrenal glands—an axis that influences brain activity and stress levels.

Japanese Honeysuckle

Lonicera japonica

Honeysuckle family: Caprifoliaceae
Perennial
Zones 4–10

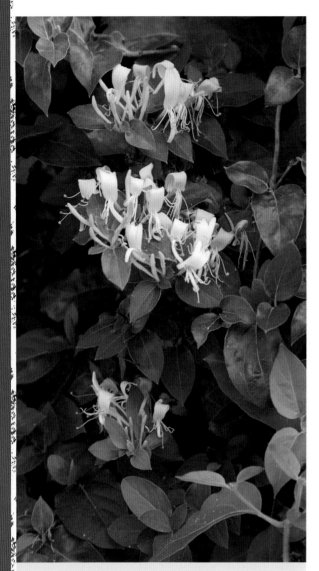

Japanese Honeysuckle (*Lonicera japonica*)

The scent of Japanese honeysuckle flowers floats through the garden with perfume that is both heady and heavy. It is similar to jasmine, except that it also smells of sweet plums and apples. Charles Darwin's grandfather described how honeysuckle "scents with sweeter breath the summer gales" in *The Botanic Garden* (1791).

The most aromatic honeysuckles are not always the showiest. *Lonicera fragrantissima* 'Repens', with purplish evergreen leaves, is highly scented and blooms in complete shade. Winter honeysuckle (*L. periclymenum*) has an especially sweet, fruity fragrance.

Japanese honeysuckle's fragrance is very relaxing. Honeysuckle flower water was once recommended to ease nervous headaches. Honeysuckle does not make a good cut flower, but it extends fragrance throughout the garden—a good place to enjoy it!

Japanese honeysuckle is covered each summer with highly fragrant cream-colored flowers. Given a trellis to climb, it creates an aromatic screen to divide the garden, cover a gazebo, or conceal old stumps. It survives best in a sheltered place.

Japanese honeysuckle is easy to cultivate; in fact, aggressive growth has caused it and *Lonicera fragrantissima* to be identified as invasive in some states. Check their status in your area before planting. *Lonicera japonica* is not fussy about soil and prefers full sun, or partial sun in very hot climates. It can survive on very little water, but flowers more profusely when given regular watering. The stems have a tendency to die back, so keep them lightly pruned.

Jasmine

Jasminum officinale

Oleander family: Oleaceae
Perennial
Zones 7-10

The delightful top scents of jasmine flowers seem to dance on heavy, base notes, creating a contrast that delights the nose. The aroma is warm, floral, and sweetly exotic, yet also a little fruity. If a scent can be seductive, this is the one. The scent permeates the garden. Coined "poet's jasmine," it is one of the most often-described fragrances in literature.

About twenty of the roughly two hundred species of tropical and sub-tropical jasmines are cultivated for fragrance. Spanish jasmine (*Jasminum grandiflorum*) blooms profusely throughout the summer. Sambac jasmine (*J. sambac*) has a fruitier scent with a touch of orange blossom perfume. Its white flowers fade pink as they mature. Both plants are hardy only to zones 9–11. Star jasmine (*Trachelospermum jasminoides*) has almost the same flowers and exotic fragrance, giving it similar properties. However, jasmine connoisseurs know the difference. I grow it in large wooden planters so it twines on trellises up around my windows. The fragrance is strong during the day, compared to true jasmine's evening scent. Once its roots are well established, it may survive in zones 6 and 7 if well mulched for the winter. It will freeze to the ground, but then come back the following spring.

Jasmine is stimulating and maybe a little hypnotic. It helps overcome insomnia and depression, and takes the edge off anger. It also eases a headache. The uplifting fragrance is used for happiness in Iran, where its name means "heavenly joy." That sounds appropriate, since it also has an age-old reputation as an aphrodisiac. Studies at Srinakharinwirot University in Nakhon

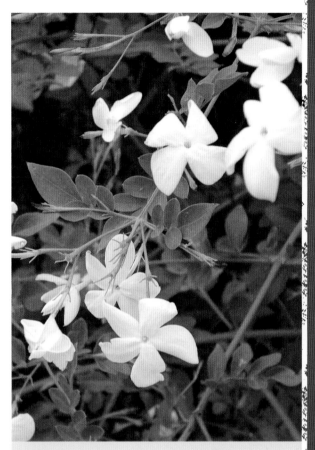

Jasmine (*Jasminum officinale*)

Nayok, Thailand, showed that jasmine was stimulating enough to slightly increase breathing rate and blood pressure. Participants felt more alert and vigorous after inhaling the scent. Volunteers in other Thai university studies said the fragrance was fresh and made them feel more active. At the University of Vienna in Austria, jasmine acted much like peppermint in increasing mental accuracy, vigilance, visual awareness, and pleasant emotions. It also helped participants take less time to do brain-related activities. When computer workers smelled jasmine, errors were reduced by one-third. Energizing beta brain waves were stimulated in studies sponsored by the Japanese fragrance firm, Takasago.

Tuscan brides are crowned with the flowers. Chinese and Indian women wear the flowers on their hair and wrists in the evening, when jasmine emits its fragrance. Chinese gardens have long been devoted solely to jasmine cultivation for scenting perfumed oils, wines, tea, garlands, and bracelets. Aromatics have been added to tea since the Song Dynasty (AD 960–1279). To make jasmine-flavored tea, add a couple of fresh or dried flowers to a pot of green, black, or herb tea. Just six flowers flavor a pot of rice. In the seventeenth century, jasmine was the most sought-after fragrance to perfume gloves.

It is no surprise that many perfumes, such as Joy by Jean Patou, contain jasmine. The essential oil is expensive, so chemists have tried to reproduce the fragrance, but the harsh-smelling synthetics always demand a touch of the true oil to soften them. Like the ancient Persians, you can infuse sesame oil with the flowers for an exotic body oil.

Jasmine adds beauty, fragrance, and charm to any garden. In India, it is called "moonlight of the grove" because the starlike, white flowers bloom at night. The plant needs to be supported on a trellis or perhaps a garden bench, or grown in large patio containers. It needs fairly rich soil with regular watering and feeding. However, pamper it too much and it will produce less scent. Prune back old stems in the fall, right after blooming is finished. The following year's flowers appear on the new shoots. Propagate it by cuttings or layering. Some gardeners are able to winter over jasmine indoors, but others treat it as an annual.

Juniper
Juniperus communis

Cypress family: Cupressaceae
Shrub
Zones 4–10

The pungent, peppery, camphorous scent of juniper is somewhat smoky. It carries some of the sharp turpentine scent of pine, yet is more complex and acceptable. It is distinctly the scent of wooden pencils being sharpened. The berries have the sweetest woody aroma, while the needles lean more toward sharp turpentine.

Juniper is one of the most popular landscaping plants in the western United States, ranging from trees to hedges to creeping varieties for rock gardens. All carry juniper's characteristic aroma. Leaf colors range from gray and silver to green and yellow variations, which fit into different garden landscapes. Ground cover junipers vary in height from just a few inches to a couple of feet tall. *Juniperus communis* 'Kalebab' is an example of an intermediate-sized plant that is ten to fifteen feet tall, with various colored needles that make it seem to glow. There are also a number of smaller, aromatic prostrate and dwarf versions, such as *J. communis* 'Compressa'. Creeping juniper (*J. horizontalis*) is a popular North American species, with over a dozen cultivars that grow between six and twelve inches tall.

The scent of juniper is a natural wake-up call to counter mental fatigue and physical debility. Volunteers at Hiroshima Prefectural Women's University in Japan preferred inhaling juniper or cypress to keep them mentally alert after, rather than before, a long workday. That may be because inhaling juniper also has a sedative effect, due to a component called cedrol, according to the Biological Science Laboratories of Kao Corporation in Tochigi, Japan.

The smoke carries the highly antiseptic essential oil into the air. Native Americans and

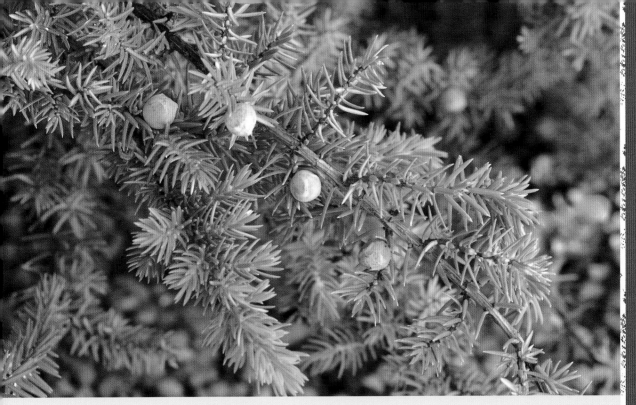

Juniper (*Juniperus communis*)

Chinese residents in the southwest Shaxi area burn juniper branches so that the smoke will ward off contagious diseases and negativity during healing ceremonies. Europeans once used juniper in the same way. It was found mixed with frankincense in Belgian funeral pots from the twelfth to fourteenth centuries. During World War II, the French returned to burning juniper branches in hospital wards when supplies of antiseptics ran low.

The berries give gin and juniper schnapps distinctive flavors and scents. Gin's association with juniper is so well established that its name is derived from *genièvre*, the French term for juniper berry. In Finland, the berries are used to make traditional ale, and for aromatic containers that preserve butter and cheese. Juniper also scents a number of colognes for men. The berries give potpourri scent and color.

Juniper has varieties that come from North America, Europe, and northern Asia. The shrub gives height to garden landscaping. Its flat, blue-green leaves create deep shadows that contract nicely with just about any garden plant. This is enhanced when dusty-blue berries cover it from fall into winter. The berries, which are technically small cones, take a year to mature, so a plant bears them in both ripe and unripe stages. Juniper tends to spread out; start trimming it when it is still young if you want it contained. Keep in mind that pruning back an old juniper too far leaves gaping holes in the shrub.

Juniper shrubs kindly grow where little else will. They prefer acidic soil, but manage in almost any poor soil. They require very little water, developing root rot if over watered. They are usually planted in full sun, but tolerate some shade. The tough seeds need a hard freeze before they will sprout. Dry the berries on a screen or in a shallow bowl and hang the branches.

Korean spice viburnum

Viburnum carlesii

Moschatel family: Adoxaceae
Shrub
Zones 4–6

The fragrance of Korean spice viburnum is most often referred to as spice cake. In the garden, the air around the shrub becomes intoxicating with floral depth. This combination of carnation and spice is reminiscent of clove pink, yet more complicated and even more intense. It only flowers for a couple weeks in late spring, but such fragrant weeks those are! Plant one near a window, and the aroma will flood the house. It is no surprise that another name for this shrub is fragrant viburnum. Some gardeners claim it as their favorite aromatic plant. The smell of cloves is known to be both energizing and relaxing. As with clove pinks, the scent is joyful and helps overcome mental fatigue, nervousness, and poor memory.

Viburnum ×*carlcephalum* 'Cayuga' has comparable fragrance, but better mildew resistance. It was introduced by the United States National Arboretum. *Viburnum carlesii* 'Compactum' is a dwarf that tops out at about four feet tall. Fragrant viburnum (*V.* ×*carlcephalum*) and the hybrid, *V.* ×*juddi* are contenders with Korean spice as the most aromatic. *Viburnum* ×*burkwoodii* 'Mohawk' joins the competition with its distinctly clove-scented white flowers. The jury is still out, so plant several and judge for yourself. Be wary of some species. Arrow wood viburnum (*V. dentatum*) is very attractive, but the flowers smell absolutely foul.

Korean spice viburnum presents a visual sensation every spring. This bushy, seven-foot-tall deciduous shrub has copper-colored leaves when young. Very attractive, round clusters of blushing pink buds gradually give way to strongly scented, pale pink flowers. They are followed by oval black fruits that are enjoyed by wild birds. The cut stems can be brought indoors and forced to produce a bouquet of fragrant flowers.

The five- to eight-foot-high, rounded shrub grows in full or partial sun with a moderate amount of water. It will be happiest in moist, acidic, well-drained soils in full sun, but tolerates semi-shade, various soil types, and some drought. Unfortunately, this species has trouble with mildew, bacterial leaf spot, and borers, not to mention the viburnum leaf beetle residing in New England. Keeping older branches cut back encourages fresh, new growth. Be sure to discard the old stems.

Lamb's ears

Stachys byzantina

Mint family: Lamiaceae
Perennial
Zones 4–9

Lamb's ears smell as soft as they look with a gentle, pretty scent of mint and chamomile, which has been compared to an herby version of apple and pineapple. It is the tasty fragrance of sweet herb tea when you lift the lid of the teapot. This is a favorite plant of children, who love the fuzzy, aromatic leaves and fragrance, as well as the name!

Lamb's ears' relative, wood betony (*Stachys officinalis*), is better known for being an herbal relaxant, but lamb's ears also has this quality. It is interesting that the smell is so close to chamomile, since both plants have a long history of being given to children to relax them.

Children once were given a lamb's ears leaf to hold near their nose and enjoy the subtle scent as they drifted to sleep. The leaves also make fragrant, fuzzy bandages and lend their soft fragrance to sleep pillows and potpourri. Like

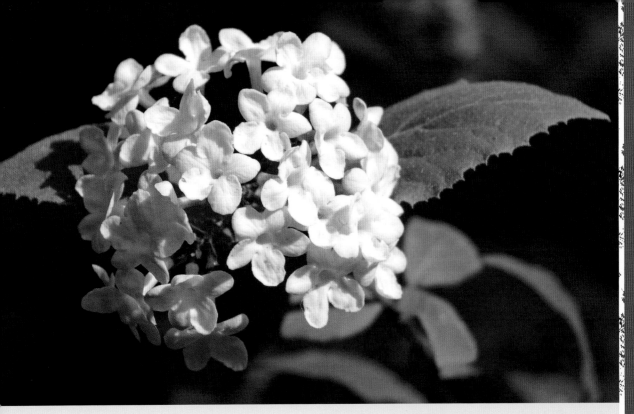

Korean spice viburnum (*Viburnum carlesii*)

chamomile, it makes a tasty herb tea to ease nervous tension. It flavors a famous mole verde sauce from Oaxaca, Mexico.

The aroma of *Stachys byzantina* is so faint that it may seem an odd choice for the fragrance garden. However, it is ideal to edge a pathway or fall over the top of a garden wall where children, as well as adults, can stroke and smell it. It makes an interesting ground cover. The attractive, fuzzy gray flower stalks grow about a foot tall and are dotted with tiny purple flowers that are pollinated by honeybees, bumblebees, and hummingbirds.

The plant hails from Turkey and Southwest Asia and tolerates poor conditions and drought. However, it does much better when given fairly rich soil with good drainage. It grows in sun or partial shade. To harvest the leaves, pick them individually to dry them on a screen or in a paper bag.

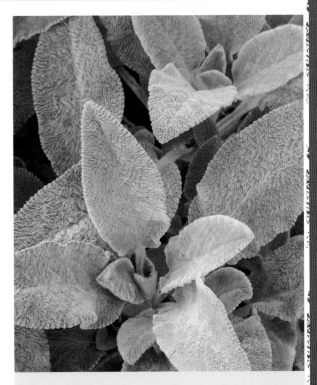

Lamb's ears (*Stachys byzantina*)

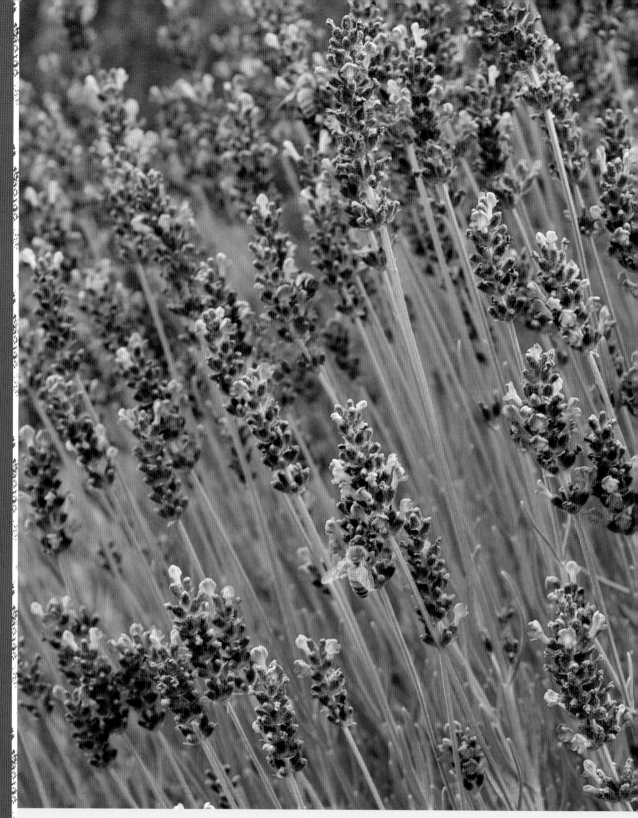

'Hidcote' lavender (*Lavandula angustifolia* 'Hidcote')

Lavender

Lavandula angustifolia

Mint family: Lamiaceae
Perennial
Zones 5–8

The aroma of lavender (sometimes called English lavender) is herbal and sweetly floral, with rich balsamic undertones and a hint of spice. However, it is not just another pretty scent. In the background, a sharp, camphorous note resembles a soft version of rosemary. I have loved lavender's fragrance since I was a child, first encountering it in my grandmother Irene's dresser, where lavender sachets scented her clothing. The wonderful fragrance that floated out of that drawer was a bouquet of flowers and herbs that smelled a little like my grandmother herself. She was born in the Victorian era, when Queen Victoria filled the royal apartments with lavender's aroma.

There are over forty species and another four hundred varieties of lavender—enough to confuse even the lavender lover. When you are shopping for lavender plants, do your homework. A good book to sort it out is *The Lavender Lover's Handbook*, by Virginia McNaughton. Your decision will depend on whether you are seeking the most fragrant or colorful lavender, or a certain size or flower structure. *Lavandula angustifolia* 'Rosea' tests with one of the strongest fragrances. *Lavandula angustifolia* 'Maillette', with green foliage, has extremely fragrant violet-blue flowers on long stems that are distilled commercially, thanks to their high content of essential oil. Nurseries commonly sell shorter-growing varieties that are compact and do not fall on neighboring plants; for example, 'Munstead', 'Compacta Nana', and 'Hidcote' are dwarf cultivars around a foot tall or less. 'Jean Davis' and 'Twinkle Purple'

are slightly taller. So is 'Hidcote Giant', which is probably the most fragrant of the bunch. Since lavender grown from seed varies, there is some confusion over these names. There are so few true 'Munstead' plants that aromatic plant specialist Dr. Arthur Tucker of Delaware State University would like to see them all designated simply as 'Compacta'.

There are also many different aromatic species. Spike lavender (*Lavandula latifolia*) has tall, branched stems that produce many somewhat camphorous flowers. French lavender (*L. dentata*) has a lighter lavender scent mixed with lemon, and sports green, square-toothed leaves. My favorite is a hybrid, *L. ×ginginsii*, known as Goodwin Creek Grey and developed by my friend, Jim Becker, although it needs winter protection even in zones 8 and 9. Sweet lavender (*L. hetrophylla*), probably a French and English cross, is a fast grower with lavender-scented leaves. The scent is a unique, harsher mix of lavender with lemon and pine. Spanish lavender (*L. stoechas*) smells the most strongly of camphor. The interesting, square flower head is topped with two little petals. These last two are only hardy to zones 7 to 10.

Lavandin (*Lavandula ×intermedia*) is a cross between spike and English lavenders that produces abundant flowers and yield and is the source of most lavender oil. The scent tends to be a little flatter and less sweet than English lavender, causing some lavender connoisseurs to shun it. However, a lavandin plant can yield nearly three times more essential oil than lavender and tolerates more acidic soil. My appreciation for lavandin grew after visiting Provence, where French growers compare the aromatic characteristics of their lavandin varieties as if they were fine wines. *Lavandula ×intermedia* 'Impress Purple', 'Edelweiss', and the slightly camphorous, spicy 'Provence' had the strongest aromas when tested. 'Grosso' is one of the most productive of the highly fragrant lavandins. 'Super' has a milder, camphor-like fragrance and large, violet-green flower heads. 'Alba' produces long spikes of fragrant, white flowers. Give it excellent drainage and do not water it from overhead.

One of the most studied aromatics, lavender has become the poster child for science-backed aromatherapy. It is used when people are feeling down or burned out, to address nervousness, exhaustion, insomnia, depression, and general irritability. It has a balancing action that both relaxes and stimulates the mind, depending on the dose and probably what the individual needs. Renaissance herbalists described this as "raising the spirit" and "comforting the braine" and recommended sticking sprigs under a hat to cure a nervous headache. Centuries before them, Abbess Hildegard of Bingen wrote that a lavender bath after a walk assured a good night's sleep. Research shows that about ten minutes of inhalation can ease headaches, pain, depression, confusion, premenstrual syndrome, anxiety, memory problems, aggression in Alzheimer's patients, and feelings of dejection. Volunteers in a 2000 study at Chiba University Graduate School of Medicine in Japan said lavender made them feel more comfortable, cheerful, and natural. In this and other studies, activity in the active alpha brain waves decreased, indicating relaxation. Lavender may also help prevent heart disease since it lowers cortisol stress levels and increases blood flow through the heart. In some cases, lavender-scented hospital rooms lull hospital patients into restorative sleep with fewer painkillers and without side effects. Deep sleep is increased while active rapid-eye-movement sleep is decreased. Mothers at the University of Miami in Florida who gave their infants lavender-scented baths smiled and relaxed more. Their babies cried less and slept more deeply. Patients waiting for their dental appointments at King's College Dental Institute in London were less nervous when they smelled lavender. Several

Japanese studies indicate that lavender is not only relaxing, it also makes the mind sharper and more alert.

More than thirty different types of lavender essential oils are traded on world markets. In blending aromatherapy products, lavender is invaluable because it softens harsher scents and brings down over-the-top sweetness. It scents body care products, soaps, and deodorants. The name lavender comes from the Latin lavare, which means "to wash." In ancient Rome, it was added to washing water. For centuries, laundry has been scented by being dried on lavender bushes. Medieval washing women were even referred to as "lavenders." It is no longer popular in the kitchen, but lavender tea and cookies are an instant hit at garden parties.

The dried flowers scent potpourri, sachets, and pillows. Simple, small lavender pillows once calmed fussy babies and fancy lace pillows resided in Victorian parlors to revive swooning women. Lavender also went into Victorian smelling salts. Lavender pillows and lavender wands (made by weaving ribbon around the flowering stalks) were often held by mothers in birthing rooms. Many travel with a lavender pillow to ensure a good night's sleep when away from home. Charles VI of France is said to have sat on lavender-stuffed cushions. A seventeenth-century English folk song begins "Lavender's blue, dilly, dilly," and a stanza of John Keats' poem "The Eve of St. Agnes" contains the line "and still she slept an azure-lidded sleep, in blanched linen, smooth and lavender'd."

In the garden, choose companion plants that bloom at the same time, such as pastel shades of yarrow or red or pink roses. Keep it trimmed back, especially in wet climates, to prevent rot. You may want to try the French practice of shaping the shrubs into a dome every fall to increase the bloom and keep the plant from becoming leggy. This may be emotionally difficult, but cutting off the first year's flowers strengthens the

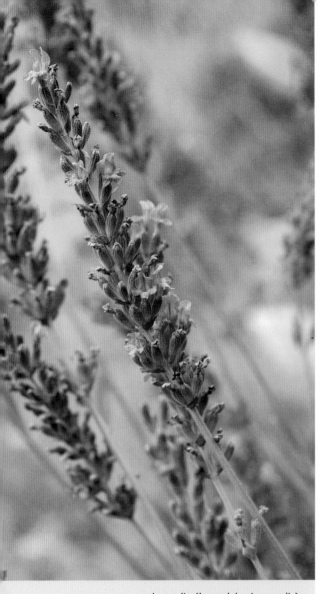

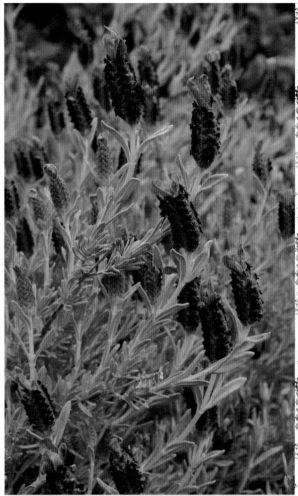

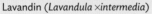
Lavandin (*Lavandula ×intermedia*)

Spanish lavender (*Lavandula stoechas*)

future plant. Tiger swallowtail butterflies and bumblebees pollinate the flowers.

Lavender prefers a Mediterranean climate with well-drained, alkaline soil, sparse rain, and plenty of sunshine. It seems partial to growing in rocks. When I first saw lavender growing wild on the rocky hillsides of the mountains of the Provence region of France, I understood. It also grows best at over fifteen hundred feet altitude,

where I have seen it growing wild. Lavender propagated from seed varies, so it is usually propagated from cuttings.

Lavender is harvested just before the buds open and the scent is released. When the first petals open off the tiny flowers, it is ready. Cut off the long stems just above the leaves. Lavender flowers in early summer, but usually blooms again if it is cut after first flowering.

Lemon

Citrus ×limon

Citrus family: Rutaceae
Tender perennial
Zones 9–11

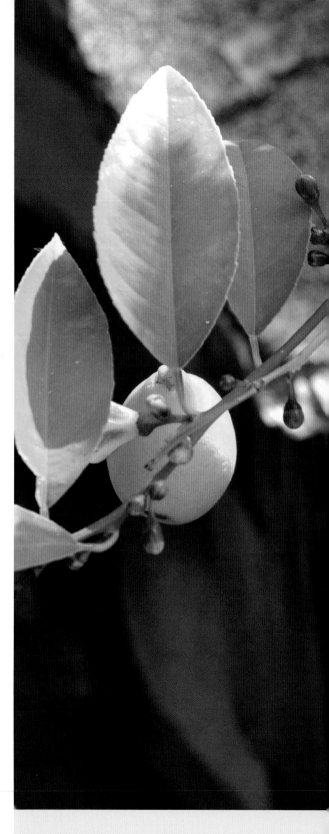

Lemon tree smells sweeter than it tastes. The aroma of freshly sliced lemon is a familiar, refreshing contrast of sharp acidic and sweet fruit. Think of sweet, balsamic vinegar heavily infused with honey. The peel, which is the source of lemon essential oil, smells similar, but is slightly bitter.

Meyer lemon (*Citrus ×limon* 'Improved Meyer') is a disease-resistant variety that handles temperatures down to 20 degrees F, slightly lower if covered. The fruit is sweeter and has a thin skin that turns yellow when it is ripe, so don't pick it too soon. It is available as a fifteen-foot tree or a dwarf that is half that size, while standard trees can reach twenty feet. Lisbon lemon (*Citrus ×limon* 'Lisbon') is adapted to both cold and high heat.

Lemon is uplifting, pure, and clean. Lemon-scented dish soaps take advantage of this to give the illusion that they clean better. Aromatherapy enlists lemon's fresh aroma to improve self-esteem, relieve depression, and as a general feel-good scent. Scientific research shows that lemon's aroma acts through the nervous system and brain chemistry to counter anxiety and stress, and slightly lower blood pressure—a sign of relaxation. In one study, it enhanced the participants' general mood. Preliminary research at institutions that include Italy's University of Siena and Yamaguchi University in Japan suggests that lemon's aroma relieves depression, anxiety, and pain by enhancing tryptophan in the brain. The refreshing scent is probably why lemons symbolize life in Europe and are said to protect against disease. In India, which is

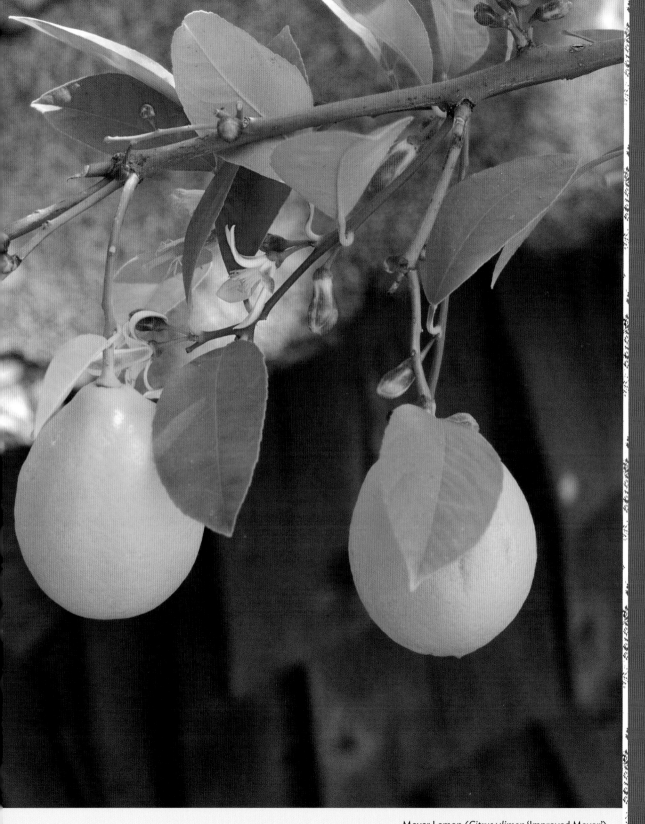

Meyer Lemon (*Citrus* ×*limon* 'Improved Meyer')

possibly their country of origin, lemons represent purification of the body and mind and elimination of negative thought patterns.

Lemon is a culinary treat, but also a household disinfectant that fights bacterial and fungal growth while making the house smell fresh and inviting. Prepare non-toxic, all-purpose cleaner by mixing a quarter teaspoon of lemon essential oil with one cup vinegar and one cup water.

Lemon trees are attractive in the garden with their large leaves, flowers, and fruit for most of the year. They are frost sensitive, but hardy strains survive in a protected spot, such as next to a building. My neighbors have a very festive tree because they keep it warm with Christmas lights! Dwarf trees grow in a well-drained, three-by-three-foot container. My 'Improved Meyer' tree lives in a large pot on a south-facing deck where it can be wheeled under a protective roof. Healthy plants survive cold weather better, so fertilize trees and spray kelp and fish emulsion foliar on the leaves in the fall.

Citrus trees need full sun and very well-drained soil. They should be well composted three times a year. Water established trees about once a week and those growing in pots at least twice a week; more often when the weather is hot. In clay soil, the surface should dry out between waterings. Only prune deadwood or overlapping branches, keeping in mind that the most fruit is produced on bottom branches.

Lemon balm
Melissa officinalis

Mint family: Lamiaceae
Perennial
Zones 4–8

Lemon balm does not easily release its fragrance into the air, but lightly press a leaf, and the scent is delightfully lemony and herbal. The aroma is lighter than lemon and more fleeting. It smells like sweet herbal tea served with a slice of lemon.

Golden lemon balm (*Melissa officinalis* 'Aurea') has yellow-green leaves. Variegated lemon balm (*M. officinalis* 'Variegata') is green to pale yellow with blotchy colorations. Both have lemon balm's fragrance and properties. *Melissa officinalis* 'Lime Balm' has a light lime fragrance that is mostly disguised by lemon.

Lemon balm's aroma is uplifting, yet calming. It helps quell nervousness, depression, anger, fear, and insomnia. The eleventh-century healer, Avicenna, recommended it to elevate a bad mood. Research centers, such as the University of Ottawa in Canada, are investigating how lemon balm improves mood by acting on brain neurotransmitters, such as GABA.

Carmelite nuns made lemon balm the main ingredient in their Carmelite complexion water, which was splashed on the face to treat headaches and nervous system problems. Eau de Mélisse des Carmes in France and the German Klosterfrau Melissengeist are still produced for the same purpose. I love a cup of relaxing lemon balm tea and use the leaves in salad or desserts. The delicious honey from the plant is delicate and distinctly lemony. The genus name, *Melissa*, is Greek for "bee." The scent and taste of the dried leaves diminishes with time, so harvest a fresh crop every summer.

Lemon balm's bright green leaves stand out nicely next to those of deeper colors, such as peppermint. Avoid placing lemon balm near strongly scented plants that may overpower it, such as sage. Lemon balm dies back after seeding in late summer, so a solid bed is not the best choice for year-round garden design. Instead, you can plant it here and there near a pathway where garden visitors can enjoy the fragrance, but not be bothered by the flurry of honeybees it attracts.

Although it seeds like crazy, this two-foot-tall shrub does not spread by runners or fall on its neighbors. The seedlings are easy to weed. One of the easiest plants to cultivate, *Melissa officinalis* grows wild throughout most of the United States as a garden escapee. It is drought resistant, but grows fuller if watered regularly and given fairly rich, well-drained soil. Lemon balm handles semi-shade to full sun, although too much sun turns the leaves pale, especially with the golden and variegated cultivars. Hang the stems and the thin leaves will dry quickly. Once dry, strip leaves from the stem.

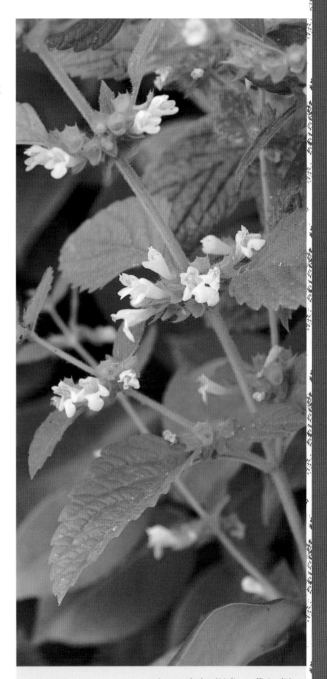

Lemon balm (*Melissa officinalis*)

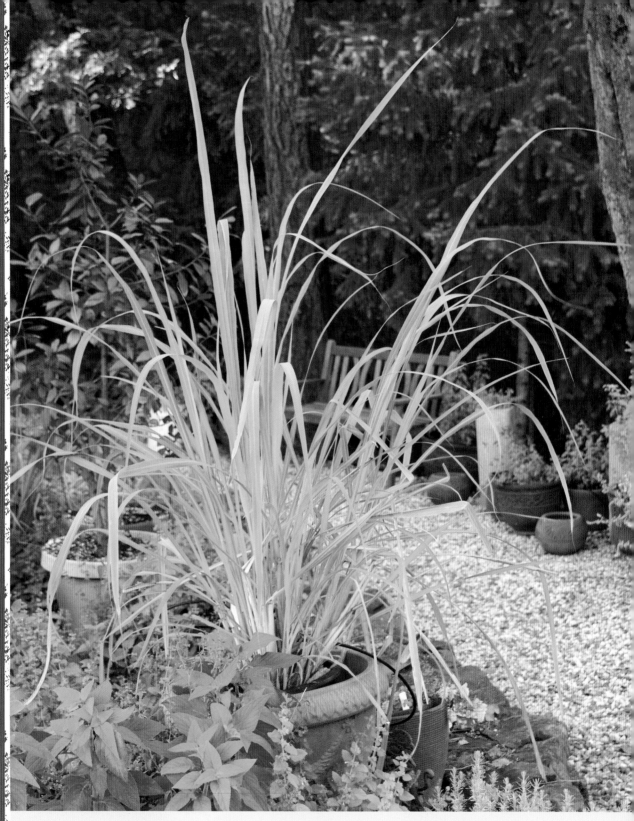

Lemon grass (*Cymbopogon citratus*)

Lemon grass

Cymbopogon citratus

Grass family: Poaceae
Tender perennial
Zones 10–11

The delightfully fresh fragrance of lemon grass leaves is distinctly lemon, but also somewhat grassy, making it more interesting than pure lemon. It is the essence of sipping sweet lemonade on a hot day while sitting on a lawn of freshly mown grass. This is also the delicious aroma of Thai coconut soup and the characteristic scent of Ivory soap.

Palmarosa (*Cymbopogon martini*) has a more elegant lemon grass scent with a bit of rose, reminiscent of rose geranium. It is a substitute for the more expensive rose geranium in some colognes and aromatherapy products. As with rose geranium, it is used by aromatherapists to relieve anxiety-related conditions and nerve pain. It is also a mosquito repellent. It grows in low light as a houseplant (if you like tall grasses in your house). It is not supposed to produce seed, but apparently no one told my palmarosa plant. Citronella (*C. nardus*) is a well-known relative that was first exhibited at London's Crystal Palace in 1851. It became the most popular scent for commercial cleaning products and natural bug sprays. Citronella is one of the best lemon scents to repel mosquitoes, although it is not as effective as the chemical repellent DEET. Use diluted bug sprays and do not put full-strength citronella essential oil directly on skin or on pets; it will be absorbed into the bloodstream.

Lemon grass is used to help overcome stress, nervous exhaustion, and especially sleep disorders. Similar to lemon, it also improves self-esteem. It is used to soothe nervous conditions —in Brazilian and Caribbean folk medicine as an aromatic wash, and in Chinese and ayurvedic treatment as a medicine. In India, it is infused into coconut oil and massaged into the skin to relieve pain and itching. Lemon grass works much like pharmaceutical sedatives, encouraging production of relaxation chemicals in the brain, such as GABA. Combining it with other sedative herbs such as valerian or hops increases the calming effect.

Lemon grass leaves make tasty tea and the leaf base nicely flavors soup. You probably already know the fragrance of lemon grass, as it is among the world's ten best-selling scents for soap, cosmetics, hair rinse, deodorant, and cleaning products. It often replaces more expensive essential oils, such as rose geranium, lemon verbena, and lemon balm. Even when Melissa oil from India was introduced a hundred years ago, it was made with lemon grass instead of lemon balm. The cut leaves are added to potpourri.

Lemon grass is widely cultivated in much of the tropical world, where the five-foot-tall shrubs grow in the full, hot sun. For those of us in zone 9 or colder, it becomes a reluctant houseguest in a south-facing window during the winter, moving outside to the fragrance garden for the summer. It prefers well-drained soil that is fairly rich in potassium. Too much watering diminishes the scent.

Lemon verbena

Aloysia triphylla

Verbena family: Verbenaceae
Perennial
Zones 8-10

I am in love with lemon verbena—the most beautiful and intensely fragranced of the lemon-scented herbs. Compared to lemon itself, it smells less acidic and far more sophisticated. It is delightfully fresh and not cloying. Imagine a delicious lemon dessert with honey, roses, and a touch of sweet basil. It is similar to the scent of lemon grass, but more refined.

Sweet almond verbena (*Aloysia virgata*) is so aromatic, it is also known as incense shrub. It has a unique and curious aroma of almond, honey, buddleia, and grape juice. This odd combination of scents actually smells fantastic when you can catch whiffs of it across the garden during its long summer blooming season. The bees and butterflies love it. The shrub looks a little straggly and can grow to eight feet tall. Oreganillo (*A. wrightii*) is suitable for hot climates as a mid-sized ground cover, although it hates humidity. Smelling and tasting much like slightly harsh oregano, this native of the southwestern United States and northern Mexico found its way into regional cooking. It's a robust herb with a sharp bite and some heat, featuring flavors of oregano, lemon, licorice, and a slight hint of mint. It is a source of nectar for native solitary bees and is food for the rustic sphinx moth.

The soothing fragrance of lemon verbena improves both concentration and sleep. It helps stop disruptive dreams. Plant lore links it to love. It was once said that wearing a sprig of it attracts love to you.

After being introduced to eighteenth-century Europe, lemon verbena quickly found its way into perfume. Today, Givenchy's Very Irresistible is based on it. Lemon verbena body care products are very popular for their fresh, lemon-herb fragrance, although many are actually scented with the less-expensive lemon grass. In its native South America, lemon verbena flavors liqueur and food. It's my favorite tea to serve during herb garden tours. Add an innovative, Victorian touch to a dinner party by scenting finger bowls with a few leaves.

I don't mind the plant's undisciplined growth. If you prefer a tighter look, then gently prune it in the fall or shape it against a wall. It looks stunning accented in the center of a bed in a pot or in the ground and surrounded by shorter plants. The bees are charmed by its little panicles of pure white flowers. Honeybees and butterflies pollinate them. The leaves dry into attractive curls that maintain fragrance for years in potpourri. It gives the landscape a sense of depth because you can see through the shrub to the garden beyond it.

Lemon verbena is a tropical South American plant that wants well-drained, good soil in full

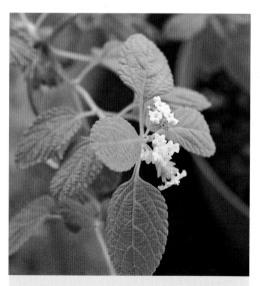

Oreganillo (*Aloysia wrightii*)

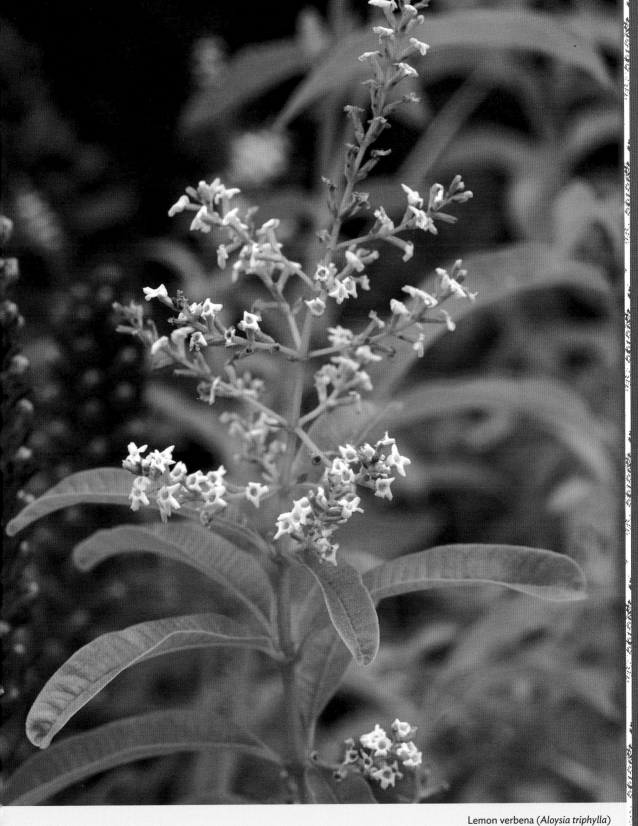

Lemon verbena (*Aloysia triphylla*)

sun. It is drought tolerant, but does best when it completely dries out in between regular waterings. It will grow in a greenhouse if the temperature is around 55 degrees F. In zones 8 and even 9, plants usually need to be large and well established to make it through the winter. I completely cover my bushes since they are deciduous in these zones, and they survive without sunlight until spring. I know gardeners in Maine's zone 5 that severely cut the plant back and transplant it into moist sand to spend the winter indoors, then transplant it back into the spring garden. This is a lot of work, but once you grow lemon verbena, you'll always want it gracing your fragrance garden. It can be tricky to grow from seed or cuttings. Harvest lemon verbena by stripping off the leaves by hand in the fall garden. If you want to cut it back, this is a good time to do so; take the leaves in the process. Place them on a screen where the thin leaves will dry quickly.

Lilac

Syringa vulgaris

Oleander family: Oleaceae
Perennial
Zones 3–7

Lilac flowers yield the sweet, powder-like, slightly spicy aroma of old-fashioned perfume. It hints of jasmine, which is in the same family. There is nothing in spring like large clusters of fragrant lilacs. Nearly every yard once had a shrub. American garden writer Louise Beebe Wilder said in *The Fragrant Garden* that in the 1930s, "To drive down country lanes during lilac time is to enjoy a continuous bath of fragrance." Lilac festivals throughout North America celebrate it every May.

Choose lilacs carefully. French hybrids have brilliantly colored, large flowers, but fragrance has sadly been bred out of most of them. *Syringa vulgaris* 'Madame Lemoine' has cascades of beautifully scented white blooms. *Syringa vulgaris* 'Marlyensis pallida' is generally considered the most fragrant, although *S. vulgaris* 'Serene' tops the rating by Arnold Arboretum in Massachusetts for the most aromatic. The Chinese lilacs (*S. oblata*), (*S. pubescens*), and (*S. ×chinensis*), are also high on their list.

The fragrance of lilac has long been known to make one happy and reminiscent. "The first whiff of their perfume in the garden is as the very heart and soul of memory," declared Victorian artist and author Eleanor Vere Boyle in *A Garden of Pleasure*. The aroma has been associated with melancholy, memories, and loss in Europe and the Middle East. Young women wearing lilacs were said to never marry and sending a bouquet signaled the end of a relationship.

Its reputation as a sleep aid has led to lilac-scented bath salts, shower products, and bed sheets. In the sixteenth century, herbalist John Gerard disagreed and complained of lilacs keeping him awake. The essential oil is produced only synthetically, and it never duplicates the real thing, so lilac is best as a cut flower. Budded tops bloom early when brought indoors. The dried flowers are added to potpourri, although their fragrance and color quickly fade.

Full sun creates clusters of lilac blooms to which bees and butterflies flock, although the shrubs do better with a little shade in very hot climates. Plant lilacs near other May bloomers, such as iris, in good garden soil. A pronounced winter chill encourages spring bloom, while heavy pruning discourages it, but thin out deadwood. To help lilacs that are overgrown, cut a few of the old stems every year. The shrubs look cleaner when spent flower clusters are removed. Cut them above points where buds form or you'll lose next year's bloom.

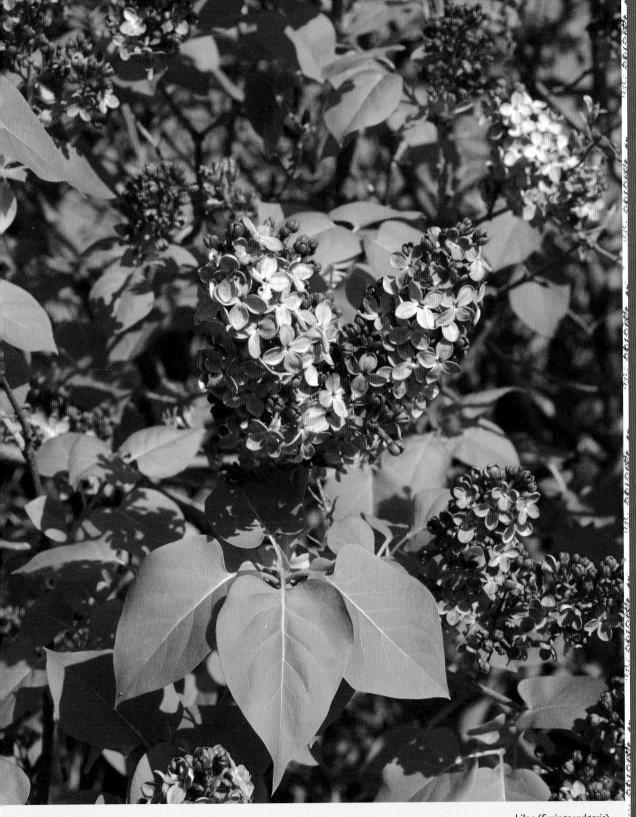

Lilac (*Syringa vulgaris*)

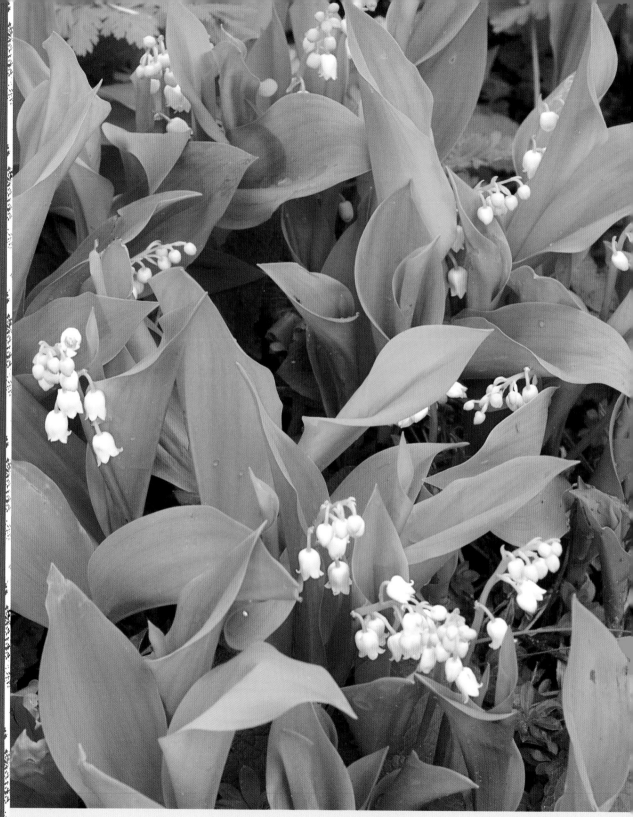

Lily-of-the-valley (*Convallaria majalis*)

Lily-of-the-valley

Convallaria majalis

Lily family: Liliaceae
Perennial
Zones 2–7

It is amazing that such a small flower produces so much fragrance. The aroma is a sweet and delicate combination of rose, lemon, and musk, thanks to compounds it shares with rose geranium. It is also a little fruity with a touch of green pea, for a compelling blend of flowers with food. Its blooms signal the return of spring. This was the favorite fragrance of Russian composer Pyotr Tchaikovsky, who said, "I love it to distraction." He dedicated the "Spring Sonata" from *The Seasons* to it. The title of his poem "Landysh" translates to "lily-of-the-valley."

Convallaria majalis 'Flore Pleno' has double petals, so it emits twice the amount of the same, lovely fragrance of its single-petaled parent plant.

Lily-of-the-valley provides comfort and improves memory and sustained concentration. The sweet fragrance, along with pure white flowers, represents innocence, purity, and happiness. The use of these symbolic flowers for weddings has been on the rise since the Duchess of Cambridge carried them when she married Prince William. Water distilled from the flowers, called aqua aurea, was used to heal the heart both emotionally and physically. They call it *muguet* in France, where Lily-of-the-Valley Festival is celebrated on the first Sunday of May. Classic perfumes inspired by the fragrance include Christian Dior's Diorissimo, which was created in 1956 by the great perfumer, Edmond Roudnitska. It is a popular scent for soaps, although they rely on a synthetic version.

Lily-of-the-valley is happiest growing as an eight-inch-tall carpet shaded by woodland shrubs. My plants are tucked around daphne, which blooms earlier, so the two scents do not conflict. Plant the bulbs in rich, moist earth in late fall in the garden, or in a pot where they can live undisturbed. Since they are poisonous, rodents won't bother them. Protect potted plants from severe winters by submerging them in loose soil, then bring them inside for an early spring bloom. Lily-of-the-valley is pollinated by bees and flies.

Marjoram

Origanum majorana

Mint Family: Lamiaceae
Perennial
Zones 7–9

Marjoram smells herby, spicy, a little warm, and sweet. It hints ever-so-slightly of camphor or a touch of rosemary. Marjoram has the aroma of herb-flavored sweet bread fresh from the oven. The exact fragrance varies depending upon the plant's genetic makeup. Marjoram is sweeter, more perfumery, and a bit softer than its sharply scented kin, oregano.

There is often confusion in identifying marjoram and oregano species since there are quite a few across the spectrum. Italian oregano (*Origanum vulgare*) has the well-known aroma of pasta sauce. Pot marjoram (*O. onites*) is a little less aromatic and sweet, but has an interesting, compact growth and flat flowers. It grows only to zone 8. Dittany of Crete (*O. dictamnus*) bears woolly-white, round leaves; aromatic, rose-purple flowers; and cone-shaped fruits. It is beautiful in rock gardens, hanging over tall pots, or in hanging baskets and used in dried flower wreaths.

Sweet marjoram's traditional use is as a calming aroma that especially deals with sadness, grief, loneliness, and irritability. Old herbalists say that it heals a broken heart, but warn that it may numb emotions so much that it can lead to feeling apathetic.

Marjoram is very sedative. Danish University of Pharmaceutical Sciences research in 2004 noted relaxing GABA activity in several plants in the genus *Origanum*. Oregano (so quite possibly marjoram) appears to encourage neurotransmitter activity in the brain to enhance mental well-being, says Switzerland's Research and Development Human Nutrition and Health in Basel.

In Greece, aromatic sprigs and head wreaths of sweet marjoram were worn as a badge of honor. Brides still wear it in their hair indicating that the couple will honor each other and as a promise to find love and happiness. A species of marjoram was probably the "hyssop" used in the Bible to make scented, ceremonial oil. Massage oil for tight muscles, inflamed areas, and emotional balance can be made by infusing marjoram leaves in olive oil.

Marjoram's green-gray leaves contrast nicely with darker plants or when planted with gray sages. Placed near the edge of a bed, its gray, soft color stands out and it can be easily pinched for use in the kitchen. It will live on a sunny windowsill if trimmed back, which will supply you with fresh marjoram for your cooking. It has tight enough growth be very attractive hanging in a basket on a sunny porch. Honeybees and little skipper butterflies pollinate marjoram's flowers.

Marjoram likes a Mediterranean climate with dry, hot days and well-drained soil that is fairly rich in nitrogen. It is not as hardy to cold temperatures as its oregano cousin, so it is treated as an annual below zone 6. Germinating the seed is easy, although young plants are fragile and subject to damping off disease or being knocked over by an overly forceful spray of water. Harvest the top sprigs and hang them to dry them.

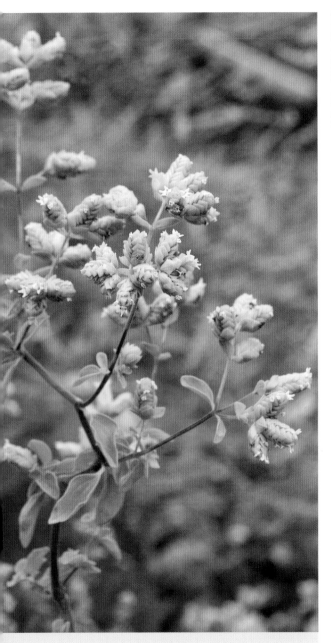

Marjoram (*Origanum majorana*)

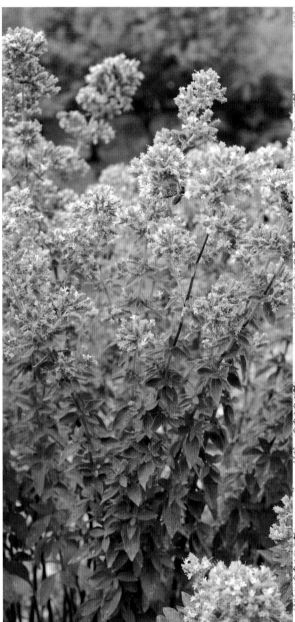

Italian oregano (*Origanum vulgare*)

Mexican marigold

Tagetes lemmonii

Aster Family: Asteraceae
Perennial
Zones 8–11

Many people find Mexican marigold's fragrance so strong that they avoid brushing against the shrub. It intensely combines aromas of pungent lemon, mint, and wormwood. Others find the pungent, bitter aroma oddly attractive in small doses, but the smell can be a bit smothering when working next to it in the garden. Marigold's common Italian names, *puzzola* and *puzzalina*, mean "smelly."

Lemon marigold (*Tagetes lucida*) or *pericón*, carries marigold's pungency, but it also has the distinct scent of tarragon, and almost its taste. It is used in cooking in its native Mexico and it is on my culinary rack. The Aztecs used it for ritual incense and Mexico's Huichol tribe favored it as a fragrant tobacco. It is easier to grow, although it is cultivated as an annual below zones 7 and 8. French marigold (*T. patula*) is the familiar garden border plant that flowers in combinations of yellows, oranges, and maroon colors. The flowers have a musty, sharp scent. The roots exude a scent that deters harmful nematodes in the soil.

In Mexico, marigolds symbolize death and everlasting life. The scent is considered protective and able to keep away negative influences both physically and emotionally. Various types of marigolds fill houses and church alters with the aroma during special celebrations, such as the Day of the Dead celebration in November. The Mayans make scented water from various species of marigold for healing ceremonies. The various types of marigold occasionally lend a special effect to high-end perfume. The smelly flowers attract mostly beetles to pollinate them.

The sprawling Mexican marigold shrub is easy to cultivate in a sunny, warm location. The biggest problem can be too much water, causing the roots to rot.

Mexican marigold (*Tagetes lemmonii*)

Mexican orange flower

Choisya ternata

Rue family: Rutaceae
Shrub
Zones 7–10

The white clusters of Mexican orange flower bear individual blossoms that look and smell like large orange flowers, giving this shrub its common name. Flowers open in late winter or early spring for a delicious two-month bloom period. Take the heady, exotic scent of orange flowers (with its subtle touch of fresh citrus) and mix it with a sweet, honey-like aroma, and you have Mexican orange. It is a scent that you can almost taste. In fact, I cannot help imagining orange marmalade and honey on toast while sitting in the shade of an orange tree in full bloom. When bruised, the dense foliage has the surprisingly musty, pungent aroma of the herb rue. Some descriptions are more polite, comparing the scent to basil or eucalyptus. However, most people find it *unpleasant*. Orange and rue may seem an odd botanical combination to find in one plant, but they are both are in the same family as Mexican orange.

Choisya ×*dewitteana* 'Aztec Pearl' is a more compact shrub. *Choisya ternata* 'Sundance' has golden leaves that make up for it bearing fewer flowers. Both cultivars have gained the Royal Horticultural Society's Award of Garden Merit. There is sometimes confusion between Mexican orange and mock orange (*Philadelphus microphyllus*). The shrubs look quite different, but their white flowers look and smell like orange tree flowers.

A 2013 edition of the journal *Phytotherapy Research* reported that the essential oil scent of Mexican orange showed signs of being an antidepressant, as well as decreasing anxiety and promoting sleep. How it affects the mind seems linked to the brain's GABA receptors.

The Mexican orange shrub makes a good seven-foot-high border plant. Since it is sensitive to wind and frost, it does best planted in a protected spot. The abundant, sweet nectar draws honeybees. Distinctive, glossy leaves make this fast-growing, deciduous bush especially attractive. A native of Mexico and the southwestern United States, it is drought tolerant, although it does best with an even amount of moisture in acidic soil, with excellent drainage. If you live in zone 5 or 6, but cannot live without it, some gardeners in colder regions manage to grow Mexican orange in a protected location, keeping it mulched through the winter. The shrub can also be grown in a large pot, although this does make it more prone to developing root rot.

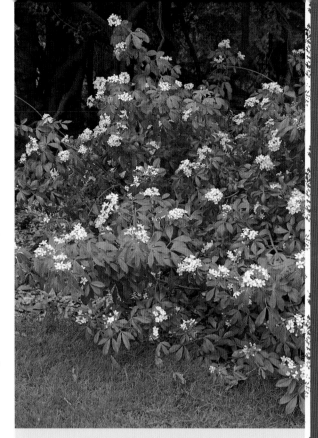

Mexican orange flower (*Choisya ternata*)

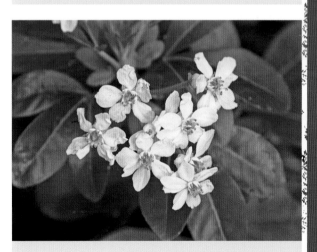

Mexican orange flower is another bloom that comes in clusters.

Mignonette

Reseda odorata

Reseda family: Resedaceae
Perennial cultivated as annual
Zones 3–11

This cottage flower is no longer well-known, but it was once a garden favorite. Its rich, powerful, musky scent makes it worthy of any fragrance garden. In French, mignonette means "little darling," although it smells anything but cute. The flowers are intensely sweet, like violets with a fruity odor and a green nuance. The aroma is that of fruit salad covered with violet flowers. Curiously, it shares some fragrance compounds with tobacco.

Mignonette has appeared in gardens since ancient times. There is only one garden species, but it has numerous, fragrant strains of hybrids. Gardeners like the hybrids since they are more robust and less straggly than the parent species, but they also tend to be less fragrant. It has always been grown more for fragrance than for its somewhat scruffy appearance and small, greenish flowers. During the eighteenth and nineteenth centuries, pots of mignonette were set on London balconies to cover street odors during hot, summer days. It was also thought to protect the inhabitants from disease. Napoleon first sent the seeds to Empress Josephine in France, during his Egyptian campaign.

In France, mignonette honey rivals that of the popular linden honey. The fragrance of the cut flowers is almost too strong to bring indoors. However, it used to be the room freshener of choice for the large homes of the French aristocracy. Mignonette is still grown for perfume in the Grasse region of France.

This flower makes a foot-tall border or terrace plant if combined with other, short plants that

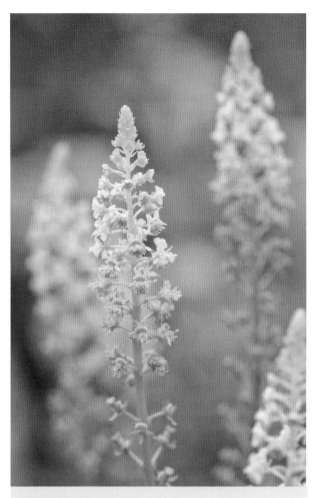

Mignonette (*Reseda odorata*)

are a little fuller. You can also follow the English tradition of planting it in a window box. It's pollinated by bees and butterflies.

For highly fragrant flowers, mignonette requires a rich, acidic, clean soil with plenty of water. Give it sun in the north, but partial sun in the south. It doesn't transplant easily and is tricky to grow in a dry, hot climate unless the soil remains damp.

Mint shrub

Prostanthera rotundifolia

Mint family: Lamiaceae
Perennial
Zones 8–11

Rub against this native of Australia, and you are met with a delicious fragrance that gives mint shrub its name. The aroma of the leaves has the bite of peppermint with an underlying sharp, eucalyptus-like scent. The plant is rich in essential oils, including the menthol compound that is found in peppermint and the cineole compound in eucalyptus.

Since mint shrub combines the aromas of both eucalyptus and peppermint, the effect on the mind is stimulating. The small, mint-flavored leaves are used in culinary dishes in place of thyme and for potpourris. Essential oil is produced from the leaves. A tea of the leaves is tasty. Australian aborigines use it to relieve headaches. It is also a mosquito repellent.

This seven-foot shrub is covered in late spring with bright purple-blue flowers. It has an attractive, airy feeling, but it can also be pruned into a hedge. The Royal Horticultural Society gave it their Award of Garden Merit. This species is listed as environmentally vulnerable by the Tasmanian government.

Mint shrub likes sandy, well-drained soil on the edge of a rainforest, but it handles clay soil and can be very drought resistant. It needs at least a few hours of direct sun a day but does best with some shade during the heat of the day. It is easy to grow from seed or cuttings.

Mint shrub (*Prostanthera rotundifolia*)

Mock orange

Philadelphus microphyllus

Hydrangea family: Hydrangeaceae
Shrub
Zones 5–9

The name "mock orange" refers to how the white or cream-colored flowers look and smell so much like those of the orange tree. They bear the fruity fragrance of quince and melon, sprinkled with a generous amount of orange blossom and maybe a touch of jasmine. It only takes a few bushes to fill a summer evening with an intense fragrance that moves through the garden like scented waves. The aroma is especially strong in the morning and evening. Not everyone likes mock orange; some find it overwhelming. In fact, it has been called both the most-loved and most-hated fragrance in the garden. Herbalist John Gerard wrote in his *Herball* that he found it "too sweet, troubling, and molesting the head in a strange manner." But then, he was not fond of the scent of lilacs, either.

The use of mock orange in aromatherapy is not common, but it should be. It can affect the mind much like orange blossoms, as a mental relaxant and antidepressant.

Numerous *Philadelphus* species are native to North America, southern Europe, and southwestern Asia. The scent varies greatly among species and not all are fragrant, making this a good plant to purchase while it's in bloom. *Philadelphus* ×*lemoinei* 'Belle Etoile' has a lovely, sweet, sensational aroma that makes it a favorite of gardeners. The famous hybridizer Pierre Lemoine developed it in the early twentieth century from a cross with the European *P. coronarius*. It is noted for its prolonged flowering period and improved fragrance. *Philadelphus* ×*lemoinei* 'Erectus' and *P. argyrocalyx* lean more toward a delicious pineapple aroma with orange blossom lingering in the background. In the 1930s, the

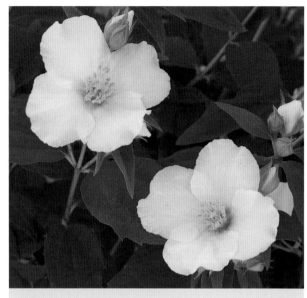

Mock orange (*Philadelphus microphyllus*)

Arnold Arboretum at Harvard University described the number of species and varieties that had crept into the nursery trade as bewildering. *Philadelphus coronarius, P. tomentosus,* and *P. zeyheri* were the species they considered most fragrant.

Mock orange flowers are enjoyed as flavorful and aromatic tea. A synthetic reproduction of the fragrance goes into a number of perfumes and colognes. The flowering branches can be cut and the lower leaves stripped off to bring the delightful fragrance in the house.

The shrub provides a good background border in the fragrance garden, although it is fairly nondescript until it bursts into bloom. A native of California and some parts of Mexico, it is tolerant of drought. It prefers well-drained sandy or clay soil in full sun. It will grow in light shade, although it may not bloom as much. It can get leggy, but you can remove old, twiggy growth after flowering, leaving the most robust canes. Cutting it down to ground level causes it to regrow much fuller.

Myrtle
Myrtus communis

Mint family: Myrtaceae
Perennial
Zones 8–10

Myrtle's shiny, stiff leaves must be well crushed to release the aroma, but it is well worth the effort. They smell of spice and balsam, with a strong herb or green note, and barely detectable camphorous undertones.

Dwarf myrtle (*Myrtus communis* 'Compacta') and *M. communis* 'Microphylla' reach only a few feet tall. Variegated dwarf myrtle (*M. communis* 'Variegata') has white-edged leaves, but tends to be slightly less hardy. 'Boetica' is an extremely fragrant, four-foot-high dwarf plant with gnarled branches, a popular selection in the desert's zone 4.

Myrtle, or *myrtos*, means "plant of love" in Greek and is associated with Aphrodite, the goddess of eternal love and beauty. Myrtle head wreaths given to poets suggested that their fame would never die. Myrtle was the main scent in complexion water called "angel's water" that doubled as a sixteenth-century cologne. It is still used in several modern perfumes. Myrtle was a favored plant in the scented gardens of Baghdad, Granada, and Damascus for both its small, attractive white flowers and its fragrance.

Myrtle's foliage is dense enough to be shaped into a hedge or topiary. When selecting a garden spot, keep in mind that it is a small tree, reaching six to twelve feet in height. The flowers are pollinated by honeybees and wind, then followed by blue-black berries. Almost any soil will do for growing myrtle, as long as it is very well drained. It grows in full or partial sun.

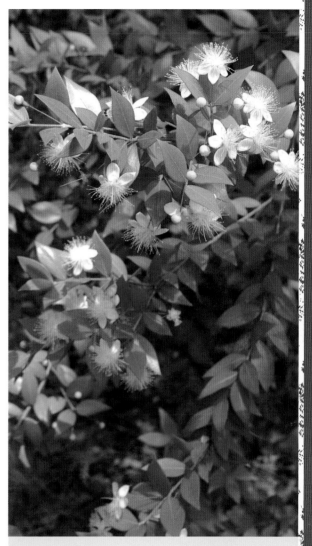

Myrtle (*Myrtus communis*)

Oleander

Nerium oleander

Dogbane family: Apocynaceae
Shrub
Zones 8–11

This evergreen is attractive all year, blooming from late spring to fall. The fragrant flowers have a lovely, strong scent of vanilla and baby powder.

In *Enquiry into Plants* (c. 300 BC), the early Greek botanist Theophrastus said that the root's fragrance works like wine to make "the temper gentler and more cheerful." Oleander appears on the Roman wall murals in Pompeii.

It needs sun, but tolerates poorly drained, salty soil and drought, so it is often used in public landscaping in dry climates. Polka-dot wasp moth caterpillars feed on the pulp surrounding the leaf veins. When crow butterfly larvae feed on the toxic leaves, they become unpalatable to birds.

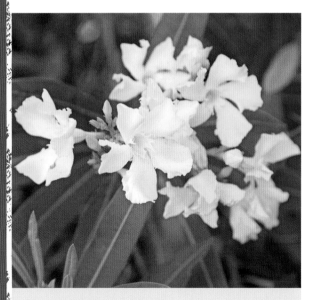

Oleander (*Nerium oleander*)

Oriental lily

Lilium orientalis

Lily family: Liliaceae
Perennial
Zones 4–10

The scent of a lily transports me to a moss-covered grotto, filled with delicious-smelling flowers. Lily has sweet, floral high notes scented with honey, but it is the additional, hauntingly musky aromas that make the fragrance truly distinctive. Oriental lilies, with outward-facing, white to pink petals, are summer bloomers. Just one flower can overpower an entire room with intoxicating, spicy perfume. *Lilium orientalis* 'Stargazer' is a favorite with its deep, spicy aroma and stunning flowers. You may find yourself with telltale pollen on your nose from poking it deep into the flower for the full aroma. Not everyone feels the same about them, though. Dutch breeders are actually developing *less* aromatic oriental lilies for those whose noses are offended by the intensity.

Madonna lily (*Lilium candidum*) has a touch of honeysuckle to its aroma. One of the oldest species, it earned a well-deserved Royal Horticultural Society's Award of Garden Merit. White lilies symbolized innocence and virtue in ancient Egyptian, Greek, Roman, and Minoan Art. *Lilium* 'African Queen' has almost a citrus tang. Golden ray (*L. auratum*) is the "queen of lilies" in Japan and produces as many as thirty magnificent flowers on each stem. *Lilium speciosum* may be the most intensely perfumed of all, and a wedding favorite. Trumpet-type lilies generally have highly fragrant, yellow and orange flowers. *Lilium* 'African Queen' is an example. It emits a rich, tangerine-apricot fragrance. *Lilium leucanthum* var. *centifolium* is richly aromatic. Asiatic lilies have little or no scent. A breeding program trying

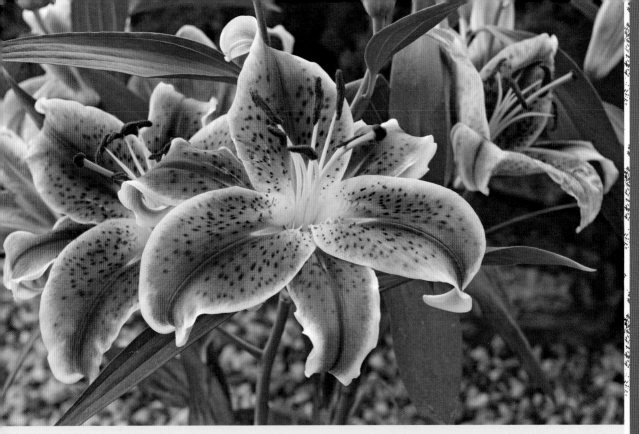

Oriental lily (*Lilium orientalis*)

to endow them with some fragrance created *L. lankongense.*

Lilies represent passion, both religious and sensual. In Roman mythology, Venus (the goddess of love), became jealous of lily's purity and beauty. Highly scented lily petals were strewn on church floors and along religious processions to inspire pure devotion. Even Flaubert's Madame Bovary is overcome by a "mystical lassitude" from the scent of flowers—surely lilies—during a religious rite. Lily is one of the four most popular florist flowers. Its use in bridal bouquets and bridal veils goes back to the ancient Greeks and Romans. Expensive perfumes contain small amounts of the pricey essential oil.

Pollinating hummingbirds, moths, and butterflies, including the tiger swallowtail butterfly, hover over lily's long flowers, planning their entry. The dramatic presence of either a single lily or masses of them brings out the visual best in a garden. Yellow and pink yarrows complement lily's colors and do not interfere with its aroma. Tall lilies look impressive in front of shrubs like viburnum. A classic combination is lily backed by climbing honeysuckle or rose to create a living potpourri of fragrance. Try 'Stargazer' with gray artemisias. Lilies in pots can conveniently be placed where you enjoy the fragrance or to fill a landscaping hole, and then moved once the plants die back.

Orris root

Iris germanica var. *florentina*

Iris family: Iridaceae
Perennial
Zones 3–9

In the garden, orris root looks like any ordinary iris. But, dig it up and the rhizome smells deliciously like violets. Unlike most dried plants, the aroma improves and becomes more intense as it ages. It is especially good after three years; I harvested some two decades ago that still smells like a bouquet of violets. The essential oil is expensive, but less than true violet flower oil. The bloom has a different, sweet, floral scent that is fairly light unless you grow a bank of them.

Sweet Dalmatian iris (*I. pallida*), with purplish-white flowers, is also distilled into violet-scented essential oil for perfume. The white cemetery iris (*I. albicans*) is often confused with orris root because it also has fragrant white flowers and rhizomes.

Since the aroma is so much of violets, orris root works on the mind in a similar way to encourage relaxation and temper anxiety and anger. The dried rhizome is carved into rosary beads that release their fragrance when handled. Teething sticks are still occasionally made from it for babies. People once chewed slivers of orris root to sweeten their breath with violets. It flavors gins like Bombay Sapphire and Magellan, and a Moroccan herb blend called *ras el hanout*.

The main use for the dried root is a fixative to retain potpourri's scent. It is usually finely cut since using powdered root makes potpourri look dusty. The powdered root can also be used as a dry shampoo that absorbs excess oil and dirt while scenting the hair with violets. In Elizabethan times, orris root powder was mixed with anise to perfume clothing. The violet scent of orris root became a popular scent for perfume and body care products, often replacing violet itself. Y by Yves Saint Laurent and Vol de Nuit by Guerlain are perfumes that are based on orris root. Its use declined after a synthetic violet-scented compound called irone was isolated. The new compound smells closer to violets than orris root. After complaints about orris root causing skin sensitivities surfaced in the 1990s, its use as a potpourri and body care ingredient also declined.

Orris root's white flowers, with yellow beards at the base of the petals, look stunning with other late spring flowers and deeper-colored iris. They are pollinated by bees and butterflies. Plant orris root in informal groupings to create a cluster. Iris has been in cultivation since at least 1400 BC. Originating from Yemen and Saudi Arabia, it appears in a wall painting of the Botanical Room of Tuthmosis III in the Temple of Amun at Karnak in ancient Thebes dated around 1426 BC.

Orris root is easy to grow and transplant and not fussy about the type of soil. Bury the rhizomes so that they are just below the soils' surface. If they are too deep, they produce more leaves and fewer flowers. Division of the rhizome is the easiest way to propagate them. It is best to divide them every three to four years anyway, since they are heavy feeders that produce fewer and fewer blooms in the center. Each individual flowering section only lives three to five years. The rhizomes are ready to harvest in three years. The tradition is to let them age for a couple years after they are harvested, to scent products such as potpourri because aging them develops their violet-like aroma.

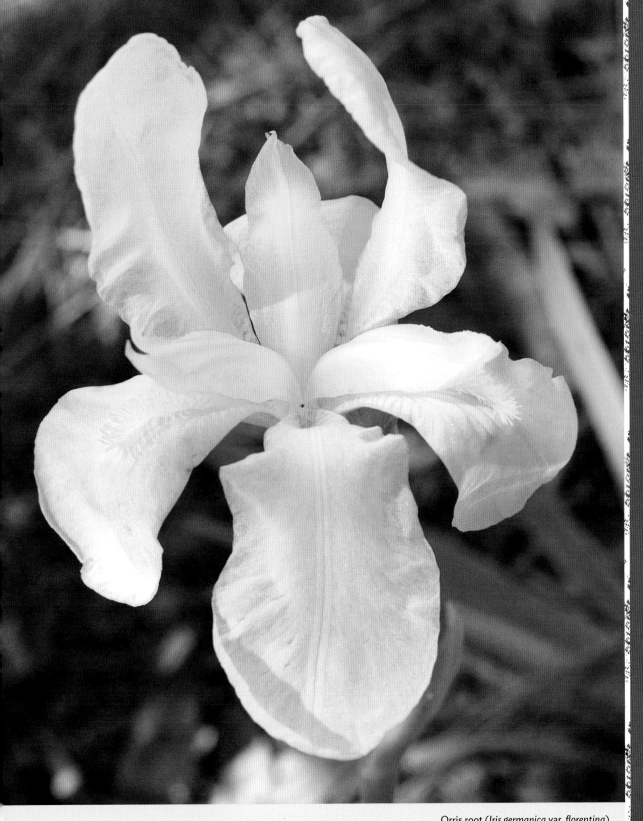

Orris root (*Iris germanica* var. *florentina*)

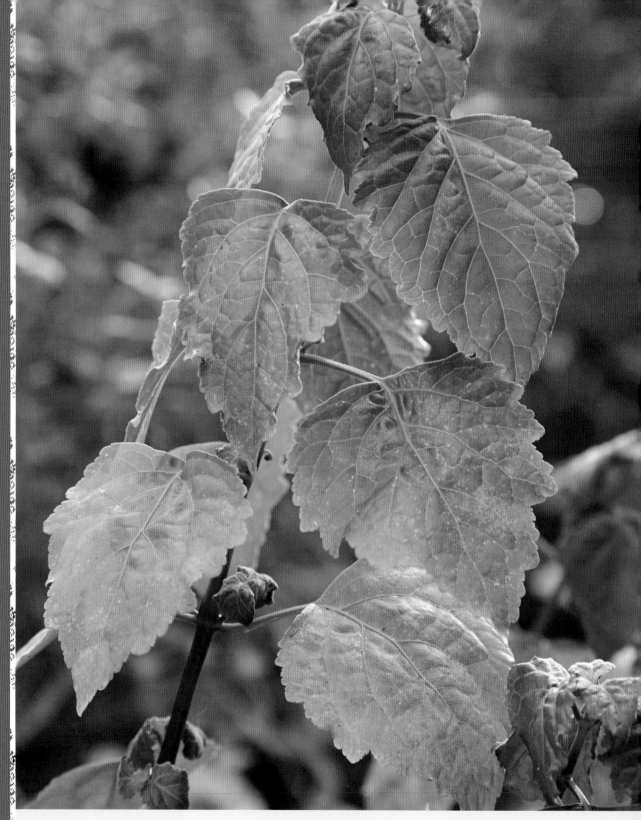

Patchouli (*Pogostemon cablin*)

Patchouli
Pogostemon cablin

Mint family: Lamiaceae
Tender perennial
Zones 10, 11

The heady, exotic smell of patchouli leaves is rich and musty. Its perfume seems to be created from the unusual combination of sweet, damp earth, rotted wood, exotic tree resin, and a hint of rosemary. Many find it complex and wonderful, but not everyone appreciates such an earthy blend. Plenty of people compare it to a musty closet. Do not expect patchouli to smell like it came out of the bottle. It develops balsamic and myrrh-like overtones when dried, fermented, and distilled into essential oil. The resulting oil becomes so rich and thick as it ages that it takes on a molasses consistency and color and a sweet, deep, resinous vanilla fragrance. My forty-year-old patchouli oil smells nothing short of heavenly.

Java patchouli (*Pogostemon heyneanus*) has a similar, but much lighter scent that is not as full or deep. It is grown in its native India more for medicine than fragrance, but sometimes finds itself made into an inferior essential oil. It shares thirteen aromatic compounds with true patchouli, but they are in different concentrations. False patchouli (*P. benghalensis*) has almost no scent and slightly hairy leaves. Both species are sold as patchouli in the United States.

Patchouli helps counter depression, insomnia, and nervousness. Aromatherapists recommend it to improve focus and to feel grounded. The Japanese fragrance company Shiseido found that it encourages relaxation, slowing down sympathetic nervous system activity as much as forty percent. In addition, patchouli has a long-standing reputation as an aphrodisiac. However, it only increases ardor if the individual likes its aroma!

Those who dislike patchouli find it difficult to believe patchouli is in Asian-style perfumes such as Tabu and Shocking. It also lends its fragrance to hair conditioners, soaps, and high-end tobacco. In India, the dried leaves are laid among clothing, silks, mattresses, woolen shawls, and rugs to deter insects. Europeans learned to recognize imitation Asian scarves made in Scotland and England because they lacked patchouli's characteristic aroma. My wool scarves and sweaters smell amazing after being stored with patchouli sachets instead of mothballs. Patchouli also makes potpourri last longer. Along with camphor, it scents India ink, probably originally as a preservative. It smells good and who knows? It may inspire the resulting calligraphy.

Patchouli lovers are often surprised to learn that they can grow the plant. The green-purple leaves contrast nicely next to lighter shades of green. My plants spend winters in a sunny window, then go outside into filtered sun for the summer. Patchouli prefers temperatures of at least 60 degrees F with some humidity. My only complaint is that it is more subject to insect damage than my other fragrant plants. Harvest the uppermost leaves off the stems and dry them on a screen or in a colander to enhance their fragrance.

Peppermint

Mentha ×piperita

Mint family: Lamiaceae
Perennial
Zones 3–9

Crush a peppermint leaf and the powerful, fresh scent makes your nose tingle. It is a delightful mix of herb and spice aromas with a dash of black pepper, highlighted by menthol's sharp aroma. This is the familiar scent of peppermint breath fresheners, mouthwash, toothpaste, and candies. Peppermint causes dual feelings of hot and cold. Roll a leaf and stick it in your mouth. When you inhale, it creates a cooling sensation, while making your tongue warm. Chewing a leaf is the best way to experience peppermint as the aroma goes to the back of the throat and up into the nose.

Peppermint comes in an array of different scents. *Mentha ×piperita* f. *citrata* 'Chocolate' is pure candy with its combination of peppermint and chocolate. Grapefruit mint (*M. ×piperita* f. *citrata* 'Grapefruit') is a definite citrus. *Mentha aquatica* 'Lime' and the large-leafed 'Citrata' lend strong citrus-mint scents and flavors to fruit and desserts—there is even a 'Banana' cultivar. Ginger mint (*M. gentilis* 'Variegata') has a spicy fruit scent and flavor, plus leaves flecked with gold. Spearmint (*M. spicata*) contains less menthol, so does not provide peppermint's zing. It is lighter and more playful. The woolly, two-toned leaves of apple mint (*M. suaveolens*) smell fruity and are favored in the kitchen. The sweet, minty smell of pennyroyal (*M. pulegium*) is more heavy and pungent. Corsican mint (*M. requienii*) smells like crème de menthe. It makes a fragrant ground cover for a shady area. For an appreciation of the variety in the genus, see *Mints*, by Barbara Perry Lawton.

Roman scholar Pliny advised wearing mint crowns to improve concentration and "exhilarate" the mind. The leaves were strewn about Roman banquet halls and rubbed on tables to inspire good appetite and conversation. Pharmacies used to sell menthol cones that evaporated into the air to make headaches disappear. Studies in Germany and elsewhere show that a tiny drop of peppermint essential oil placed on each temple works just as well. You can also crush leaves from your garden and inhale. Just the aroma of peppermint increases appetite and helps prevent nausea. Peppermint sharpens attention, focus, and memory without producing caffeine jitters, because it works through the mind instead of the adrenal glands. Numerous studies at Northumbia University in the UK and elsewhere show that inhaling peppermint for thirty seconds every five minutes improves memory and mood, and makes it easier to identify complicated computer patterns more accurately. A University of Vienna study found peppermint's scent to be both stimulating and pleasant. Volunteers had better accuracy, vigilance, and visual perception, and performed mental tasks faster. Due to the strong smell of menthol, the scent can help one come out of shock.

Mentha ×piperita is one of the few plants cultivated for essential oil in the United States, especially in Oregon and Michigan. Most of the essential oil goes to flavor gum and mouth fresheners; a small amount gives colognes an aromatic lift.

Peppermint looks good growing with its fellow mints, although they do all die down in the winter to leave an empty-looking patch. It is one of the easiest plants to cultivate, provided it has rich, moist soil. It does well in the rich soil typically used for growing vegetables. If grown in pots, feed it compost a couple times a year. It produces more fragrance when grown in soil that contains sufficient amounts of boron and zinc. The plant does not produce viable seed, but makes up for that by sending out aggressive runners, so you may want to contain it. Cuttings and root divisions make for easy propagation.

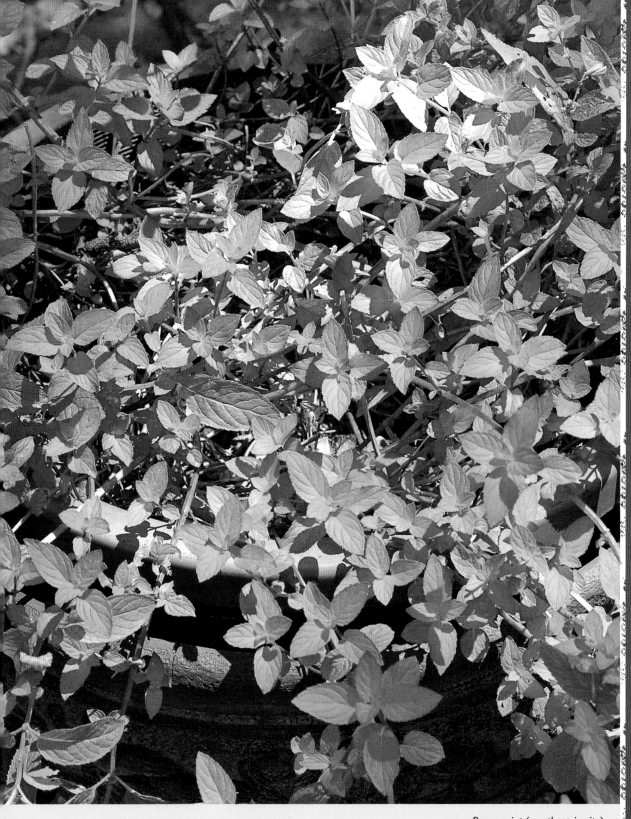

Peppermint (*mentha ×piperita*)

Phlox

Phlox paniculata

Phlox family: Polemoniaceae
Annual
Zones 4–9

The sweet, honey-vanilla scent of summer phlox smells old-fashioned, perhaps because it is a bit musty. Imagine eating a fruit salad while sitting in a Victorian parlor next to rose and violet potpourri.

Phlox can be moderately or highly fragrant, depending upon the variety. *Phlox paniculata* 'Blue Paradise', 'Bright Eyes', 'Junior Dream', 'Nicky', 'Orange Perfection', and 'Tiara Flame' are a few cultivars favored by gardeners as aromatic. Sweet William (*P. divaricata*) is commonly sold in nurseries for its colorful blue, pink, and white flowers, but is not very fragrant.

In the Victorian language of flowers, summer phlox symbolizes an offering of love and souls united. As a result, highly scented phlox varieties are chosen as wedding flowers. Simply planting phlox in your garden is said to encourage family unity and harmony. That alone might be reason enough to edge a patio with them or grow them in planters next to the house. Since the aroma is said to assure sweet dreams, pots of phlox could be near a chaise lounge or a garden swing. If only they kept their scent better when dried, phlox could stuff dream pillows.

The showy flower clusters have decorated many country-style gardens. Deadhead spent blossoms regularly to keep plants blooming. Besides their fragrance, phlox flowers bring an assortment of pollinators to your garden. Phlox's deep, narrow throat seems designed for a butterfly's long, curled proboscis. Painted ladies, swallowtails, and sulfurs are a few of the butterflies that feast on the nectar, as do moths and

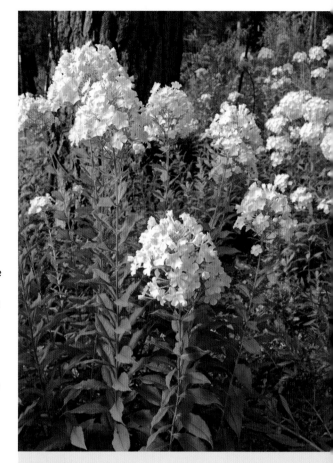

Phlox (*Phlox paniculata*)

long-tongued bees that are able to reach into the flowers. Try planting phlox with low-growing moss phlox (*Phlox subulata*).

Most nurseries have a limited selection, so you may need to order fragrant phlox online. It is best to purchase plants since they do not always come true from the slow-to-germinate seeds. The native habitat is marshes so give them plenty of water, avoiding overhead watering, which encourages powdery mildew. These hardy plants handle heat if mulched.

Pineapple sage

Salvia elegans

Mint family: Lamiaceae
Perennial
Zones 8–10

The leaves of this sage are wonderfully sweet and fruity. They smell strongly of pineapple, although many people cannot guess the scent until they are told. Then pineapple is all they can smell. There is also an underlying herby, green scent along with the common scent of sage, but with less of the musty bitterness of culinary sage. The fragrance is easy to describe because it smells like a pineapple lightly flavored with culinary sage.

Salvia elegans 'Tangerine', also known as tangerine sage, has the distinctive fragrance of melons mixed with oranges. This shorter cultivar makes a nice, mid-height ground cover. Peach sage (*S. dorisiana*) looks similar, but has a unique peach aroma. This plant is very frost sensitive. Peruvian sage (*S. discolor*) sports nearly black flowers against silver foliage with a very pungent scent. Grape-scented sage (*S. melissodora*) has small, gray-green leaves on a robust plant with spectacular, periwinkle blue flowers that smell, and taste, like little grapes!

Pineapple sage makes good tea and food flavoring if you do not mind an underlying bitterness of sage. It does not taste like pineapple! Sweeten it by mixing it with lemon balm and peppermint.

This five-foot-tall plant provides the fall garden with a blast of color. The eye-catching, tubular, bright red flowers are favorites of hummingbirds. Long-tongued bees and bumblebees reach into the extended flowers to pollinate them. Plant it with other late bloomers. Keeping spent stalks pinched back extends the bloom.

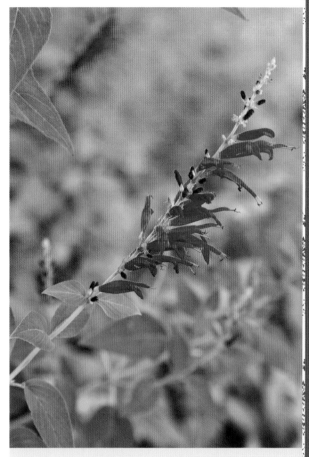

Pineapple sage (*Salvia elegans*)

Unlike many sages, it will tolerate partial shade. This tropical sage has thin leaves, but it is still somewhat drought tolerant. It is deciduous in cold climates, so well-established plants will winter over if brought indoors. Even in zone 8, it often needs to be well mulched, although it may not have time to develop flowers before the frost. In my zone 9, it never gets as bushy as it does in Southern California gardens.

Poet's daffodil

Narcissus poeticus

Amaryllis family: Amaryllidaceae
Perennial bulb
Zones 3–9

Poet's daffodil smells euphoric to the point of being hypnotic. One whiff and you will understand. The aroma that hovers over the patch is elegant and richly floral with smooth, almost animal-like undertones that make it more intense than sweet. Just a few cut flowers scent an entire room. True to its name, its fragrance has been praised in poetry and literature. Homer wrote, in *Hymn to Demeter,* that "its roots grew forth a hundred blossoms, fragrant with the sweetest smell. The broad sky above and the whole earth, and swell of the salt sea laughed."

The genus *Narcissus* contains so many species, they have been divided into several groups. Pheasant's eye (*N. poeticus* 'Recurvus'), in the fragrant poeticus group, is perhaps the most strongly scented variety. The name comes from its yellow center, defined by an orange ring. Paperwhite (*N. papyraceus*), with the small, clustered white flowers of the tazetta group, is one of the very fragrant narcissus cultivars grown in France for perfume. Jonquil (*N. jonquilla*) also has small, fragrant flowers and is in the jonquil group. The most fragrant narcissus tend to have the smallest flowers and to be the oldest varieties.

Most of the many cultivars have little fragrance.

The word narcissus is derived from the Greek *narke*, meaning stupor and related to "narcotic." The heady scent is, indeed, very relaxing. It is also considered an aphrodisiac. In Greek mythology, Aphrodite, goddess of love, stood in a sea of narcissus so the aroma would seduce the god Paris. However, ancient Egyptians hung wreaths of the flowers at funerals. The association with death may be because the aroma lasts only a few days after the flowers are cut.

In my town, a blast of daffodil scent and golden color along the highway announces that spring has arrived. Plant the bulbs in fall in good soil and dappled light. They are poisonous, so rodents do not bother them. After they flower, keep the leaves on until they brown so they nurture the bulb in anticipation of next year's bloom. Unlike tulips, daffodils keep increasing and blooming year after year with little care except an annual fall feeding. Divide them every few years, replanting bulbs right away since they don't store well. If you have potted narcissus, bring some containers indoors in late winter to fool them into an early bloom.

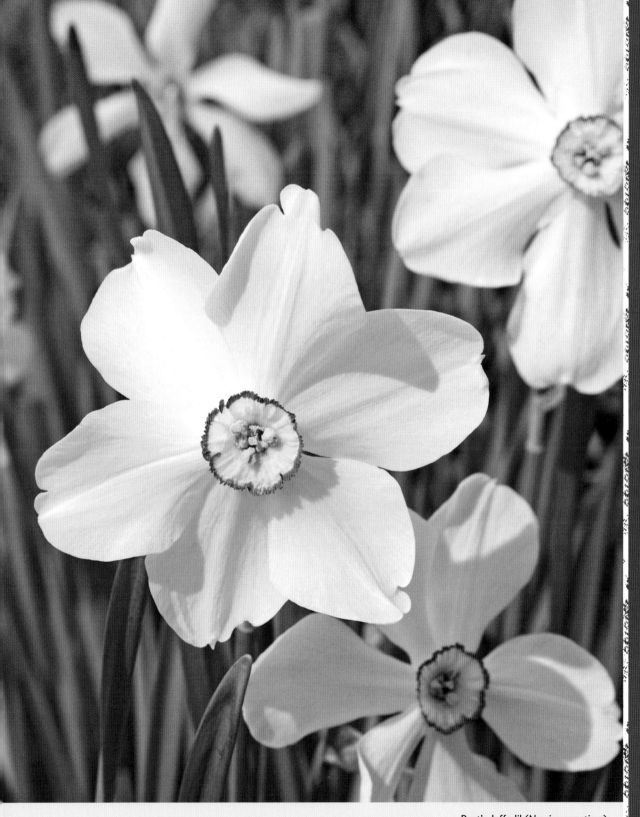

Poet's daffodil (*Narcissus poeticus*)

Primrose

Primula vulgaris

Primrose family: Primulaceae
Perennial
Zones 5–10

Flowers of primrose (also called English primrose) bring their sweet, lemon candy scent to early spring. They can lean toward fruity apple or apricot, and definitely spice, depending on the particular plant. Smelling almost good enough to eat, they could be a dish of lemon yogurt on fruit, covered with honey and sprinkled lightly with cinnamon. Their fragrance has been compared to daphne, although their fragrance is not as intense. Twentieth-century Scottish botanist and garden writer Peter Coats loved them. He found the fragrance more evocative than roses, with "the power given to few other flowers to transport one back over the years to childhood." Turn to yellow-flowering English primrose over blue or red for the most fragrance.

Tibetan cowslip (*Primula florindae*) is probably the most fragrant of the few hundred primrose species. The flower heads nod in the breeze to fill the air with their sweet, fruity scent. This late bloomer is noticeable for its attractive, heart-shaped leaves. Himalayan cowslip (*P. sikkimensis*) produces an especially sweet perfume. Orchid primrose (*P. vialli*) has very fragrant, violet-blue flowers. A perennial, it is usually treated as an annual since it does not winter over very well. Common cowslip (*P. veris*) is a familiar country garden flower discussed in old herb books. Although the flowers come in an array of attractive colors, the hybrids sold today are only lightly scented.

The aroma of primrose is used to instill happiness. It calms and steadies the nerves and relieves sadness. Fifteenth- and sixteenth-century English herbalists, such as John Gerard, prescribed it to treat nervous disorders. It was

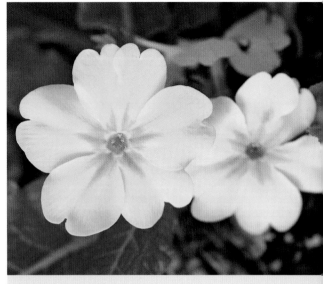

Primrose (*Primula vulgaris*)

used to help stop procrastination and to increase productivity, as well as courage. The fragrance could supposedly inspire one to express love for another, or to at least send a primrose bouquet. Primrose flowers do make a sweet, short-stemmed arrangement. European spring celebrations were once abundant with primrose wreaths and bouquets, with festival attendees wearing the floral crowns.

The low-growing primrose is most fragrant and colorful as a mass planting, or highlighted in a rock garden. It nicely edges pathways or any border with other colorful flowers, and can call attention to a shady part of the garden or patio when planted in pots. Primrose attracts butterflies, moths, long-tongued bees, and other pollinating insects that are able to reach into its tubular flowers.

I like having a planter filled with primroses on the deck off my house, where I can easily enjoy the fragrance, and also keep the soil moist. Mix them with other shade-loving plants such as violets and pansies, or just let the different primrose flower shades work together. They prefer a cold winter and are hardy and easy to grow in cool, moist, alkaline soil with good drainage.

Rockrose

Cistus ladanifer

Rockrose family: Cistaceae
Perennial
Zones 7, 8

The sticky leaves of rockrose are so strongly scented that the perfume-like fragrance is left on your hands after touching them. The balsamic scent is musky and heavily resinous with a sharp, wood-like scent of cedarwood, along with something that is almost spicy. It has also been described as smelling leathery. A hot day lifts the scent into the garden.

White rockrose (*Cistus hybridus*), with white flowers that have a yellow center, is one of the most widely grown of a number of species. It has a lighter fragrance.

The fragrance of rockrose is emotionally elevating and promotes mental focus, yet it relaxes the mind and nervous system enough to improve sleep. These contrasting characteristics make it suitable to enhance both study and meditation. Aromatherapists find that it also helps with overcoming grief or shock. Shepherds used to drive their goat herds through rockrose shrubs to collect the sticky resin on their wool, and then wash it out. You may prefer the more modern approach of boiling the leaves and twigs to cause the resin to float on water.

An essential oil called cistus (after the plant's genus) is distilled from rockrose. When aged, it is known as labdanum, which is richer and sweeter, with the deep headiness of high-end perfume. The fragrance is a woodsy version of church incense mixed with good perfume. It takes me to an undefined place that temporarily stops time. It smells much like an expensive fragrance ingredient called ambergris, which it replaces in perfumes such as the popular Amouage and Jazz. Labdanum is considered an aphrodisiac and also

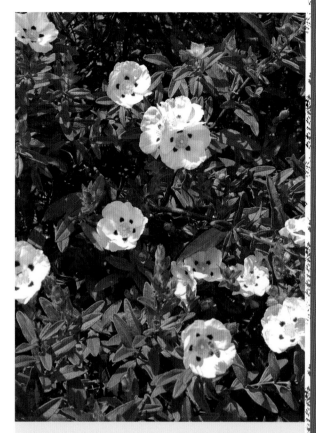

Rockrose (*Cistus ladanifer*)

scents solid "amber" perfumes from India and the Middle East.

A popular landscaping plant, rockrose blooms all summer and the leaves remain fragrant throughout the year, although they are strongest in the summer. This shrub sprawls over a large area unless it is kept trimmed for a fuller, tighter look. Plant it with other shrubs or tall-growing sunflowers, since it grows over smaller plants. It is often used to cover dry banks and prevent erosion. Bees, bumblebees, and beetles are its pollinators. Rockrose likes a well-drained soil in full sun. Very drought resistant, it tolerates poor, acidic soil, and extreme heat or wind, but is sensitive to a heavy freeze.

Rose geranium

Pelargonium graveolens

Geranium family: Geraniaceae
Tender perennial
Zones 10, 11

As the name implies, rose geranium smells very rosy, although it has more herbal and woody tones and lacks the pure, sweet, rich high notes of rose. It is difficult to describe, because your nose touches on different aspects of the fragrance with each whiff, leaving your sense of smell unsure where to go next. Imagine sitting at a cedarwood table that's been freshly polished with lemon oil; a vase on the table is filled with roses and sprigs of rosemary. That should give you some idea of the fragrance that greets you when you pinch a leaf. The species name, *graveolens*, means "strong-smelling" in Latin.

Scented geraniums should really be referred to as scented pelargoniums, to differentiate them from true geraniums in the same family, says pelargonium specialist Robin Parer of Geraniaceae nursery. Pelargoniums, originally from South Africa, captured the imagination of the British nursery world. The resulting hybridization since the seventeenth century increased the number of varieties to over six hundred. The result is a cornucopia of aromas that can be categorized according to their fragrance. *Pelargoniums*, by Diana Miller, can guide you through them. Skeleton rose (*P. radens*) offers attractive foliage along with remarkable rose scent. 'Pretty Polly' and 'Little Gem' smell so much like rose mixed with almonds, they remind me of marzipan dessert. 'Torrento' has a more lemony scent spiked with ginger.

One system of classification divides plants into groups according to their scent. Peppermint geranium (*Pelargonium tomentosum*) in the mint group is one of my favorites, with its large, fuzzy leaves. Apple geranium (*P. odoratissimum*) in the fruit group is, indeed, apple-scented. Cinnamon geranium (*P.* 'Asperum') is a rosy, spice-scented hybrid. Nutmeg geranium (*P.* 'Concolor Lace') is an example of the spice group. Its lacy leaves are scented like filberts. *Pelargonium* 'Lady Plymouth', with attractive, white-margined green leaves and a distinct eucalyptus scent, is in the pungent group. Oak-leaved geranium (*P. quercifolium*) has palm frond–like leaves covered with long hairs. These hairs are dotted with oil glands that yield a balsamy, incense-like fragrance.

Rose geranium aroma relieves anxiety, depression, and stress. While the fragrance is generally considered sedative and helps insomniacs, it can also energize someone who feels fatigued. Simply sniffing a leaf regulates blood pressure by a few points down or up, indicating a balancing action. It is used to help someone who has mood swings or is easily angered. In pelargonium's native South Africa, young Zulu men wear face cream made with night-scented flowers from *Pelargonium luridum*, reportedly to attract women.

Rose geranium's sweet scent and anti-stress properties make it perfect for massage oil. It is so complex, it smells like a professional blend all by itself. Geranium makes a slightly less effective mosquito repellent than citronella, but smells far more pleasant. Rose geranium, also sold as "geranium," is the only one of the selection that is typically distilled into essential oil for commercial sale. It goes into body care products, soap, and potpourri. A compound called geraniol is isolated from rose geranium by the pharmaceutical industry to help manufacture synthetic rose oil.

Rose geranium's sprawling leaves stand out next to almost any plant in the garden. Grow it in the ground around other drought-resistant plants such as sage and lavender, or in a pot. When grown with other scented geraniums, it looks particularly nice against the assortment of

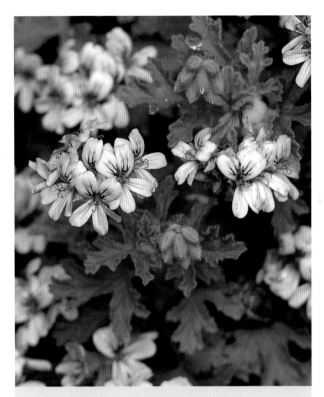

Rose geranium (*Pelargonium graveolens*)

interesting leaf shapes and colors. It is beautiful cascading out of a hanging basket. Fasten pots directly to the side of a sunny garden shed, or use plant stands to create a living wall. The flowers are pollinated by butterflies and beetles.

Plant scented geraniums in full sun and allow them to dry out between waterings. The aroma, amount of essential oil, and plant mass are increased by the use of white or black plastic mulch, as well by adding manure and potassium to the soil, according to Brazil's Universidade Federal de Sergipe. Adding magnesium, such as Epsom salts dissolved in water, also improves their growth. I had beautiful, lush mounds of scented geraniums in my Southern California coastal garden because they do best when day-time temperatures are around 75 degrees F and 50 to 60 degrees F at night. Most upright scented geraniums send out long branches that eventually make them look leggy. If you prefer a bushier look, prune the stem back once it has produced five nodes (leaf junctions).

To maintain a collection, Robin Parer of Geraniaceae says it is best to take cuttings before winter. Fortunately, cuttings root easily and the pruned-back plants will grow out from lower stems. If you live where you need to bring the plants indoors over the winter, do so before it gets too cold, then give them plenty of light and good air circulation. You can grow them in a very bright window that has a minimum of four hours of sun a day. An alternative is to suspend grow lights a foot above the plants to give them a full day's light.

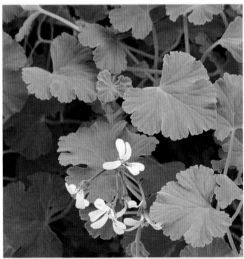

Nutmeg geranium (*Pelargonium* 'Concolor Lace')

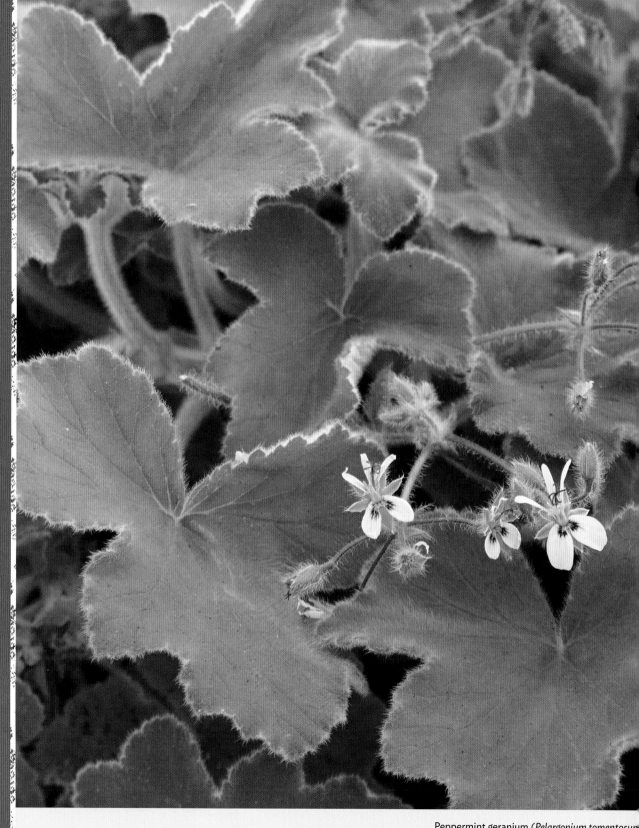

Peppermint geranium (*Pelargonium tomentosun*

Rosemary

Rosmarinus officinalis

Mint family: Lamiaceae
Perennial
Zones 5–9

Rosemary leaves have a powerful, herby, sharp, and slightly woody fragrance that includes a hint of freshly cut cedarwood and a good bit of camphor. This is the fragrance of distant memories, like opening a cedar chest in which woolens, keepsakes, and lavender sachets are stored. There are only slight aromatic variations among upright, prostrate, and dwarf forms and white or blue flowers. However, rosemary chemotypes are uniquely different. The camphor type is sharp enough to cause most people to pull back when they smell it. The verbenone type is my favorite because its lemon verbena–like scent overrides the camphor. The cineol type has a pungent and bitter lemon scent.

Rosemary's aroma improves mental perception and memory and is said to instill confidence. This extends to remembering good dreams and dispelling nightmares. Wearing sprigs in the hair and inhaling smoke from the burning leaves was once recommended to prevent brain "weakness." The old French name for rosemary, *incensier*, refers to its use as church incense to replace expensive frankincense. Rosemary is also associated with remembering vows. It is interesting that Anne of Cleves wore a golden circlet of precious stones that was "full with twigs of rosemary" when she married Henry VIII of England. The fragrant sprigs remain a part of bridal crowns, presented to wedding guests, and, where old traditions survive, slipped into wine or champagne before toasting to good health. It may serve to test the groom, since any man indifferent to the aroma was said to be incapable of true

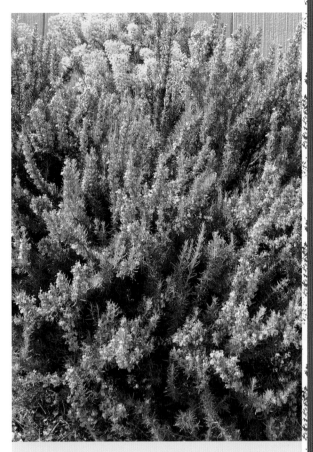

Rosemary (*Rosmarinus officinalis*)

love. Rosemary has been placed in tombs since ancient Egypt, as it was with Shakespeare's Juliet. The playwright also has Ophelia say that famous line from Hamlet, "There's rosemary, that's for remembrance."

Study volunteers at Western Oregon University found rosemary helped relieve fatigue, tension, anxiety, and confusion. It enhanced alertness by stimulating the brain's beta waves at Thailand's Chulalongkorn University in Bangkok. At the same time, it decreased levels of the stress hormone, cortisol. Japan's Meikai University

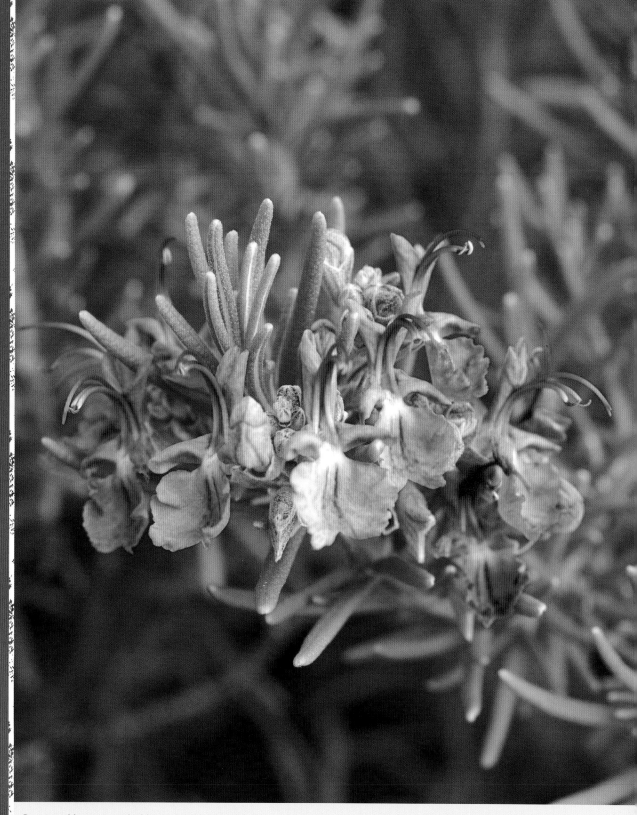

Rosemary blossoms can be blue, purple, pink, or white.

School of Dentistry found that inhaling rosemary for just five minutes caused cortisol and stress levels to drop and protected the body from the detrimental effects of long-term stress. The aroma reduces pain nearly as effectively as lavender or rose.

Several studies, such as one presented at the British Psychological Society's 2013 conference, show that rosemary helps with memory and mental work such as math, without being overstimulating. Medical researchers say that rosemary is a perfect candidate to help treat and perhaps even help prevent forms of dementia, such as Alzheimer's disease. Cineol, the main compound in rosemary, prevents an enzyme from breaking down a brain neurotransmitter involved in memory and other mental processes.

Rosemary's ability to improve the mind and prevent dizziness ties in with its long-standing use as a hair rinse. Rosemary-infused Hungary water for the hair and complexion was immensely popular from the fourteenth to the nineteenth century. It is said to have made one queen so young and vibrant that a much younger prince married her. It probably helped her memory, too! Rosemary also scents soap, eau de cologne, and body care products. Rosemary was stuffed into pouches and hollow walking stick heads, and placed on judge's benches to ward off the plague and typhoid. It does happen to be a powerful antiseptic. Smoldering rosemary boughs were carried through French hospitals to disinfect the air until the twentieth century, and again during World War II when medical supplies ran low.

Flowering time for rosemary depends on the selection; some are winter bloomers. Spring and summer blossoms attract bees. The needle-shaped leaves provide an interesting texture next to other plants. Rosemary looks good and grows well with other sun-loving Mediterranean plants, such as lavender and thyme. The plant can be trimmed into shapes or trained against a wall. My preference is to have it cascade over a wall, because it makes a natural fence that shows off winter blooms. The ancient gardens of Algiers in Morocco were once edged with rosemary.

Grow it in dry, well-drained soil in full sun. Rosemary can be a challenge to grow in zone 5 when temperatures drop below –10 degrees F, and needs to be well-mulched. Gardeners like Deb Soule in Maine dig it up in October and keep it indoors in large pots until mid-April. She warns against keeping plants near a wood stove, to prevent dry soil. When you want to dry rosemary leaves, hang sprigs or place them on drying screens or in baskets.

Rue

Ruta graveolens

Citrus family: Rutaceae
Perennial
Zone 6

Just as rose geranium has a species name, *graveolens*, that means "strongly scented," such is the case with rue. Indeed, the entire rue plant smells so pungent that it is not for the faint of heart. It is punctuated by a heavy spice scent. Deep in the background is a sharp citrus, a tribute to its citrus family. It would readily be voted the least favorite scent on my garden tours. After all, the mythological basilisk's breath caused plants to wilt and stones to crack, but had no effect on powerfully scented rue.

Rue represents patience and endurance, probably because both the scent and the plant are so long-lived. It has been said to smell strong enough to ward off almost anything, from bad vibes to infectious disease to jilted lovers. This reputation as a protector led to its use as aromatic holy water. The flowering stems were cut after the bloom's cup-like petals captured morning dew. The lightly scented water was then shaken over parishioners as a blessing, to protect them from emotional or physical harm. The plant became known as the herb of grace and the herb of repentance. It was so important in ancient times that Jewish law declared no tithe could be imposed upon it.

Bitter as it is, southern Europeans add sprigs of rue to flavor bottles of grappa and raki, which are made from spent wine grape skins. Just that little bit of rue provides a strong aftertaste that is certainly potent enough to ward off any disease. Rue is an ingredient in four thieves vinegar, along with the equally strong-scented garlic, wormwood, and rosemary. The thieves are said to have drunk this concoction and poured it over themselves until they reeked of the pungent herbs. They used the vinegar to protect themselves during the plague as they robbed abandoned homes. Like many of the time, the judge in Charles Dickens's *A Tale of Two Cities* has a rue bouquet to prevent infectious disease. Rue was also carried in the streets to cover odors. In *Gulliver's Travels* by Jonathan Swift, Gulliver must stuff rue in his nose when he returns to the streets of England.

The plant looks unique with its gray, almost shiny leaves shaped like a clover leaf, providing a nice contrast with almost anything planted next to it. Place it away from pathways so that garden visitors do not grab it. Having that strong oil on their hands can ruin their experience with other fragrances in the garden. Bees are attracted to rue's flowers, as are giant swallowtail and painted lady butterflies.

Rue grows easily in dry, well-drained soil and enjoys a long life, although it doesn't like to be moved once it is established. I once lost a couple rue plants to transplanting—then two seedlings appeared to replace them. Rue produces its own herbicide that restricts growth of nearby plants, so group rue plants together. Some gardeners have a skin reaction after touching rue and being in sunlight; you may want to wear gloves when working around it.

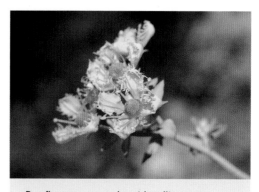

Rue flowers are popular with pollinators.

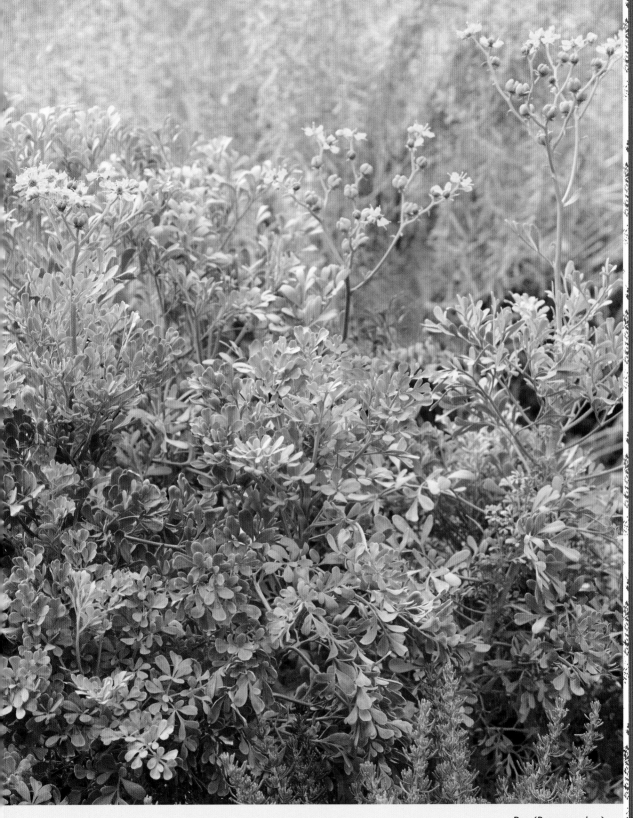

Rue (*Ruta graveolens*).

Sage

Salvia officinalis

Mint family: Lamiaceae
Perennial
Zones 5–9

The fragrance of culinary sage leaves is sharp, herby, and spicy combined with some muskiness. This is the delicious aroma of freshly toasted sage bread, and the traditional turkey dressing that fills the house at Thanksgiving. It also makes the garden aromatic on a hot day.

The genus *Salvia* includes nearly one thousand species, making up a whopping one-sixth of the highly fragrant mint family. However, only a few stand out for their fragrance. *S. officinalis* 'Berggarten' has a broader leaf than culinary sage and a little softer sage scent. It does not set seed.

Spanish sage (*Salvia lavandulifolia*) smells like sage and lavender combined, which makes it resemble rosemary. This tender perennial tolerates an occasional temperature drop to 20 degrees F. Compounds in the essential oil may inhibit an enzyme that is involved in Alzheimer's disease, according to research from London's King's College. Cleveland sage (*S. clevelandii*) is highly fragrant from fifteen feet away. It tops the sage aroma with a sweet perfume and has attractive, aromatic seedpods. This plant easily self-hybridizes and it can require a discerning eye to tell them apart. *Salvia* 'Betsy Clebsch' is named for the author of *The New Book of Salvias*. They all grow to zones 7 and 8. White sage (*S. apiana*) has a musky, heavy, beautiful scent that blankets Southern California hillsides when plants are in bloom. The Latin name *apiana* refers to the many bees that are attracted to the flowers.

The aroma of culinary sage increases memory and alertness. It helps in recovery from nervous or physical exhaustion and long-term stress. The sixteenth-century herbalist John Gerard said, "It is singularly good for the head, brain . . . it quickeneth the senses, memory." It was also recommended to heal grief.

Scientists have found that the aroma of sage does slow short-term memory loss. They think this is due to potent antioxidants that block a brain messenger associated with memory loss that plays a role in degenerative brain diseases, such as Alzheimer's.

Culinary sage lends its scent to soap and some aromatherapy products. It adds a fragrant touch to dried arrangements and wreaths, although it does get brittle. The aroma of white sage fills Native American sweat lodges when the leaves are placed on heated stones inside. The leaves are also wrapped into smudge sticks that are burned during ceremonies. Use sage freely in cooking, but be careful with its essential oil, which concentrates thujone, a compound generally considered toxic at high levels.

Grayish sage looks good contrasted with green-leafed plants and colorful flowers. When in bloom, it makes an impressive display next to other flowering plants such as lavender. *Salvia* is also dramatic in moon gardens, where leaves seem to glow on moonlit nights. Hummingbirds are attracted to sage's blue flowers, as are bees. Sage likes a hot, dry, Mediterranean climate. Dry it by hanging the stems.

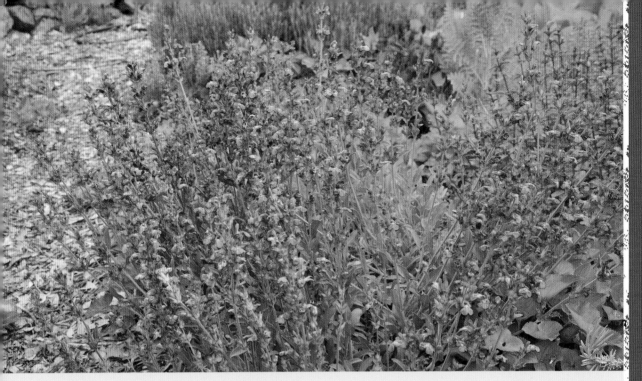

Sage (*Salvia officinalis*)

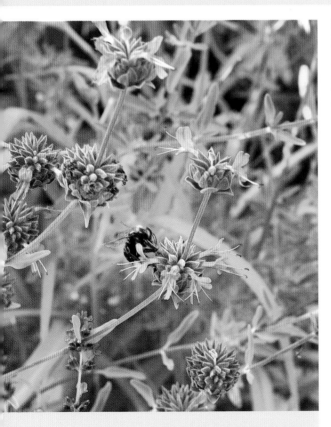

Cleveland sage (*Salvia clevelandii*)

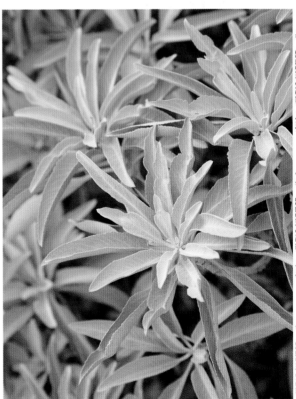

White sage (*Salvia apiana*)

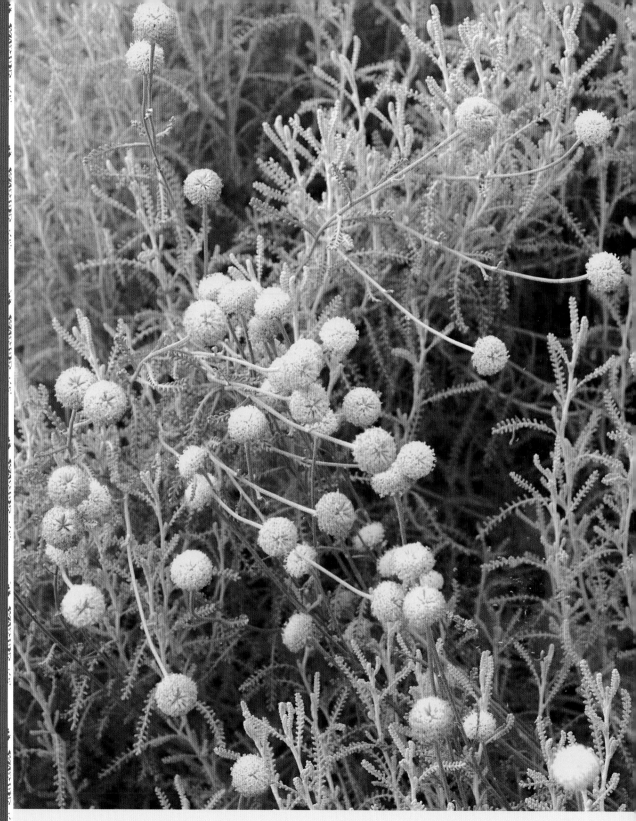

Santolina (*Santolina chamaecyparissus*)

Santolina

Santolina chamaecyparissus

Aster family: Asteraceae
Perennial
Zone 6

Santolina leaves combine the aroma of sweet lavender with the bitterness of Roman chamomile, the nose-crinkling pungency of wormwood, and a certain underlying mustiness. The species name *chamaecyparissus* means "like cypress," although the scent is not as rich or pungent as cypress. It reminds me more of walking into a vintage clothes closet hung with fragrant lavender sachets. The aroma does not permeate the air far, but surrounds individual plants on a hot day.

Santolina chamaecyparissus 'Nana' is a dwarf that received the Award of Garden Merit from the Royal Horticultural Society. Green santolina (*S. virens*) has slightly less aromatic foliage. *Santolina rosmarinifolia* resembles rosemary with a fly-away hair look, but still smells like santolina.

Santolina aroma is so relaxing, it can be difficult to concentrate while working around the plants in the garden. It is surprising to find such a musty, pungent scent in fine perfume, but small amounts lend an appealing feature. The leaves maintain their scent, so can be used in potpourri. Even though they dry brittle, add a few sprigs to herbal and holiday wreaths for the gray color and aroma. Place small cotton bags filled with dried leaves among wool clothing and inside grain jars to repel clothes and grain moths.

The mounding growth makes santolina grow into an attractive ground cover that is accented with small, bright yellow flowers. The feathery leaves turn shades of orange and brown, and provide a lovely mix of color and scent when planted next to gray-green thyme or plants with dark green leaves. Elizabethan-style knot gardens use santolina as one of the plants that create the illusion of being braided into an elaborate pattern. The plant sprawls, so cut it back to keep it bushy.

Santolina produces seed, and the stems very readily sprout by layering or cutting. Grow it with other Mediterranean plants in full sun and well-drained, dry soil. It is used to cover dry hill landscapes in hot climates.

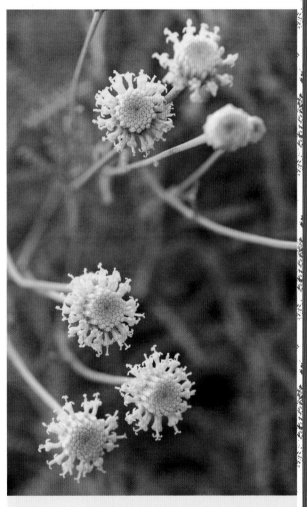

Yellow Santolina flowers have a unique shape.

Southernwood

Artemisia abrotanum

Aster family: Asteraceae
Perennial
Zone 5

Southernwood produces a pungent, bitter, and decidedly musty aroma that is characteristic of its wormwood relatives. However, *Artemisia abrotanum* is sweeter and more agreeable. A hot day or simply brushing against the leaves brings out a scent that manages to be biting and sweet at the same time. This contrast is what makes it so aromatically attractive. Imagine opening the drawer of an antique dresser sweetened with sachets of rosemary, lavender, and wormwood and you'll have an idea of the fragrance.

Its other common name, lad's love, is from its association with bittersweet love. A Finnish bridal song compares the humble-looking southernwood and its year-round scent to the fleeting fragrance of a beautiful lily: "I'll give to him . . . more sweetness than he'd dream without me— more than any lily could. I, that am flowerless . . . lad's love, green and living yet." Simply put, southernwood's bitter scent reminds us that there is more to a relationship than good looks and a captivating perfume.

Like its wormwood kin, southernwood increases alertness. Women churchgoers would carry little bouquet of both these herbs and the sweeter lemon balm to stay awake during long services. Potent bundles of southernwood, wormwood, rue, and rosemary were also carried into town to fend off infectious disease. Southernwood was used in a disinfectant bath, which must have been appropriate in an era when people rarely bathed. The leaves go into a porous bag that is placed in bathwater. While it is too harsh a scent for a relaxing bath, it may ease muscles made sore after working in the garden. *Artemisia abrotanum* makes an excellent moth repellent for the clothes closet. In old England, it was nicknamed *garderobe*, meaning to guard, or protect, clothing. Put dried leaves into small sachet bags with lavender flowers, and place them in drawers and closets. This gives the closet, as well as the clothes, a nice, herby aroma. While the upper class chose expensive sweet flag for their floors, common people used southernwood from their gardens to spread on floors as an aromatic strewing herb to cover odors and repel bugs.

Southernwood's feathery leaves show off their texture when planted next to sage or other broad-leafed plants. Its yellow-trimmed green leaf color contrasts nicely with gray wormwood. The sprawling branches do tend to fall over surrounding plants, but they are flexible enough to be repositioned.

This drought-resistant plant is probably from the Mediterranean. It likes dry, well-drained soil and a limited amount of water. It withstands prolonged freezing and has been planted in the dry Southwest to rehabilitate rangelands and old mining areas, to stabilize soil, and to protect native seedlings. Southernwood rarely produces seed, but the stems sprout by layering or cuttings.

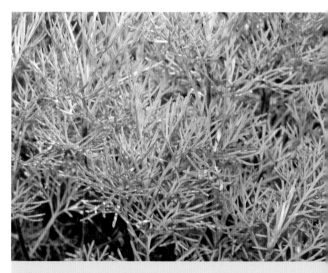

Southernwood (*Artemisia abrotanum*)

Stock

Matthiola incana

Mustard family: Brassicaceae
Perennial, usually grown as an annual
Zones 7–10

Stock is perhaps the most clove-scented of all flowers. It was once called stock-gilloflower because it smells so much like clove pinks, or gillyflower carnations. Its penetrating, spicy, clove-like scent is mixed with the sweet muskiness of lily, making it smell like a bouquet of lilies and clove pinks. This aromatic combination once made stock a popular cottage-style garden flower, as well as a clove-tasting garnish.

Yet, stock's fragrance is somewhat elusive, seeming strong one moment and vague the next. Francis Bacon observed this in his seventeenth-century essay, *Of Gardens*, commenting that the scent of its flowers "is far sweeter in the air, where it comes and goes like the warbling of music, than in the hand." I agree with him that stock's aroma is more appealing when it is wafting across the garden than when it is held up close.

Matthiola longipetala leans more toward the scent of lilac than cloves. Virginia stock (*Malcomia maritima*) was moved to a different genus, but is still called a stock. It bears unimpressive flowers that droop downward, but wait until evening when the slightest breeze picks up the nighttime fragrance. These are plants to have near an open window on a hot summer night.

The smell of stock is both emotionally relaxing and energizing, so it offers the best of both worlds. It lessens mental fatigue and nervousness, while improving a poor memory. Folklore says the aroma also inspires love and passion. The genus name is after Pietro Matthili (1501–1577), physician to Roman Emperor Maximilian II, who prescribed stock for "matters of love and lust." Studies show that the clove-scented com-

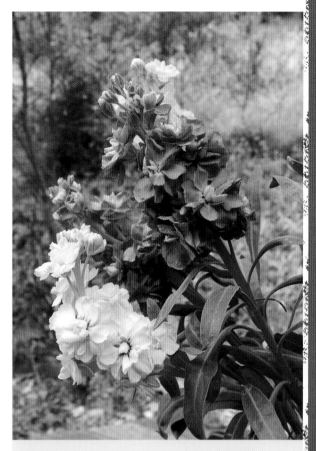

Stock (*Matthiola incana*)

ponent, called eugenol, may indeed mimic love by producing a happiness response. According to research from the Indian Institute of Technology at Banaras Hindu University in Varanasi and elsewhere, eugenol reduces stress by moderating neurotransmitters in the brain and reducing the adrenal cortisol levels that increase during stress. However, researchers warn that cloves' scent may have the opposite effect if it reminds you of a dentist's office, where eugenol is often used for its numbing effect.

The flowers are usually white but can include red to purple shades. They are pollinated by both bees and butterflies. Stock fell out of favor when modern gardeners started going more for the visual impact than the fragrance. Granted, they have that straggly character of plants from the mustard family, and look best tucked in among other plants or in a pot of mixed flowers. In regions with cool weather, stock is often grown as an annual by sowing the seed in succession from spring to early summer, to make the plants appear less messy.

Stock is particular about its growing conditions. Even though it is found on cliffs and dry lands in the Mediterranean and southern Africa, it needs cool daytime weather (under 80 degrees F) and relatively warm nights in order to flower. In any zone, plant stock in full sun early in the season, before the weather gets too hot. In zones 8 and higher, grow it as an early winter or spring flower. Since the plants need very good drainage, they are good candidates for a raised flowerbed or a window box with fertile soil.

Sweet-box
Sarcococca confusa

Boxwood family: Buxaceae
Shrub
Zones 7–9

The tiny white flowers of sweet-box are hidden among waxy leaves, yet they manage to perfume the entire winter garden. It never ceases to surprise me each year when I unexpectedly catch that first whiff of intense fragrance on a blistery cold February day. The shrub grows under my bedroom window, which I happily open on the warmest winter days to welcome the aroma indoors. Gardeners most often describe the fragrance as vanilla, yet that fails to capture all the floral notes it presents, including jasmine, honeysuckle, and lavender—along with a pinch of intoxication.

Sarcococca confusa is aptly named since it is indeed confusing even for many nurseries to tell it apart from S. *ruscifolia*. Both species broadcast the same, amazing fragrance. They look almost identical, except the small, attractive, round fruit of S. *confusa* is red, while S. *ruscifolia* fruit is black. Christmas or Himalayan box (S. *hookeriana* var. *humilis*) is a shorter shrub that is equally as fragrant.

Sweet-box is not usually regarded as an aromatherapy scent, but it is thought to possibly be an antidepressant. It also combines all of the aromas of an aphrodisiac. This is convenient, since it tends to be in bloom around Valentine's Day!

This Asian evergreen loves shade, so it grows well under trees and overhangs. It tolerates some sun where summers are relatively cool. My sweet-box does not seem to mind the hour or so of intense late-afternoon sun it receives in the summer. If trained when young, it can be grown against a wall and shaped into an espalier, with branches fanning out to create patterns. It can also be left to form into a dense bush and can make an informal hedge. It pairs nicely with other fragrant shade-loving shrubs (such as daphne), as long as it can expand out several feet and not overpower smaller shrubs.

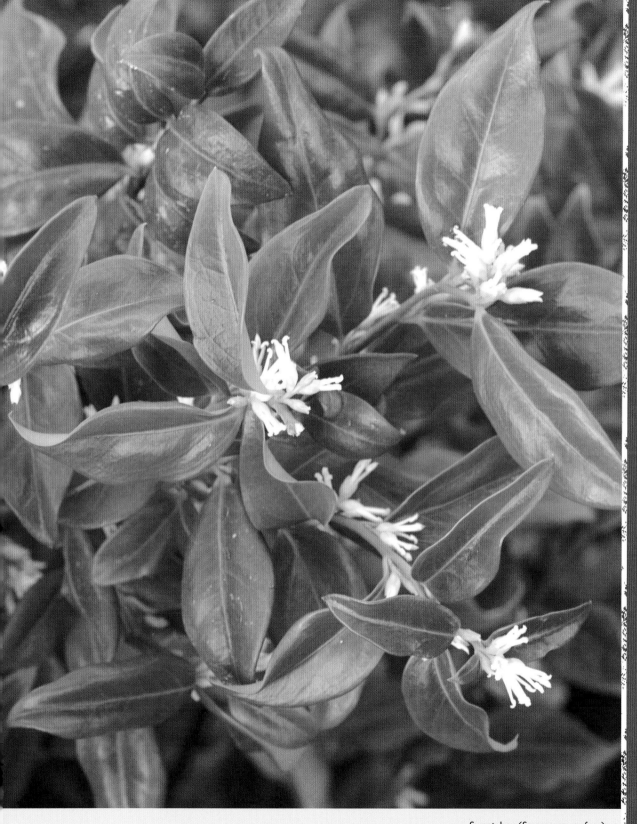

Sweet-box (*Sarcococca confusa*)

Sweet flag

Acorus calamus

Sweet flag family: Acoraceae
Perennial
Zones 4–9

The heavy, spicy scent of sweet flag blends buttery, sweet, and musk-like aromas with cinnamon and ginger notes. Plus, there is a surprising, subtle tang of bitter tangerine. This complex mix creates strong perfume in the leaves and especially in the rhizome. Just digging it up releases the aroma into the air; lightly crushing it makes it more intense. An underlying nuttiness becomes more prevalent as the rhizome dries.

Indian sweet flag is found in temperate India, Europe, eastern North America, Australia, and South Africa. American sweet flag grows from North America to Siberia. *Acorus calamus* subsp. *angustatus* is from eastern and southern Asia. Even though these varieties are from different parts of the world, they share a similar fragrance.

The plant's aroma is deeply relaxing, yet it heightens attentiveness. This dual action brings the central nervous system into balance and encourages restful sleep. It also helps with learning and recalling facts. Sweet flag is one of three plants most frequently cited to treat forgetfulness in the *Zhong Hua Yi Dian*, the *Encyclopedia of Traditional Chinese Medicine*. Preliminary evidence from Shaanxi University of Traditional Chinese Medicine indicates that the aroma improves the ability to learn and memorize facts. Studies at the Department of Oriental Neuropsychiatry at Dongguk University in Seoul, Korea, suggested that it enhances the activity of the central nervous system and GABA, a brain chemical involved in relaxation. Sweet flag also seems to prevent neurons from overfiring and to improve mental function via neurotransmitters

such as dopamine, serotonin, and adrenaline. In ayurvedic and Tibetan medicines, the rhizome is dried, powdered and burned as incense to strengthen the nerves and mind and to help one stay awake. Inhaling the aromatic fumes is prescribed for reversing memory loss, melancholy, anxiety, nightmares, and even the effects of ingesting hallucinogenic plants. Native American Dakota warriors found that sweet flag kept them calm, alert, focused, and fearless. The Cheyenne toss the rhizomes onto hot rocks in their sweat lodges and the Penobscot and other tribes still scent their homes with it. It has long been used to enhance contemplation, meditation, and prayer. The prophet Moses provides anointing oil in the Old Testament of the Bible (Exodus 30:23), with sweet flag as an ingredient. An insecticide powder made from the rhizome kills ants and fleas.

Sweet flag once flavored Benedictine, Chartreuse, and absinthe liqueurs, as well as gin, beer, the famous Stockton bitters, Dr. Pepper soda, and even tobacco. That is, until the United States Food and Drug Administration (FDA) banned it from use in food after finding that the Jammu type of Indian sweet flag contains a potentially carcinogenic beta-asarone—although there is very little of the compound in European sweet flag and none in the American variety. The International Fragrance Association restricts its use in body care products since essential oils are absorbed through skin and there is no regulation on which type of sweet flag is used. Sniffing the oil or growing the Jammu type is perfectly safe. Small amounts still scent and flavor Dutch chewing gum and tooth powder, and a crystallized candy form was sold in pharmacies to relieve indigestion.

Sweet flag is one of the longest-lasting fragrances and helps potpourri endure when used in place of orris root. When King Tutankhamun's tomb was opened in the 1920s, the alabaster jars

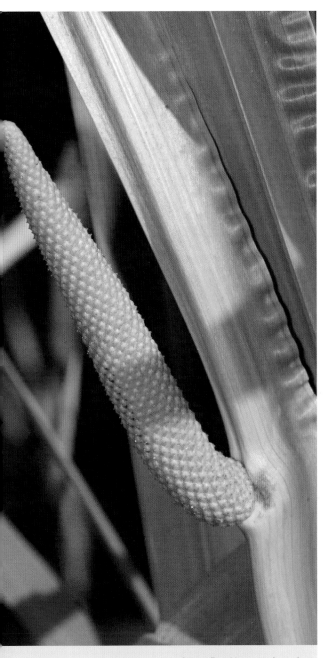

Sweet flag (*Acorus calamus*)

buried with it for over 3000 years still held a faint aroma of sweet flag. This may be the first recorded fragrant plant. The Egyptian *Medical Papyrus VI* mentioned it around 1300 BC and King Solomon grew it in his famous garden in the tenth century BC. Worldwide, sweet flag has long been considered an aphrodisiac. Modern American poet Walt Whitman describes the "aromatic, pungent bouquet" as a metaphor for love and physical desire in the "Calamus" poems in his *Leaves of Grass*.

The long, sword-like leaves of sweet flag are interesting, and a slender flower stalk juts out at a forty-five degree angle from the side. Sweet flag likes partial shade and rarely flowers unless it is planted in wet ground. Try growing it in a tub in the garden to contain the spreading rhizomes and to keep the soil moist. It looks especially nice planted along the edge of a pond or creek with other water-loving plants, although the resulting matted roots can make harvesting a messy business.

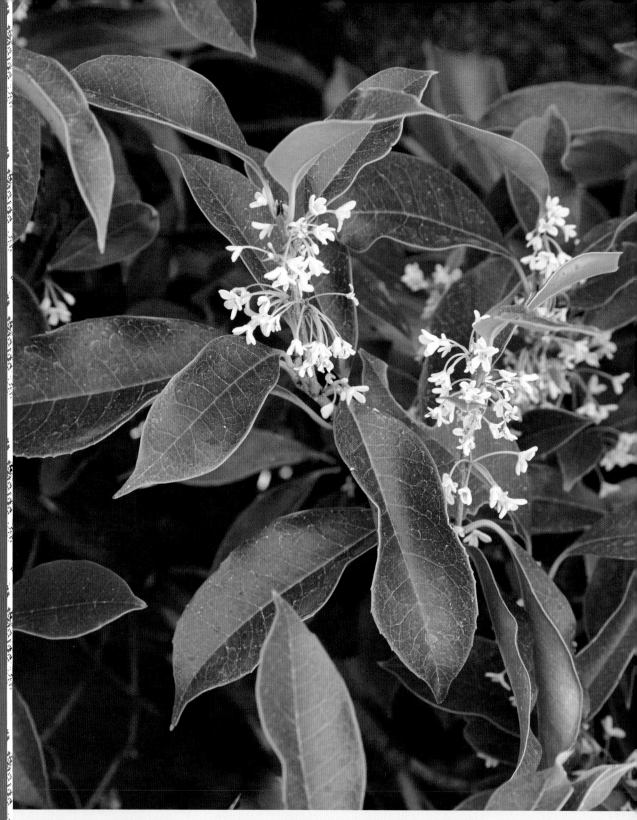

Sweet olive (*Osmanthus fragrans*)

Sweet olive

Osmanthus fragrans

Olive family: Oleaceae
Perennial
Zones 8, 9

The small, white flowers send out a strong, sweet, creamy aroma that is clearly of apricots, but also much more. The fruity-floral fragrance also has woody undertones, with a subtle but rich, leathery aroma and a touch of spice. It has been described as mouth-watering. The genus name *Osmanthus* even means "fragrant flowers."

The various cultivars are all very fragrant. *Osmanthus fragrans* 'Liuye Jingui' has red-yellow flowers with a scent that hints of violets. *Osmanthus fragrans* 'Gecheng Dangui', with orange flowers, is even more distinctly floral. The cream-colored flowers of *O. fragrans* 'Houban Yingui' have an additional, slight herbal scent due to compounds it shares with basil. In China, *O. fragrans* 'Gecheng Dangui' is considered to have the most delicate and elegant scent.

Traditional Chinese medicine defines the aroma as comforting and relaxing, recommending it to calm nerves and reduce fears. A study reported in a 2013 *Scientific Report* article showed that it produces a mild sedative effect, apparently by affecting neurons in the brain's hypothalamus. The scent even shows some potential in decreasing the motivation to eat.

Sweet olive symbolizes riches and good fortune in China. As a result it has often been planted in courtyards and temples. Tourists flock to Hangzhou every autumn to get a whiff of the masses that have been blooming there since the Tang Dynasty (AD 618–907), when poet Zhiwen first described the fragrance. They line the road to Lingyin Temple.

A pricey sweet olive absolute is used in perfumes. Facial creams and perfumed hair oil made from sweet olive blossom have been used since ancient times. The dried flowers, often mixed with roses and fragrant spices, is still also used in baths and clothing sachets.

The flowers lend their almond-like, floral aroma and flavor to pastries, soups, vinegars, wines, liqueurs, candied flowers, jams, sticky rice cakes, *dim sum* dishes, and very fragrant tea— all of which are medicinal. The flowers are combined with chrysanthemum, as well as black *pu-er* teas produced in China. The red flowers are prized not only for their aromatic flavor, but for the colorful swirls they impart to cakes. A Chinese tradition preserves the flowers by grinding them with licorice and salted plums or ginger and salt. A small amount is then diluted to make an aromatic soup.

Osmanthus fragrans is typically twelve feet tall, but can grow larger—or be kept smaller when contained in a pot. The dense, compact growth allows this shrub to be shaped into an espalier. It prefers shade, but tolerates some sun and a range of soil conditions, even heavy clay.

Sweet pea

Lathyrus odoratus

Pea family: Leguminosae
Annual

As its name implies, sweet pea's fragrance is indeed very sweet. It also has an underlying, deeper aroma that almost smells balsamic. A vase with just a few sweet peas fills a room with a delicious, light, airy scent that does not over-power. Twentieth-century perfumers Steffen Arctander and William Poucher both accurately describe the aroma as a supersweet blend of orange blossom, hyacinth, and wild rose. Arctander adds that it also recalls the scent of freesia. To me, it smells like a garden in full bloom with a flowering orange tree in the back corner.

However, due to the florist's quest for larger flowers, longer stems, and an astounding array of colors, modern sweet peas have not retained much of their precious fragrance. In *Popular Flowering Plants*, twentieth-century novelist Harry L. V. Fletcher discussed "the great lament of the sweet peas, which lost their perfume." Now breeders are creating plants that boost both large flowers *and* the original, strong scent. Sweet pea's species name, *odoratus*, even means "fragrant." Charles Unwin spent his life hybridizing sweet peas into amazing colors for his company, Unwin Seeds. When he began, around 1914, much of the scent had already been bred out of the flowers. It was not until many years later, when someone presented him with a highly scented sweet pea from a cottage garden, that he smelled the old stock. He said, "Until that moment, I never fully realized why sweet peas were so named."

Lavender and light pink sweet pea flowers tend to be the most aromatic, with scarlet shades the least fragrant. *Lathyrus odoratus* 'Cuthbert-son' usually has highly scented, deep pink to white flowers. 'High Scent' smells fragrant from yards away. Its white, bluish-edged flowers on long stems make it a favorite among florists. 'Annie B. Gilroy' is an exceptionally sweet-scented heirloom cultivar. 'Old Spice' is the best-suited of the highly fragrant sweet peas for hot weather. 'Matucanas' is the cultivar closest to the original Sicilian wildflower. Its flowers are small, but the scent is intoxicating. Perennial sweet pea (*L. tuberosus*) is sometimes distilled for cologne. It has beautiful, vivid pink flowers, but be forewarned that the long taproots can be invasive.

The Victorian definition of sweet peas says that they create "blissful pleasure." Old-fashioned versions are fragrant enough for potpourri and aromatic corsages and bouton-nieres. An expensive sweet pea essential oil is produced for high-end perfume. The commonly used sweet pea scent is synthetic and to me, smells nothing like either the old-fashioned or modern sweet pea.

The fragrance of old-fashioned sweet peas makes them worthy of any garden. They quickly cover an empty space with their vines and spots of color. Provide something on which they can climb or let them cascade from a large, hanging pot that provides ample room for their roots. Plant them where they will not be overpowered by a strongly scented plant, such as jasmine. Sweet peas are pollinated by bees, butterflies, and moths.

Nurseries usually sell sweet pea plant mixes, but you probably need to purchase seed to grow the highly scented varieties. Soak the seeds before planting and they will come up readily. The seedlings may need to be protected from birds and other critters. Pinch back the tops so that they branch out. They require plenty of water, even though their ancestors grew under the hot, Mediterranean sun. Nowadays, heat causes mod-ern sweet peas to die back, so they are considered a spring flower except in regions where summers are cool. They do not benefit from a rich diet of fertilizer, but feeding them monthly keeps them strong so they last a little longer.

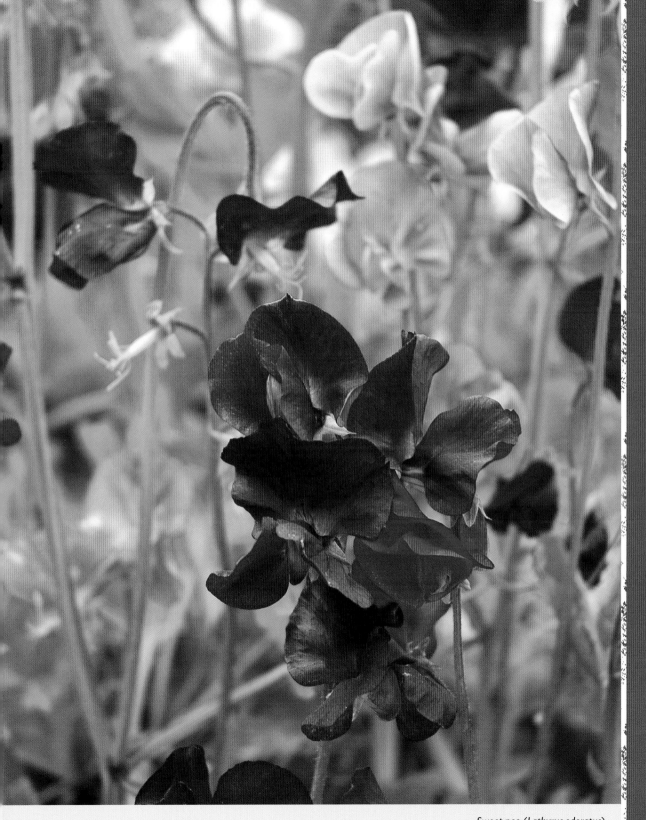

Sweet pea (*Lathyrus odoratus*)

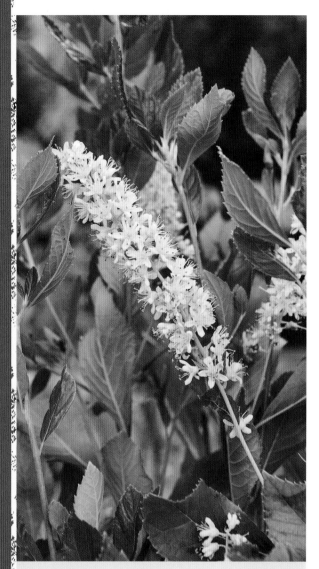

Sweet pepperbush (*Clethra alnifolia*)

Sweet pepperbush
Clethra alnifolia

Clethra family: Clethraceae
Shrub
Zones 7–11

The name sweet pepperbush comes from the spicy scent of its flowers and the fruit, which resembles black peppercorns. This complex combination of clove, heliotrope, rose, and honeysuckle inspired another name, summersweet. Not everyone agrees which aroma—spicy or floral—predominates in the mix. My vote is for honeysuckle-clove. No matter how you perceive it, the result is a haunting aroma, especially in the evening. It resembles an old-fashioned perfume so much that you might imagine that a woman wearing a long, lacy, white dress and carrying a parasol just walked by. The scent does have aspects of some of the most popular personal fragrances of the early 1900s.

Preliminary studies suggest that the scent of sweet pepperbush has anti-anxiety and antidepressant properties. That makes perfect sense, considering that the aromas of rose and clove have those benefits as well.

The essential oil is not produced commercially for use in cosmetics or aromatherapy. However, other essential oils have been blended together to mimic the fragrance in perfume, such as with the popular Brazilian scent, Clethra. The fragrance is also attractive to bumblebees.

This deciduous native of eastern North America grows ten feet tall and spreads very slowly by way of suckers. The tiny, bright white or pink flowers create an attractive display against dark green leaves. The leaves turn golden brown in fall. The shrub likes fairly rich, slightly acidic soil that stays moist. It prefers partial shade, but adapts to sun—except in areas like mine where the summer is very hot.

Sweet woodruff

Galium odoratum

Citrus family: Rubiaceae
Perennial
Zones 5–9

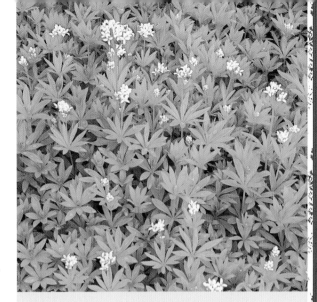

Sweet woodruff (*Galium odoratum*)

Sweet woodruff leaves smell delightfully of the green, fresh sweetness of newly mown hay. The two do share a vanilla-scented compound called coumarin. Sweet woodruff adds a touch of muskiness. The old French name *muge-de-bois,* or musk of the woods, does it justice. This woodsy aroma combined with vanilla creates an interesting and surprisingly wonderful contrast. You could say that the leaves make you feel as if you are eating vanilla ice cream while sitting on a freshly mown lawn, with the cut grass drying in the hot sun. Crushing the fresh leaves releases the wonderful aroma, but coumarin increases when the leaves are dried, producing a much more potent vanilla scent.

The fragrance of sweet woodruff is emotionally comforting and is associated with new beginnings. As a result, it plays a role in spring celebrations, especially in Germany, where the leaves are sometimes woven into head wreaths and church garlands. Sweethearts often give each other sprigs of the leaves to wear. Traditional May wine, or *maitrank* in German, is flavored with sweet woodruff. It's a wonderful addition at springtime potlucks. To make your own May wine, add a couple handfuls of the dried leaves to a bottle of white wine. Let it sit for two weeks, then strain. Sweeten to taste.

Before the era of clothes fresheners, sweet woodruff leaves were laid among linens to make beddings smell fresh. They also scented snuffs. Eighteenth-century men tucked the circular whorl of leaves in the back door of their pocket watches so that when they opened the door, the pleasing aroma was released. The leaves also scent potpourri. Dry them carefully to maintain the best scent.

Sweet woodruff's whorled leaves make a decorative ground cover. In the spring, the plant is covered with small white flowers that are pollinated by bees and flies. The scented leaves are fragrant year-round. They do not produce much scent unless walked upon, so grow sweet woodruff next to walkways where it can creep into the path. Grow it with other aromatic ground covers that can handle some shade, such as Roman chamomile and germander; these three plants create a beautiful combination. Show them off in a planting under a bench, birdbath, or garden statuary. I grow it with aromatic daphne bushes.

A shade plant from the forests of Europe and Asia, *Galium odoratum* prefers less light; the leaves can yellow and the flowers diminish in full sun. If your fragrance garden receives full sun, use taller plants to provide shade. Its shallow root system means sweet woodruff does well when grown in planters or in a small pot as a houseplant. If grown from seed, first freeze the seeds to stratify them. It is a fairly fast grower when watered regularly and given good soil. Dry the thin leaves on screens or lightly piled in the bottom of a paper bag.

Tansy

Tanacetum annuum

Aster family: Asteraceae
Perennial
Zones 3–9

Tansy's aroma is a mix of chrysanthemum, pine, camphor, and eucalyptus, in that order. To me, this combination smells like a liniment for sore muscles. English chef and author Allegra McEvedy more poetically describes it as "fruity, sharpness to it and then there's a sort of explosion of cool heat a bit like peppermint."

Botanists think that tansy represents a number of subgroups, or races, that have different scents. Fern-leaved tansy (*Tanacetum vulgare* var. *crispum*) is more contained and ornamental with its fern-like leaves, but still has tansy's scent. Some forms grow more like a ground cover and rarely produce flowers.

Tansy was used so much during funerals to pack into coffins and for embalming, it became associated with death. In England, tansy biscuits with caraway seeds were served during funerals. Tansy's modern claim to fame is as an insect repellent. It has been found less effective, but far less toxic, than DEET-based pesticides to kill flies, ants, ticks, and other pests. Dried tansy leaves act as an insect repellent when laid around the base of cucumbers, squash, roses, and berries in the garden. Planted alongside potatoes, it can wipe out Colorado potato beetles. The leaves are still placed on some country house windowsills and hung in doorways and stables to repel flies. Before the days of refrigeration, meat was rubbed and packed with the leaves to preserve it and keep flies away. Tansy leaves also were placed on floors as a strewing herb and flea repellent. A popular 1940s mosquito repellent contained tansy, fleabane, pennyroyal, and alcohol. Some beekeepers burn the dried leaves in their bee smokers when they are calming the hive.

The aromatic compound myrtenol, derived from tansy, is used as a beverage preservative, flavoring, and fragrance. Nineteenth-century Tennessee whiskey magnate Jack Daniel was said to enjoy a crushed tansy leaf in sweetened whiskey. The United States FDA currently permits tansy as a flavoring in alcoholic beverages, such as Chartreuse, provided that the compound thujone (toxic at high levels) is removed. Also abundant in wormwood, thujone over-sensitizes brain activity and can lead to convulsions. Sue Perkins, the star of the BBC food series *The Supersizers*, developed tansy toxicity when the show was exploring the Restoration era and she ate too many tansy-seasoned cakes, which was a popular dish of that time. Just touching the plant can cause a skin reaction, but only in a few, sensitive individuals. Perhaps surprisingly, Irish folklore suggests a tansy and salt bath to ease joint pain.

Tansy comes from northern Europe and western Asia. It was a favorite of Emperor Charlemagne, who had it planted in all the medieval monasteries under his western European rule. Modern gardeners often consider it invasive, but it is attractive in the fragrance garden if grown in a contained bed. The tall, flowering stalks fall on neighboring plants and can be tied together, although they will twist and curl into a strange-looking arrangement. Tansy flowers are pollinated by bees, flies, and wasps. It is used to trap insects because it mimics an insect pheromone.

Give tansy plants full sun. They produce lush growth in well-drained soil with some moisture, although they tolerate a variety of soil conditions. Tansy readily propagates from cuttings, especially if the heel of the stem (where it roots into the ground) is included. The easiest way to dry tansy is to hang it.

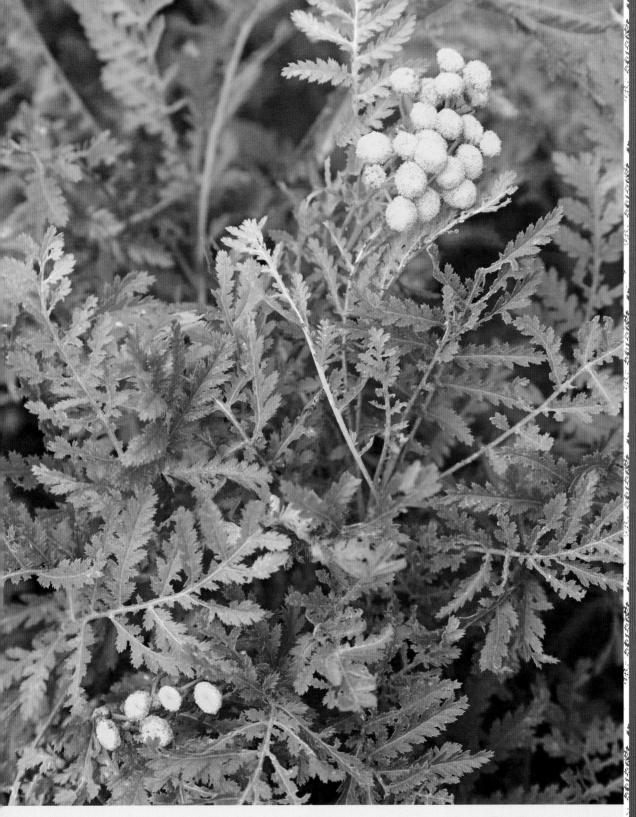

Tansy (*Tanacetum annuum*)

Thyme

Thymus vulgaris

Mint family: Lamiaceae
Perennial
Zones 4–5

Thyme's strong aroma is sweet, sharp, very herby and "green." The Scottish poet Robert Burns sang its praises, and author Rudyard Kipling considered it the "perfume of the dawn in paradise." The Greeks complimented someone by saying that he or she smelled of thyme. It often seems more medicinal to the modern nose since it is the aroma of chest vapor rubs, cough drops, gargles, and mouthwashes that contain thyme or its primary aromatic compound, thymol.

An estimated three hundred fifty species, plus cultivars, offer the thyme connoisseur many diverse scents. There are thymes scented like lavender, oregano, spice, lemon, and camphor. It is no surprised that there is some confusion over their nomenclature. Thyme is subdivided according to scents produced by different aromatic compounds. The geraniol and linalool types have gentle floral aromas, while the thymol and thuyanol types smell harsh. French thyme (*Thymus vulgaris* 'Narrow Leaf French') is most of what we see in gardens and on our culinary shelves. *Thymus citriodorus* 'Fragrantissimus' smells like orangey-rose geranium, while *T. vulgaris* 'Orange Balsam' has a spicier scent. Of the many species, lemon thyme (*T. citriodorus*) and its variation *T. citriodorus* 'Lime' are popular in nurseries. Nutmeg thyme (*T. praecox* subsp. *articus*) makes a spicy ground cover between stepping-stones. The aroma of Pennsylvania Dutch thyme (*T. pulegioides*) resembles pennyroyal. Mother of thyme (*T. serpyllum*) comes in different combinations of camphor, spice, and spearmint scents. Mastic thyme (*T. mastichina*), smelling strongly of eucalyptus and lavender,

scents soaps and shampoo. It is only hardy to about zone 8. A fragrant thyme lawn can be grown with short, dense varieties, such as creeping thyme (*T. praecox*), woolly thyme (*T. pseudolanuginosus*), and mother of thyme (*T. serpyllum*). Caraway thyme (*T. herba-barona*) is a favorite because the springy mounds do not easily dry out in hot climates.

Thyme's aroma relieves memory loss and depression and, some say, melancholy and mental instability. Data gathered by the University of Foggia in Italy suggests that carvacrol, one of the aromatic components in thyme's essential oil, influences neuronal activity through the brain's neurotransmitters to increase well-being. The strong scent has been associated with courage. A thyme-flavored beer soup was said to help overcome shyness. The Scots drank wild thyme tea to inspire bravery and vigor, and Roman soldiers bathed in thyme-scented waters. Court ladies sent their knights off with thyme embroidered on their tunics. A sprig placed under the pillow is said to banish nightmares, and grant courage to face them. Benedictine monks added thyme to their therapeutic elixirs. The sprigs were carried in flower posies to mask odors and ward off disease. Romans burned the dried leaves to fumigate their homes and placed fresh thyme on the floor to deter bugs.

Thyme attracts so many honeybees, it appears to vibrate from the commotion. A famous honey from Mount Hymettus, near Athens, Greece, is famous for its intense aroma of wild thyme. Thyme essential oil is used in beehives to control the varroa mites responsible for massive beehive deaths.

Thyme is the perfect ground cover for rock gardens, as an edging in border gardens, alongside and in pathways, and as a fragrant lawn. Growing a thyme lawn requires maintenance. It is easier to grow the plants among stepping-stones. It looks particularly beautiful cascading over a retaining wall. A bank filled with different thyme

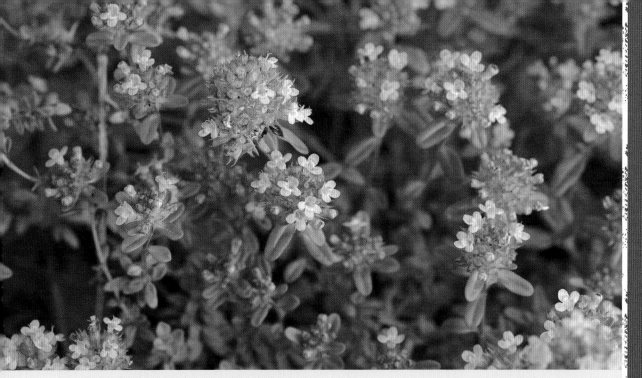

Thyme (*Thymus vulgaris*)

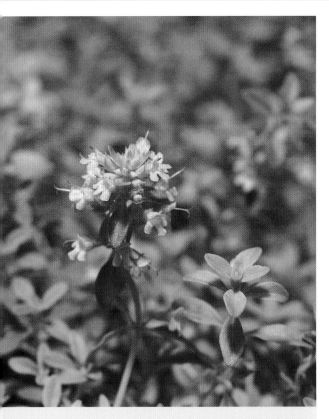

Lime thyme (*Thymus citriodorus* 'Lime')

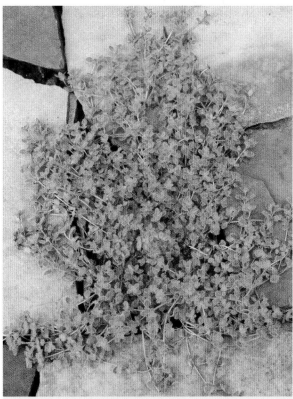

Woolly thyme (*Thymus pseudolanuginosus*)

ground covers displays a variety of colors, textures, and scents. Thyme can also fill in areas between other sun-loving plants, such as lavender and sage.

Give thyme the well-drained, light, and rather dry soil favored by Mediterranean plants. The fine root system makes it more difficult to transplant than most herbs. Even well-established plants can be damaged if the ground freezes and heaves. A layer of sand on the soil's surface helps to prevent frost damage.

Trumpet flower

Brugmansia versicolor

Nightshade family: Solanaceae
Tender perennial
Zones 10–12

Trumpet flowers smell so intensely sweet that it is hard to resist sticking one's face into the huge, eight- to ten-inch blossoms and taking a deep breath. The scent is thick, heavy, and impossibly fragrant, especially in the evening. Its exotic scent is difficult to describe—an aromatic combination of lilies and narcissus, but with a touch of muskiness and orange blossom (the flower contains several citrus compounds). One plant can produce two hundred fragrant flowers—enough fragrance to fill a backyard, plus half the surrounding block! Some of the most aromatic walks I have taken were on warm summer evenings in coastal California towns where trumpet flower is plentiful.

Several hybrids and numerous cultivars have been developed from the various species as ornamental plants, creating intensely fragrant variations. *Brugmansia* ×*candida* has immensely fragrant white flowers. *Brugmansia suaveolens* has larger leaves, but slightly less-fragrant flowers. Red angel's trumpet (*B. sanguinea*) has a disappointing lack of scent, but tries to compensate with stunning flowers.

When ingested, the plant is toxic, with mind-altering properties; the fragrance may follow suit. The heavy aroma has a reputation for producing vivid (sometimes erotic) dreams in its native South America. It is even rumored there that women who smell the fragrance in the evening are more easily impregnated. I do know that the trumpet flower outside my office window seems to inspire my writing!

Since trumpet flower's size and fragrance dominate the garden, plant this beauty away from other fragrant, late summer bloomers, or you will not smell anything else. It can reach fifteen feet under perfect conditions, so give it space. Shelter the large, thin leaves from strong wind. The pale flowers are showy on moonlit nights. Trumpet flower is the main source of food for clearwing butterfly larva that store alkaloid compounds and turn into unpalatable butterflies to predators. Moths pollinate it in the evening, when its fragrance increases.

My trumpet flower drinks a couple gallons of water daily in the summer, so this is a good plant to have on a drip system! It is shocking to see how easily the thin, huge leaves droop when they dry out. As with many tropical plants, trumpet flower is a very heavy feeder, so give it rich soil and fertilize it throughout the growing season to assure a good bloom. Hot, direct summer sun burns the leaves, so keep it in filtered light unless you live where there is abundant summer cloud cover. I manage to grow trumpet flower in a pot on a south-facing, covered deck in zone 9. Once the leaves completely die in early winter, I cover the plant with protective nursery cloth and keep the soil moist. This is a high-maintenance plant for me, but I cannot imagine living without it.

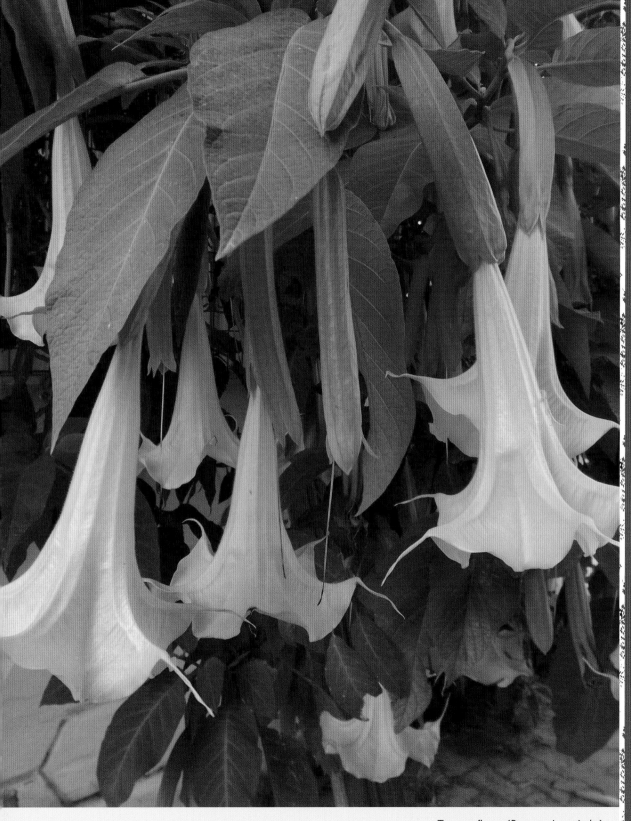

Trumpet flower (*Brugmansia versicolor*)

Tuberose

Polianthes tuberosa

Agave family: Agavaceae
Perennial
Zones 7, 8

Tuberose flowers have a wonderfully complex fragrance that is perfume in itself. The aroma smells exotic, heady and so sweet that some people complain that it's too sugary. English poet Percy Shelley called it "the sweetest flower for scent that blows." Despite its name, tuberose is closer to a fine jasmine or gardenia perfume than roses. The fragrance of jasmine is blended with honey, sweet vanilla, and a faint hint of orange blossom. There is also a musty, tobacco-like undercurrent along with grape jelly and wintergreen. This odd combination does share aromatic compounds with tuberose. The tobacco, grape, and wintergreen scents are very subtle, but cause some people to dislike tuberose. It smells like eating a grape jelly and vanilla ice cream float made with Dr. Pepper soda (that is flavored with wintergreen), while in a greenhouse filled with exotic flowers, and having someone walk in smoking a pipe. As I said, the aroma is complex. It is recorded that the scent of hundreds of pots of tuberose perfumed the air so strongly in the gardens of the Grand Trianon during the reign of Louis XIV, that it sometimes forced the court inside.

Polianthes tuberosa 'The Pearl' produces twice the scent due to its double petals. This is the most common tuberose sold as a cut flower. Tuberose is both stimulating and relaxing, helping to treat insomnia, depression, and excessive anger. Like jasmine, it seems more hypnotic than sedative. In the Indian ayurvedic tradition, tuberose inspires serenity and creativity and is an aphrodisiac, worn often as a wedding garland. The scent is so powerful that young women in India and Europe were once told not to inhale its erotic perfume after dark, for fear that it might corrupt their morals.

Tuberose is one of the few flowers that produce fragrance after being picked, making it an especially long-lasting cut flower. Over nine pounds of the buds are needed to produce just one ounce of essential oil, making it a costly ingredient for perfume. However, many perfumes are dominated by tuberose, including classics such as Fracas, White Shoulders, Chloé, and Christian Dior's Poison, as well as more recent scents Tubéreuse Criminelle, Carnal Flower, and Flor Azteca. Tuberose is related to agave, extracts of which also scent perfume.

The pure white flowers clustered around an upright stem are particularly fragrant in the evening. Its East Indian name, *ratkirani*, translates as "queen of the night." In the garden, find a spot that you frequent in the evenings or that is near an open window to fully enjoy the scent. Plant tuberose away from other potent evening bloomers (such as flowering tobacco), where you can enjoy its singular fragrance. When it blooms in the evening it is pollinated by moths.

Curiously, this Mexican native has not been recorded as growing in the wild, but the popularity of its fragrance has kept it flourishing in cultivation. The plant needs very little light, so it makes a great houseplant. Plant the tubers in containers and cover with three inches of soil, then provide plenty of water during the growing season. Repot tuberose about every four years. In zone 9 and colder, the bulbs should be dried off and stored, then replanted in spring to grace the garden with blooms, year after year.

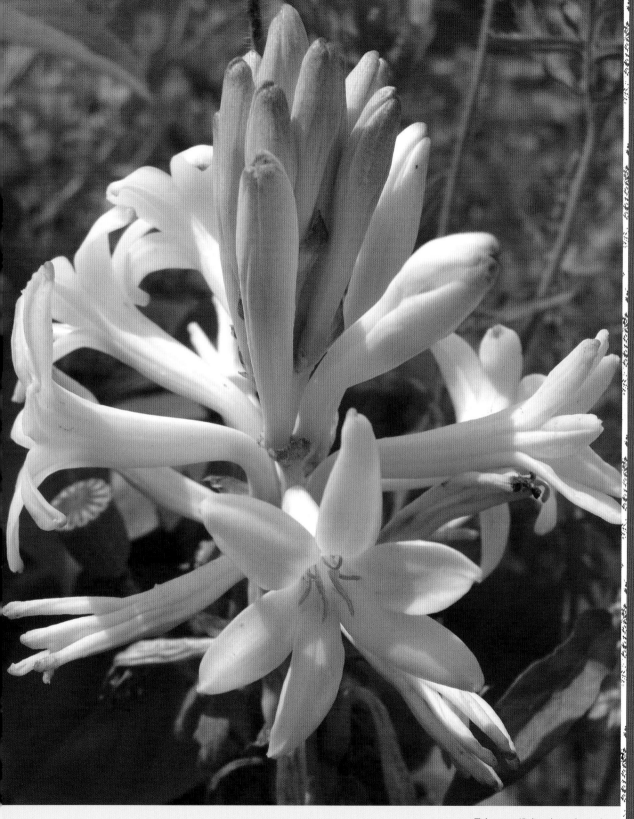

Tuberose (*Polianthes tuberosa*)

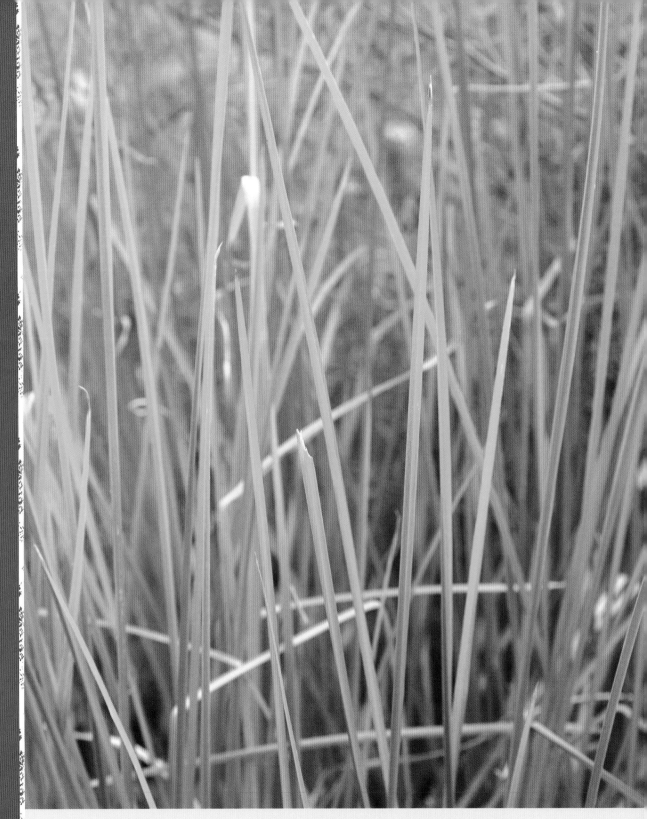

Vetiver (*Vetiveria zizanioides*)

Vetiver

Vetiveria zizanioides

Grass family: Poaceae
Tender perennial
Zones 9–11

Vetiver, with sharp, grass-like leaves that dry and curl, will never be voted the most picturesque specimen. The aboveground plant has no scent, so it gives little hint of the aroma that exists beneath. It is only when the roots are dug that their deep, rich fragrance is revealed. Perfumers accurately categorize it as woodsy and masculine, but it is much more. The heavy balsamic scent is so deeply earthy and musky that it is reminiscent of rich garden soil. It reminds me of digging deep into rich, composted garden soil on a warm summer day, surrounded by a garden in full bloom. If earth had a perfume, this would be it; however, this is not a scent for everyone. Once harvested, vetiver's aroma matures, becoming deeper, richer, and a little sweeter. When distilled, the essential oil actually becomes thicker. The oils I have had for several decades barely pour from the vials and have amazing fragrance, with added hints of vanilla and molasses.

In India, vetiver massage oil is called the "oil of tranquility" and recommended for anyone who feels nervous, anxious, or overly sensitive. However, researchers at Japan's Kyushu University reported in the scientific journal *Biomed Research* that small doses of vetiver fragrance actually stimulated the nervous system, causing faster reaction times in the brain. Just a few sniffs by participants enhanced their computer work. It seems to improve our eyes' ability to differentiate between objects. It is also said to cool down heated emotions. Indian screens called *khus-khus tatties* are woven from vetiver's thin roots, to place over doors and windows. They are sprayed with water to release the scent and cool the room. A vetiver fan can cool during summer's heat.

A touch of vetiver gives perfume a deep note that rounds out softer and more floral scents. It has been scenting men's cologne since British India began importing in the nineteenth century. Famous Victorian-era perfumes, such as Maréchale and Bouquet de Roi d'Anglettere, were based on its aroma. Indian muslin was also scented with vetiver to deter insects.

Vetiver is not a showpiece in the garden so looks best blended with small shrubs, such as the taller, tropical sages and lemon-scented marigold shrub. Plant it away from pathways, as the leaves are sharp and offer no aroma. Vetiver is not fussy about soil conditions, but it does grow best in dry regions. In its native India, and now in the United States, the extensive root system is helping reduce soil erosion on dry, barren hills. It is not easy to dig the thin, long roots because they grow deep and become entangled. With some effort, however, the root crown can be divided into separate plants. Roots can be dried whole.

Violet

Viola odorata

Violet family: Violaceae
Perennial
Zones 5–9

One inhalation and violet flowers fill your head with their soft yet penetrating, very sweet fragrance. Saint Thérèse of Lisieux said, "The splendor of the rose and the whiteness of the lily do not rob the little violet of its scent." The aroma is powdery and some might say enchanting. Violet's aroma also is elusive, probably because our noses only perceive it for a few moments. After that, we temporarily lose the ability to detect it at all, before it returns in its full glory. After stimulating scent receptors, a compound called ionone binds to the recptors to temporarily shut them off. William Shakespeare mentioned this effect in *Hamlet* as "sweet, not lasting, the perfume and suppliance of a minute . . . " Since the fragrance is there one moment and gone the next, violets are often associated with magic in children's stories. The leaves have their own very green aroma and are distilled into essential oil.

The aroma of most violet hybrids does not compare to that of the old-fashioned versions. One exception is the double-flowered, lightly colored, and heavily scented Parma violets from the Italian town of Parma, which is famous for its perfume. *Viola* 'Swanley White', 'Neapolitan', and 'Marie-Louise' are considered the most fragrant of the Parmas. Pansies (*V. tricolor*) rarely have much scent anymore. The best fragrance comes from the old-fashioned, smaller pansies in warm colors of orange, yellow, and red. Also known as heartsease, pansy is said to mend a broken heart and remind separated lovers of each other.

Violet's scent is relaxing, helping to temper anxiety and anger. Fragrant violet bouquets were carried into European and North American cemeteries to soothe the sorrow and as protection from poisonous air. Violets were important in ancient Rome, where Pliny the Elder suggested that wearing a crown of the flowers could dispel headaches, dizziness, and insomnia. Masses of violets scented entire banquet halls to create contentment during dinner parties. Roman spa patrons were served violet water before being given a massage with violet-infused oil, then wrapped in a linen blanket. A violet and goats' milk complexion cream made by the early Celts even doubled as a love potion. Due to their fleeting fragrance and nodding flowers, violets also came to represent humility and shyness in Europe and the Middle East.

Today, there are violet-scented body care products, soaps, and colognes, although most are made with the less expensive synthetic fragrance. Violet perfume and cut flowers were the rage for centuries. In France, the delicate fragrance scents and flavors sugar, syrups, ice, honey, candies, breath fresheners, and wine. After visiting Provence, France, the violet and lavender products tucked in my suitcase engulfed the customs officials when they opened it!

Violets have become a welcome weed in my garden as an attractive ground cover. The heart-shaped leaves nicely fill in gaps. They grow well in pots and window boxes. They can become invasive, but are easy to pull out unless they invade a chamomile or sweet woodruff bed. Violets are very easy to grow in woodland conditions with filtered shade and moisture. They prefer good soil, but tolerate almost anything. Feeding them very early in the spring encourages a heavy bloom.

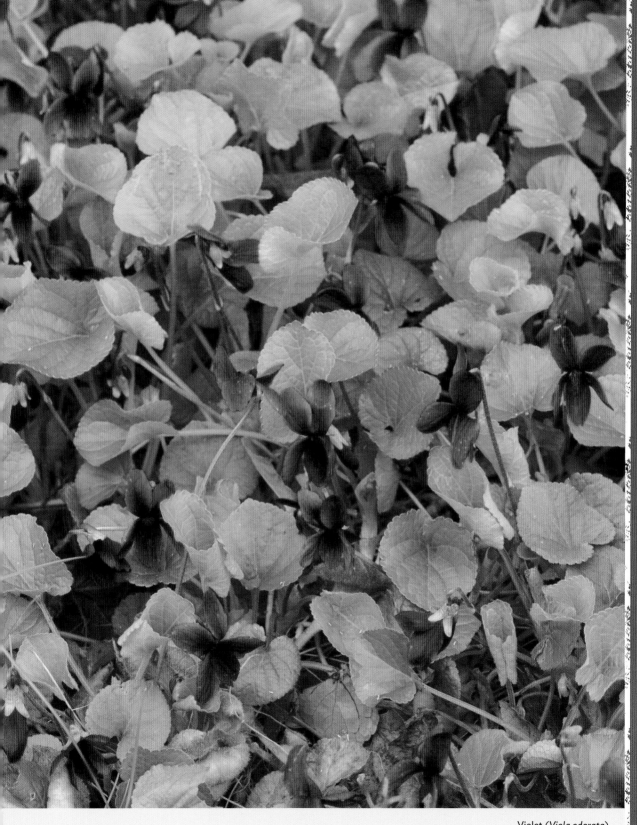

Violet (*Viola odorata*)

Wallflower

Erysimum cheiri

Mustard family: Brassicaceae
Perennial, usually grown as biennial
Zones 4–6

Wallflower's pervasive, sweet scent has the spiciness of cloves blended with a floral violet note. It smells like someone presented you with a mixed bouquet of violets and clove-pink carnations. It is no wonder that the plant is identified in French as *giroflée violier*, meaning "clove-violet"—similar to clove-pinks' old name, gilloflower, and the old English name, wall-violet. Most wallflowers sold in nurseries are so softly scented that their fragrance is more like baby powder.

Wallflowers symbolize happiness and affection, especially the devotion that survives over time and adversity. They are nicknamed the faithful flower and were carried by traveling troubadours to remind them of loved ones at home. Like other clove-scented plants, wallflowers contain the compound eugenol, which produces a happiness response and reduces stress by moderating neurotransmitters in the brain. Research at the Indian Institute of Technology, at Banaras Hindu University in Varanasi, showed that clove's aroma lessened mental fatigue and nervousness. According to China's Shaanxi University of Traditional Chinese Medicine, the scent seems to improve a poor memory. Most people find the smell of cloves very pleasant, although they appeal to women more than men. The nerve and muscle oil made from wallflowers has a pleasing, relaxing scent. An essential oil has been produced from wallflowers, but is so rare and expensive that it is only found in upscale perfumes.

Wallflower blooms are no longer as popular as they once were. However, their abundance of fragrance and jewel-like colors in the spring make them ideal for any cottage or fragrance garden.

Wallflower's short stature makes it good at the front of borders or in window boxes, where the aroma can waft into the house. An added bonus is that Baltimore checkerspot and tiger swallowtail butterflies as well as honeybees are attracted to the flowers.

This native of Turkey and the Mediterranean region likes well-drained, dry, alkaline soil that is not overly rich. If conditions are right, the flowers bloom so prolifically in the second and/or third year that the plants exhaust themselves after a few years and need to be replaced.

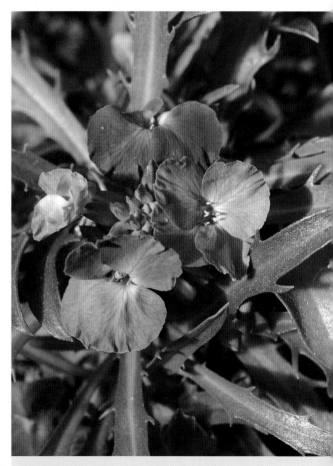

Wallflower (*Erysimum cheiri*)

Willow peppermint
Eucalyptus nicholii

Myrtle family: Myrtaceae
Tender perennial
Zones 8–10

Although a member of the genus *Eucalyptus*, willow peppermint is also called narrow-leaved black peppermint, and the essential oil is called peppermint gum, because it smells so much like peppermint. It is so sharp, you can immediately feel it in your sinuses. It reminds me of the peppermint-eucalyptus lozenges I've used for sore throats, or the vapor rub my mother used to put on my chest when I had a cold. Australia's blue forests are named for the blue haze produced by the essential oil from *Eucalyptus nicholii* floating in the air.

Over one hundred distinctly different scents have been identified in the many species and varieties. The mallee types grow only to about four feet tall. Willow peppermint's graceful, weeping stature is accented by narrow, pale green leaves. It is suited for cold climates, surviving temperatures down to freezing. However, it has to be planted in a dry climate with space for a tree that could grow twelve to twenty-five feet tall. *Eucalyptus parvula* has a strong eucalyptus scent and yields strongly flavored honey. Tasmanian blue gum (*E. globulus*), the most common eucalyptus, is a huge tree.

Both eucalyptus and peppermint are wake-up calls in the aromatherapy world. With the two scents combined, it is no surprise that this bush helps keep you alert. It helps with emotional imbalance and stress. Just a few sniffs can help with a headache or shock.

Findings presented at a conference of the British Psychological Society suggest that eucalyptol, the main compound in *Eucalyptus nicholii*, prevents an enzyme from breaking down a

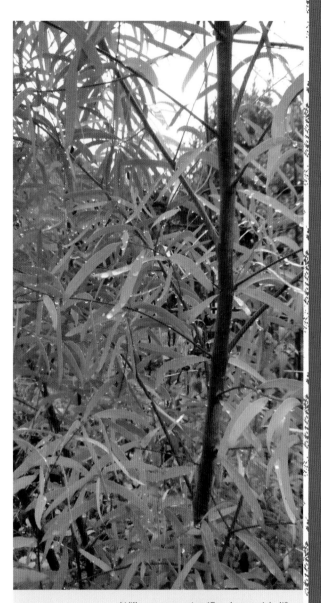

Willow peppermint (*Eucalyptus nicholii*)

memory-related neurotransmitter in the brain. Sniffing it also improves the ability to do mathematical calculations, but without being overstimulating to mind or body.

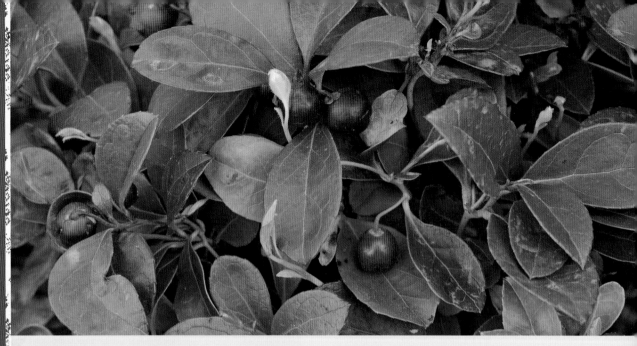

Wintergreen (*Gaultheria procumbens*)

Wintergreen

Gaultheria procumbens

Heath family: Ericaceae
Perennial
Zones 3–9

Wintergreen leaves have the aroma of anise, peppermint, and some general spiciness, all blended together. Smelling them reminds many people of wintergreen breath mints or toothpaste. To others, they carry the medicinal scent of liniments, mouthwashes, and syrups that use it for flavor—it is one of the scents and tastes in root beer. If you are familiar with the traditional men's cologne Russian Leather, then you know wintergreen's fragrance. The cologne became so popular that the Russian government kept the recipe a closely guarded secret for years, although it obviously had a distinctive wintergreen scent. It is a definite pick-me-up aroma, reminiscent of walking through a moist meadow filled with wild wintergreen. Iceland Wintergreen cologne perfumed handkerchiefs in the nine-teenth century. The essential oil is used by book-binders to keep leather soft and easier to work. It is also a popular fragrant tea, known as teaberry. Native Americans flavored smoking mixes with it. Wintergreen and birch have a surprisingly similar chemistry and aroma. Today, most so-called win-tergreen scent comes from birch trees, because they are larger and more abundant. A synthetic essential oil is based on methyl salicylate, the main aromatic compound in both plants.

Chinese wintergreen (*Gaultheria hookeri*) is a more heat-tolerant plant, and is gaining popular-ity in nurseries. Most of the true wintergreen essential oil comes from China.

Wintergreen is very attractive throughout the summer, with shiny leaves that almost look wet and white flowers that turn into bright, red ber-ries. It makes an excellent ground cover for shady areas, and the perfect companion plant for other shady ground covers, such as sweet woodruff. The plant does require a lot of water and fairly rich soil to keep it happy. Even though it has thick leaves, it prefers some humidity to match its ori-gins in the eastern and midwestern regions of North America.

Wintersweet

Chimonanthus praecox

Calycanthus family: Calycanthaceae
Shrub
Zones 7–10

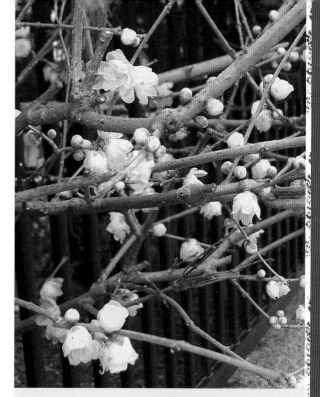

Wintersweet (*Chimonanthus praecox*)

Wintersweet (also known as Japanese allspice) is esteemed in Japan and its native China for its spicy fragrance and as an ornamental shrub. The scent contrasts hot, spicy, aromatic sensations with fresh, cool mint. That is topped with an elegant perfume that hints of orange blossom or perhaps jasmine. Wintersweet is aptly named since it does sweeten the winter air with its heady perfume. It has been infamous throughout China ever since the great Sung dynasty poet, Huang T'ing-chien, praised its fragrance.

Chimonanthus praecox 'Grandiflorus' and *C. praecox* 'Luteus' are Chinese varieties that received the Royal Horticultural Society's Award of Garden Merit. *Chimonanthus fragrans* was introduced over forty years ago to the perfume regions of Provence , France, to help supply the industry with unique materials. It has not been used much, but the expensive absolute occasionally finds its way into high-end perfume.

The flower is a traditional Chinese medicine to relieve fever and lung problems, and several other conditions. Chinese researchers reported in the *Journal of Medicinal Plants Research* that the aroma of *Chimonanthus salicifolius* may reduce anxiety and depression.The flowers are made into a highly scented tea. A popular green tea blend that contains the flower has a scent and flavor that is reminiscent of jasmine black tea. The flowers scent potpourri and sachets. The Chinese lay them among linens to scent them, much like lavender is used in the west. In addition, wintersweet makes a very fragrant floral arrangement.

The bush spends most of the year looking quite humble in the garden. Then January and February arrive and it lets loose a display of aromatic flowers. This is typically just in time for the Chinese New Year, allowing the fragrant flowers to become part of the celebration. Wintersweet takes center stage in the fragrance garden, blooming at a time when other plants are dormant and offer little competition. To make up for the lack of pollinating insects in the winter, the flower pollinates itself by having the five stamens fold themselves over the stigma. Wintersweet is prized in Chinese fragrance gardens. Growing ten to fifteen feet tall, the many stems emerging from the base are deciduous. The fragrant, small, translucent flowers borne on these leafless branches have been gracing winter gardens for over a thousand years. Wintersweet's cultivation was first described in China's twelfth-century *Fancun meipu* treatise. Give it full sun with a sufficient amount of water and the flowers will happily last for over a month. The plant adapts to either alkaline or acid soil and does require some winter cold. Propagate it through cutting.

Witch hazel

Hamamelis virginiana

Witch hazel family: Hamamelidaceae
Shrub
Zones 3–8

These deciduous ten-foot-tall shrubs have bright fall foliage, and yellow to red nodding flower clusters in winter, giving the North American species the name winterbloom. The scent is a sweet, intoxicating lemon. Ozark witch hazel (*Hamamelis vernalis*) and the intermedia hybrids from crosses between Japanese and Chinese species have the best fragrance. Witch hazel grows in full or partial sun.

Wormwood

Artemisia absinthium

Aster family: Asteraceae
Perennial
Zones 4–9

Wormwood's dry, bitter smell and taste characterize the genus *Artemisia*. The species name "absinthium" is a Roman word that even means "bitter." The nose-tickling aroma is pungent, musty, and very sharp, but with a small amount of sweetness. When the people on my garden tours sniff it, they typically pull back their nose rather than diving in for more. Yet, there is something enticing.

Other species share a similar aroma to *Artemisia absinthium*. Mugwort (*Artemisia vulgaris*) leaves are dried for dream pillows. Chinese mugwort (*A. argyi*) is dried, powdered, and formed into moxa cones that acupuncturists burn and use to treat an area with aromatic heat instead of needles. Sagebrush (*A. tridentata*) provides gardens in dry, hot climates with the pungent fragrance of western deserts. Sweet wormwood (*A. annua*), also called *quighaosu* or artemisinin, has a sweeter aroma and is beautiful in fragrant wreaths, although it is rarely used since the strong scent causes so many people to sneeze. It has gained medicinal interest as a treatment for malaria.

Researchers at Saint Louis University School of Medicine in Missouri found that the thujone compound in wormwood's essential oil stimulates brain activity; they suspect it may interact with the same receptors as marijuana. This may account for the popularity of the wormwood drink, absinthe, among nineteenth-century French expressionistic artists, such as Vincent van Gough, Henri de Toulouse-Lautrec, and Eugene (Paul) Gauguin. Vermouth and the Italian wine Cinzano owe their uniquely bitter smell and taste to small amounts of wormwood. However, its use is restricted in most countries, because thujone is considered a brain and nervous system toxin at high levels, and may induce epileptic seizures. According to Wroclaw Medical University in Poland, the thujone compound in wormwood appears to stimulate the brain by reducing GABA activity, helping the mind stay sharp and alert. The name is probably derived from the Anglo Saxon *wermode*, meaning "mind preserver." Churchgoing women once carried nosegays of it mixed with southernwood and lemon balm, to avoid nodding off during services.

Tarragon (*Artemisia dracunculus*) is a common flavoring that does not produce seed and is treated as an annual in many locations. French queen Marie Antoinette had her ladies-in-waiting wear kid gloves when they harvested it, so none of the precious scent would be lost on their hands. Wormwood's bitterness represents love and commitment through adversity. Saint Francis de Sales wrote in the seventeenth century, "To

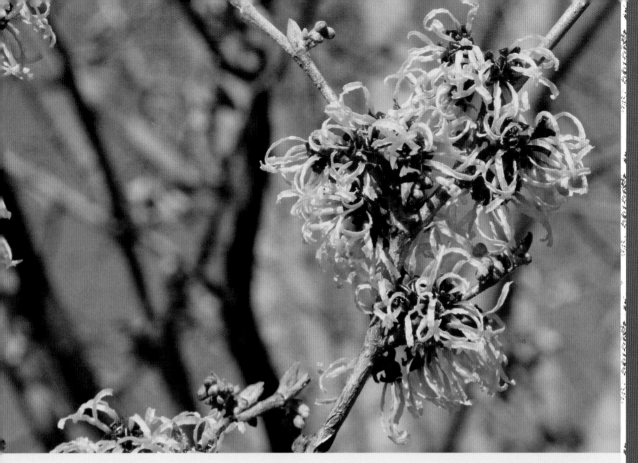
Witch hazel (*Hamamelis virginiana*)

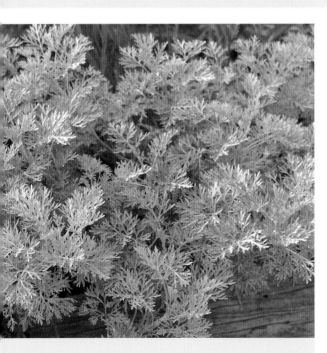
'Powis Castle' wormwood (*Artemisia absinthium* 'Powis Castle')

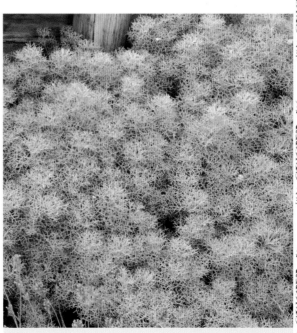
'Silver Mound' wormwood
(*Artemisia schmidtiana* 'Silver Mound')

love in the midst of sweets, little children could do that, but to love in the bitterness of wormwood is a sure sign of our affectionate fidelity."

Small amounts go into potpourri, but that is more for wormwood's attractive gray leaves than for the aroma. The dried leaves lend an attractive smell and look to herb wreaths, although they are brittle. They are also an effective moth and flea repellent, and in earlier times were spread on house floors as an insecticidal strewing herb and room freshener—although many favored the slightly sweeter southernwood. North African Bedouin tribes burn the dried leaves as incense to ensure the health of newborns, and place the rolled leaves in their nostrils as a decongestant inhaler.

Wormwood provides the garden with a contrasting gray color and interesting texture and aroma. The plant has a tendency to sprawl, so use it as the middle section in a border garden, as edging or the background to a bed of low-growing plants, or in the center of a bed as the main attraction. Plant it next to darker-colored plants, or go for a striking, all-gray section in the garden that will capture everyone's attention and seem to glow in the moonlight. Wormwood does not always produce its tiny flowers or viable seed. Propagate it through root divisions, cuttings, or especially with layering, since it readily sprouts from stems laying on the ground. The leaves, and probably the roots, exude a substance that restricts growth of neighboring plants (especially culinary herbs, such as thymes and mints), so allow wormwood plenty of space.

Yarrow
Achillea millefolium

Aster family: Asteraceae
Perennial
Zones 4–8

Yarrow's bitter aroma is reminiscent of wormwood, tickling the back of the nose. The old English name, sneezewort, is appropriate. Its pungency makes many people pull back the first time they smell it. Yarrow's aroma also contains camphor-like and musty components, along with a sense of chamomile, although any sweetness is overridden by the bitterness. The aroma of yarrow in the garden air on a hot day remains pungent, but it is far more herby and pleasant than sticking your nose into the plant.

The one hundred or so yarrow species come in a selection of colors and sizes. Many of these share the same, distinctive aroma. *Achillea millefolium* 'Cerise Queen' and *A. millefolium* f. *rosea* are rosy colored varieties, while 'Paprika' has a vivid reddish color. Fern-leaf yarrow (*A. filipendulina*) has brilliant, golden-yellow flowers on four- to five-foot stems. *Achillea* 'Coronation Gold' and 'Gold Plate' are common cultivars. Noble yarrow (*A. nobilis*) tends to be one of the most aromatic, although with a strong camphor smell. *Achillea ptarmica* has fine-toothed leaves and a touch of licorice, so it almost resembles tarragon and has been used in salads. Mace yarrow (*A. decolorans*) is less common, but has the attractive, spicy scent of that kitchen spice. Woolly yarrow (*A. tomentosa*) is short with fern-like leaves and golden flowers—ideal in rock gardens and fragrant lawns. *Achillea tomentosa* 'Aurea' is a favored cultivar.

The aroma of yarrow is linked with healing both emotional and physical wounds. It is also an insect repellent. Yarrow beer is still made

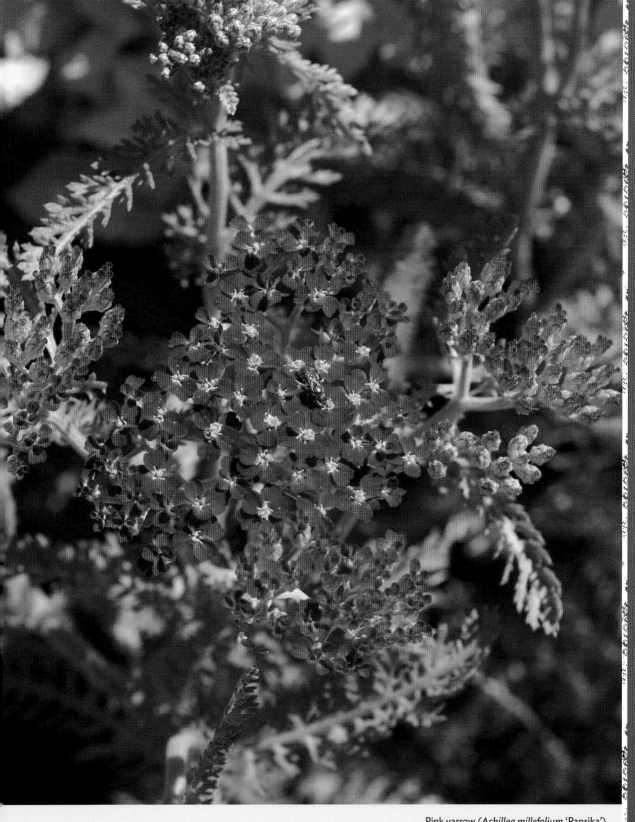

Pink yarrow (*Achillea millefolium* 'Paprika')

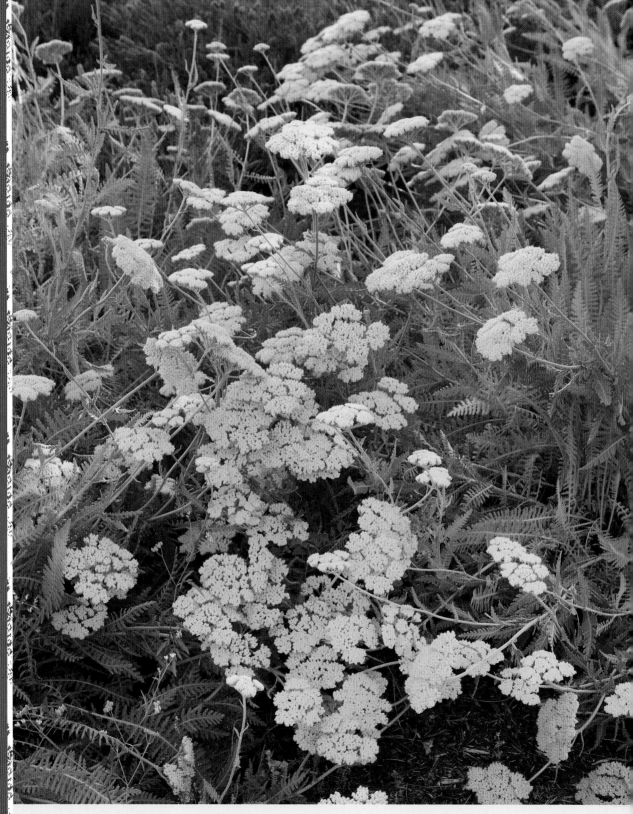

'Coronation Gold' yarrow (*Achillea* 'Coronation Gold')

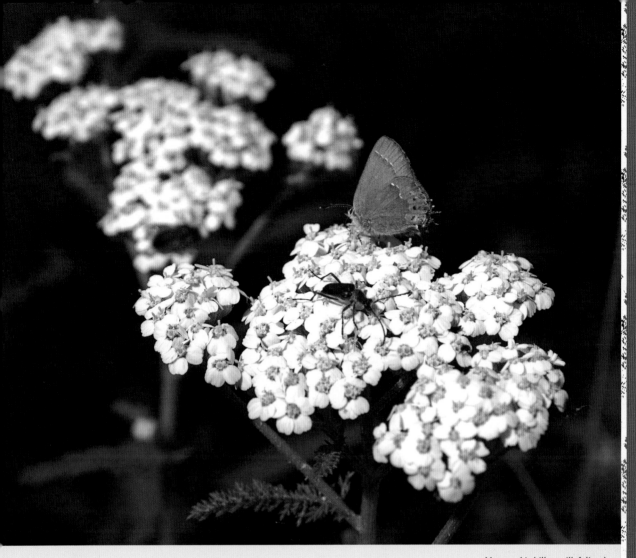

Yarrow (*Achillea millefolium*)

commercially in Sweden, where it is considered more intoxicating than beer containing hops. It scents some tobaccos and snuffs. Yarrow is striking in either fresh or dried flower arrangements.

I like to see informal, colorful clumps of yarrow, so the flat flower heads carry the eye here and there in the garden. It also makes beautiful large patches for a colorful, long-lasting display. After a few years, yarrow patches begin to die back and may need replanting. Keeping them fertilized slows this process. They are lush in rich ground, but are not fussy about soil. This may be why yarrow can be found in North America, Europe, and Western Asia. The plants tolerate some shade, but prefer sun. The plant exudes a substance around its perimeter to increase its disease resistance, as well as that of nearby plants, but the trade-off is inhibited seed germination.

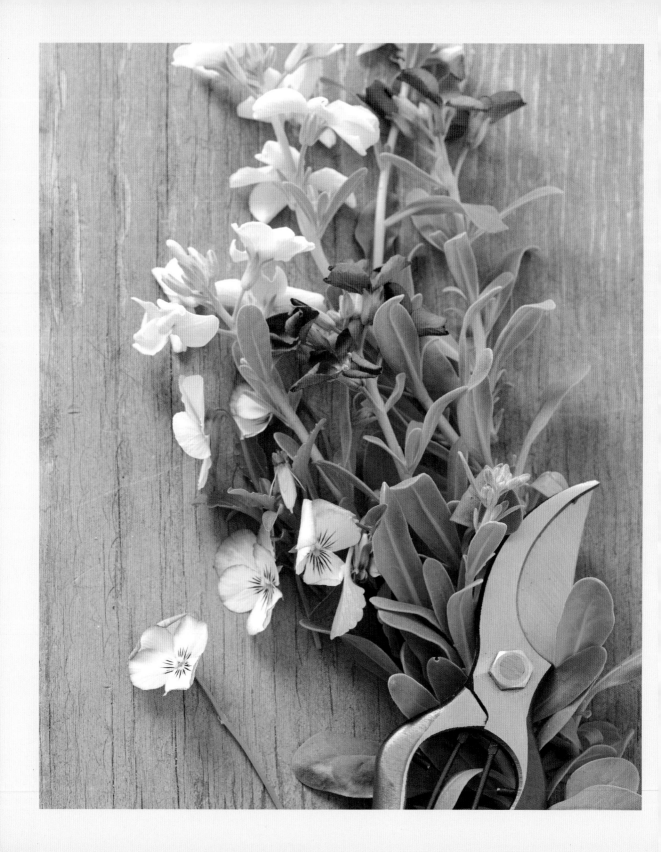

acknowledgments

Working with Juree Sondker and Julie Talbot of the Timber Press staff has been wonderful. Timber Press books have been teaching me about gardening for over two decades. Thank you to Karen Callahan and Caitlin Atkinson for photographing my garden and to Prospector and Weiss Brothers nurseries and the San Francisco Botanical Garden for allowing a photographer to ramble about. My sister, Janna Buesch, lent her wonderful knack for research backed by a passion for gardening. Herbal author and editor Beth Baugh offered helpful suggestions and constant support.

I had the pleasure of benefiting from the knowledge of extraordinary nursery people. In California, these are Rose Loveall-Sale of Morningsun Herb Farm in Vacaville, Deborah Wigham of Digging Dog Nursery in Albion, Kathy Horner of Prospector's Nursery in Nevada City, and Linnie McNaughton of Peaceful Valley Farm Supply in Grass Valley. In Oregon, they are Rebecca Chance of Dancing Oaks Nursery in Monmouth, and Rico Cech of Horizon Herbs and Jim and Dotti Becker of Goodwin Creek Gardens, both in Williams. I was also assisted by Don Mahoney, head curator at the San Francisco Botanical Garden.

A special thank-you to the gardeners and gardens that have inspired me along the way—you with your sunburned noses, dirty fingernails, and a smile on your face as you balance a potted plant on your hip. My garden hat goes off to Tim Blakely at Aura Cacia, Virginia and Louis Saso, who owned Saso Herb Gardens, and all the many good gardening folks at the International Herb Association and the Herb Society of America. Plant on! I also appreciate the support of friends and family who helped with gardens, pets, and classes as I focused on creating this book.

◁ There is nothing more rewarding than collecting some of the sweet smells of the garden.

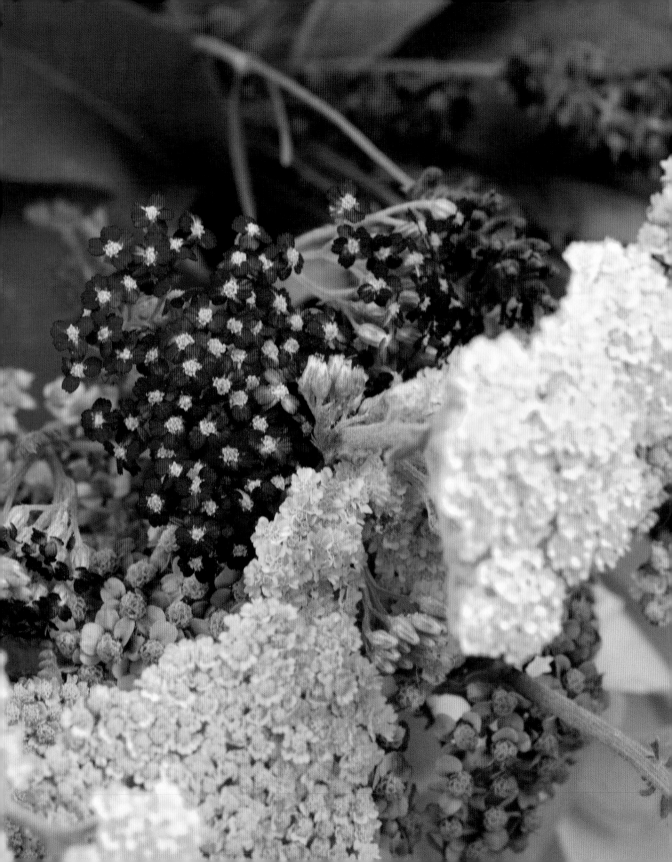

resources

aromatherapy and essential oil resources

ASSOCIATIONS, JOURNALS, AND ONLINE SITES

American Herb Association
ahaherb.com

Journal: *American Herb Association Quarterly.* Special issues on herb gardening, aromatherapy, ethnobotany, Asian herbs, and clinical herbalism.

American Herbalists Guild
americanherbalistsguild.com

United Plant Savers
www.unitedplantsavers.org

Online aromatherapy resources
Aromatherapy Today, aromatherapytoday.com

Aromatherapy Trade Council (UK), a-t-c.org.uk

Canadian Federation of Aromatherapists, cfacanada.com

Herbal Gram, herbalgram.org

holisticmed.com, www.aromatherapy.html

International Federation of Aromatherapists, ifaroma.org

International Journal of Clinical Aromatherapy, ijca.net

International Journal of Essential Oil Therapies, ijeot.com

International Journal of Professional Holistic Aromatherapy, ijpha.com

Journal of International Aromatherapy & Aromatic Medicine Association Inc. (Australia),iaama.org.au/journal/journal

National Association for Holistic Aromatherapy, naha.org

PubMed: www.ncbi.nlm.nih.gov/pubmed

BOOKS

Al-Samarqandi. 1967. *The Medical Formulary* (13th Century) Reprint. Oxford: Oxford University Press.

Atal and Kapur, eds. 1982. *Cultivation and Utilization of Aromatic Plants.* India: Regional Research Lab, Council of Scientific & Industrial Research.

Bauer, Kurt, Dorothea Garbe, and Horst Surburg. 1990. *Common Fragrance and Flavor Materials.* Weinheim, Germany: Wiley-VCH.

Beckstrom-Sternberg, Steven, and James Duke. 1996. *Handbook of Medicinal Mints (Aromathematics): Phytochemicals and Biological Activities.* New York: CRC Press.

Brenzel, Kathleen. 2000. *Sunset Western Garden Book.* CA: Sunset Books Inc.

Craker, Lyle, and James Simon, eds. 1986. *Herbs, Spices and Medicinal Plants: Recent Advances in Botany, Horticulture, and Pharmacy.* Vols. 1–3. Phoenix: Oryx Press.

Dickerson, Brent. 1999. *The Old Rose Adventurer: The Once-Blooming Old European Roses and More*. Portland, OR: Timber Press.

Dorland, Gabrielle. 1993. *Scents Appeal: The Silent Persuasion of Aromatic Encounters*. Medham, NJ: Wayne Dorland Co.

Dugo, Giovanni, and Angelo Di Giacomo. 2002. *Citrus*. NY: CRC Press.

Engen, Trygg. 1982. *The Perception of Odors*. NY: Academic Press/ Elsevier.

Genders, Roy. 1972. *Perfume Through the Ages*. NY: Putnam.

Gerard, John. 1636. *The Herball, or Generall Historie of Plants* (1597). Enlarged by Thomas Johnson.

Gilbert, Avery N., and Charles J. Wysocki. 1987. The Smell Survey Results. *National Geographic 172:* 514–25.

Grieve, Maude. 1971. *A Modern Herbal*. NY: Dover Publications.

Guenther, Ernest. 1972. *The Essential Oils*, Vols. 1-4. Malobar, FL: Robert E. Krieger Publications.

Hildegard. 1987. *Manuscript* (12th century). Reprint. NM: Bear & Co.

Hirsch, Alan. 1998. *Scentsational Sex*. Boston, MA: Element Books.

Hobhouse, Penelope. 1992. *Plants in Garden History*. London: Pavilion Books.

Kintziols, Spiridon. 2002. *Oregano: The Genera Orianum and Lippia*. NY: CRC Press.

Landing, James E. 1969. *American Essence: History of the Peppermint and Spearmint Industry in the U.S.* Kalamazoo, MI: Kalamazoo Public Museum.

Langenheim, Jean. 2003. *Plant Resins: Chemistry, Evolution, Ecology, and Ethnobotany*. Portland, OR: Timber Press.

Lawrence, Brian. 2008. *Peppermint Oil*. Carol Stream, IL: Allured Press.

Lawton, Barbara. 2002. *Mints: A Family of Herbs and Ornamentals*. Portland, OR: Timber Press.

LeGuerer, Annick. 1992. *Scent: The Mysterious and Essential Powers of Smell*. NY: Turtle Bay Books.

Leung, Albert. 1983. *Encyclopedia of Common Natural Ingredients used in Food, Drugs, and Cosmetics*. NY: Wiley-Interscience.

Lis-Balchin, Maria. 2002. *Geranium and Pelargonium*. NY: CRC Press.

Lis-Balchin, Maria. 2002. *Lavender: The Genus Lavandula*. NY: CRC Press.

Maffei, Massimo. 2002.*Vetiveria: The Genus Vetiveris*. NY: CRC Press.

Morris, Edwin. 1984.*Fragrance: The Story of Perfume from Cleopatra to Chanel*. NY: Charles Scribner's Sons.

Parry, Ernest. 1918.*The Chemistry of Essential Oils and Artificial Perfumes*. Vols. 1–2. London: Scott, Greenwood and Son.

Piesse, G. W. Septimus. 1856. *The Art of Perfumery and Method of Obtaining the Odors of Plants*. Philadelphia: Lindsay and Blakiston.

Pizzetti, Ippolito, and Henry Cocker Pizzetti. 1968. *Flowers: A Guide for Your Garden*. NY: Harry N. Abrams, Inc.

Poucher, William. 1926. *Perfumes, Cosmetics and Soaps*. NY: D. Van Nostrand Company.

Ravindran, P. N., and K. J. Madhusoodanan. 2002. *Cardamom*. NY: CRC Press.

Rimmel, Eugene. 1865. *The Book of Perfumes*. London: Chapman & Hall.

School of Salernum. 1870. *Regimen Saanitatis Salernitanum* (14th century). Reprint. Philadelphia: JB Lippincott and Co.

Stahl-Bisup, Elisabeth, and Francisco Sáez. 2002. *Thyme: The Genus Thymus*. NY: CRC Press.

Thacker, Christopher. 1979. *The History of Gardens*. Oakland, CA: University of California Press.

Theophrastus. 1916. *Enquiry Into Plants: Concerning Odours* (4th century BC). Reprint. Sir Arthur Hort, Trans. London: W. Heinemann Publisher.

Tisserand, Robert. 1988. *The Essential Oil Safety Data Manual*. Brighton, England: Aromatherapy Publications.

Tucker, Arthur and Thomas Debaggio. 2009. *The Encyclopedia of Herbs*. Portland, OR: Timber Press.

Upson, Tim, and Susyn Andrews. 2004. *The Genus Lavandula*. Portland, OR: Timber Press.

Van Toller, Steve, and George H. Dodd. 1990. *Perfumery: The Psychology and Biology of Fragrance*. NY: Springer Publications.

Wilder, Louise Beebe. 1974. *The Fragrant Garden: A Book About Sweet Scented Flowers and Leaves* (*The Fragrant Path*, 1932). NY: Dover Publications.

Williams, David. 1996. *The Chemistry of Essential Oils*. Port Washington, NY: Micelle Press.

Wright, Colin. 2002. *Artemisia*. NY: CRC Press.

botanical gardens with fragrance sections

UNITED STATES

Atlanta Botanical Garden, Atlanta, Georgia
atlantabotanicalgarden.org

Japanese, Rose, and Edible gardens. Interpretive botany, ecology, and nutrition exhibits. Fuqua Orchid Center and Orangerie with tropical and medicinal plants.

Brooklyn Botanic Garden, Brooklyn, New York
bbg.org

Japanese, Rose, Children's, Shakespeare, Herb, Native Flora gardens; lilac, magnolia, orchid, and rose collections; and the Steinhardt Conservatory Starr Bonsai Museum. The Fragrance Garden, created in 1955 by landscaper Alice Recknagel Ireys, was the first braille garden in the United States and is wheelchair-accessible.

Chicago Botanic Garden, Chicago, Illinois
chicagobotanic.org

Rose, Children's, and Native Plant gardens. The Sensory Garden is experienced through smell, sound, sight, and feel.

Cleveland Botanical Garden, Cleveland, Ohio
cbgarden.org

Children's gardens. Elizabeth and Nona Evans Restorative Garden features mints and the calming scents of lavender and geranium. Western Reserve Herb Society Herb Garden has fragrance, rose, knot, culinary, medicinal, terrace, and edible flower sections.

**Fort Worth Botanic Garden,
Fort Worth, Texas**
fwbg.org

Rose, native, and fragrance gardens.

**Golden Gate Park,
San Francisco, California**
golden-gate-park.com/conservatory-
of-flowers.html

Conservatory of Flowers, with tropical plants.

**Lewis Ginter Botanical Garden,
Henrico, Virginia**
lewisginter.org/

*Rose, Children's, Edible Display, Asian Valley,
Healing, and Sunken gardens; a semi-tropical
conservatory.*

**Los Angeles County Arboretum and
Botanic Garden, Arcadia, California**
arboretum.org

Rose and herb gardens; tropical greenhouses.

**Missouri Botanical Garden,
St. Louis, Missouri**
missouribotanicalgarden.org

*Zimmerman Sensory Garden (with scented
flowers and spicy herbs); Gladney Rose Garden;
Maze; Glass Observatory; and Kemper Center for
Home Gardening, with twenty-three display
gardens, including butterfly, children's, fragrance,
and herb gardens.*

**San Francisco Botanical Garden,
San Francisco, California**
sfbotanicalgarden.org

*Garden of Fragrance (with terraces for the
visually impaired)*

CANADA AND MEXICO

**Butchart Gardens,
Brentwood Bay, B.C., Canada**
butchartgardens.com

Rose Garden.

**Montreal Botanical Garden,
Montreal, Quebec, Canada**
espacepourlavie.ca/en/botanical-garden

*First Nations, Monastery, Medicinal Plants, and
Rose gardens, and Courtyard of the Senses that
includes fragrant plants.*

**Vallarta Botanical Gardens,
Cabo Corrientes, Jalisco, Mexico**
vbgardens.org

*Orchid and Vanilla House and tropical dry
forest biome.*

invasive plant resources

invasivespeciesinfo.gov/unitedstates/state.
shtml

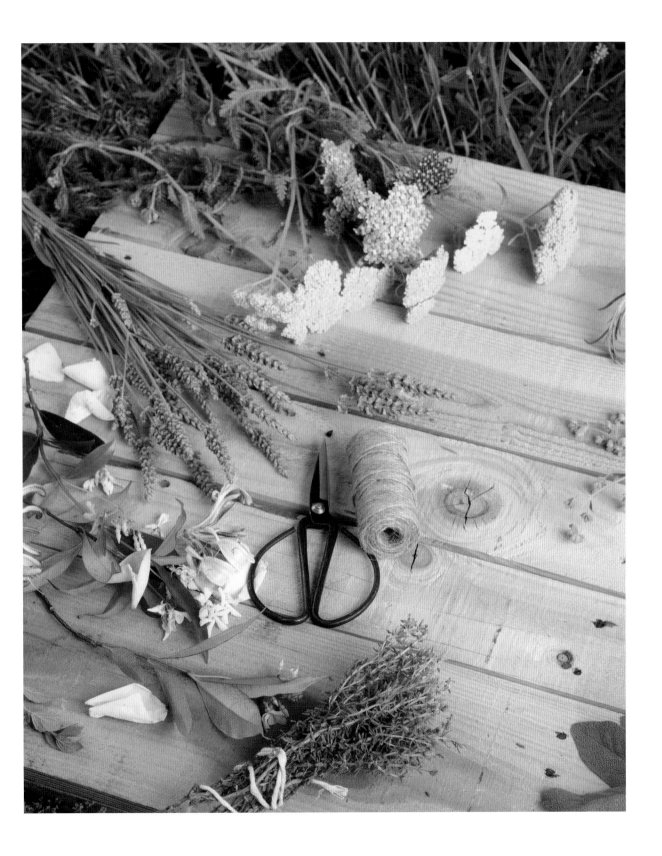

metric conversions

inches	cm
¼	0.6
½	1.3
¾	1.9
1	2.5
2	5.1
3	7.6
4	10
5	13
6	15
7	18
8	20
9	23
10	25
20	51
30	76
40	100
50	130
60	150
70	180
80	200
90	230
100	250

feet	m
1	0.3
2	0.6
3	0.9
4	1.2
5	1.5
6	1.8
7	2.1
8	2.4
9	2.7
10	3
20	6
30	9
40	12
50	15
60	18
70	21
80	24
90	27
100	30

temperatures

$°C = 5/9 \times (°F - 32)$

$°F = (9/5 \times °C) + 32$

photography and illustration credits

Photography

MychkoAlezander /iStock, page 119

Caitlin Atkinson, pages 12, 13, 17, 19 bottom, 33 left, 37 left, 42, 61 bottom right, 63, 64 bottom right, 67, 72, 97, 98, 100, 101 bottom, 103, 104, 105, 106, 108, 109, 114, 131, 143, 153, 168, 173 bottom, 192, 193 bottom, 198, 202, 207, 213 bottom, 214, 219, 221 bottom right, 230, 237, 244, 258.

Ron Bertolucci, page 61 top

bgwalker/iStock, page 126

brytta/iStock, page 233

Karen Callahan, pages 8, 19 top, 20–21, 23, 25 top, 27, 29, 31, 33 right, 35, 36, 41, 48–49, 50, 52, 53, 54, 55, 56, 57, 58, 61 left, 62, 64 top and left, 66, 68, 70, 74, 76, 77, 79, 82–83, 88, 89, 90, 94 top, 101 top, 115, 116, 120, 123, 125, 127, 130, 32, 136–137, 139, 140, 144, 148, 149, 151, 155, 156, 149, 164, 167, 171, 174, 177, 181, 182, 184, 185, 187, 189, 191, 193 top, 195, 196, 197, 199, 201, 205, 206, 209, 210, 211, 216, 218, 221 top and left, 222, 223, 225, 227, 234, 235, 239, 247, 248, 250, 253 bottom left and right, 255, 256, 257, 268

Frank Leung/ iStock, page 25 bottom

Robert Mabic/GAP Photos, page 86

Skye McNeill, page 46

Sarah Milhollin, pages 2–3, 6–7, 10, 92, 112, 260, 265

nosnibor137/Bigstock, page 81

Mary Beth Rich, page 162

shef–time/iStock, page 241

Studio Barcelona/Shutterstock, page 111

Tommy Tonsberg/GAP Photos, page 194

FLICKR

Used under a Creative Commons Attribution 2.0 Generic license
Swaminathan, page 243

WIKIMEDIA

Used under a Creative Commons Attribution–Share Alike 2.0 Generic license
Chrumps, page 173

Einwohner, page 43

Jengod, page 134

Miwasatoshi, page 129

Used under a Creative Commons Attribution–Share Alike 2.5 Generic license
Aka, page 224

Eric Hunt, page 213

Used under a Creative Commons Attribution–Share Alike 3.0 Unported license
Captain–tucker, page 45 bottom

Bff, page 152

Jean–Pol GRANDMONT, page 161

Christian Fischer, page 229

KENPEI, page 251

Si Griffiths, page 253 top

Released into the Public Domain
Albert Jankowski, page 15

Javier martin, page 169

All other photographs are by the author.

Illustrations

WIKIMEDIA

Released into the Public Domain
Otto Wilhelm Thomé (1840–1925), page 39

Jan Saenredam (1565–1607), page 45 top

index

L

labdanum, 211
lad's love, 224
lamb's ears, 68, 172–173
Larrea tridentata, 69
Lathyrus odoratus, 232–233
    'Annie B. Gilroy', 232
    'Cuthbertson', 232
    'High Scent', 232
    'Matucanas', 232
    'Old Spice', 232
Lathyrus tuberosus, 232
Laurus nobilis, 124–126
lavandin, 175, 177
Lavandula angustifolia, 117, 174–177
    'Compacta Nana', 175
    'Hidcote', 174, 175
    'Hidcote Giant', 175
    'Jean Davis', 175
    'Maillette', 175
    'Munstead', 175
    'Rosea', 175
    'Twinkle Purple', 175
Lavandula dentata, 175
Lavandula ×ginginsii, 175
Lavandula hetrophylla, 175
Lavandula ×intermedia, 175, 177
    'Alba', 176
    'Edelweiss', 175
    'Grosso', 175
    'Impress Purple', 175
    'Provence', 175
'Super', 176
Lavandula latifolia, 175
Lavandula stoechas, 175, 177
lavender, 9, 53, 56, 95, 96, 107, 109,
    115, 174–177
The Lavender Lover's Handbook
    (McNaughton), 175
lavender-rose anti-inflammation
    oil, 111
Lawrence, Brian, 78
Lawton, Barbara Perry, 204
layering stems, 87–88
leaves, 16
lemon, 178–180
lemon balm, 56, 65, 128, 180–181

lemon basil, 19
lemon bee balm, 126, 127
lemon catnip, 133
lemon grass, 182–183
lemon marigold, 192
lemon-scented basil, 122
lemon thyme, 238
lemon verbena, 53, 184–186
licorice mint hyssop, 121
light-colored flowers, 55–56
light-fragrance plantings, 53–54
lilac, 186–187
Lilium, 'African Queen', 198
Lilium auratum, 198
Lilium candidum, 198
Lilium lankongense, 199
Lilium leucanthum var. *centifolium*,
    198
Lilium orientalis, 198–199
    'Stargazer', 198, 199
Lilium speciosum, 198
lily-of-the-valley, 55, 188–189
limbic system, 14
lime thyme, 65, 239
linalool, 18, 238
Linnaeus, Carl, 14, 15
liqueurs, 42
liquid fertilizer, 75, 82, 85, 87
Lisbon lemon, 178
Lonicera fragrantissima, 168
    'Repens', 168
Lonicera japonica, 168
Lonicera periclymenum, 168
Los Angeles County Arboretum
    and Botanic Garden, 19, 66

M

mace yarrow, 254
madonna lily, 198
maggots, 26
Magnolia virginiana, 69
Maier, Kathleen, 68
Malcomia maritima, 225
manzanilla, 134
marjoram, 54, 190–191
massage oils, 111
mastic thyme, 238

Matricaria recutita, 134
Matthiola incana, 225–226
Matthiola longipetala, 225
McNaughton, Virginia, 175
mealy moths, 100
Mediterranean-climate plants, 73,
    74, 78, 80, 91
Melissa officinalis, 180–181
    'Aurea', 180
    'Lime Balm', 180
    'Variegata', 180
memory, 14, 30, 32, 34
Mentha aquatica
    'Banana', 204
    'Citrata', 204
    'Lime', 204
Mentha gentilis 'Variegata', 204
Mentha ×piperita, 204–205
Mentha ×piperita f. *citrata*
    'Chocolate', 204
Mentha ×piperita f. *citrata*
    'Grapefruit', 204
Mentha pulegium, 204
Mentha requienii, 204
Mentha spicata, 204
Mentha suaveolens, 204
menthol, 195
methyl salicylate, 250
Metropolitan Museum of Art, 42
Mexican giant hyssop, 121
Mexican marigold, 13, 192
Mexican orange flower, 192–193
Meyer lemon, 178
mignonette, 194
Milbert's tortoiseshell, 24
milkweed, 69
millefleurs, 42
Miller, Diana, 212
mint, 91
Mints (Lawton), 204
mint shrub, 195
mixed-fragrance plantings, 53
mock orange, 193, 196
A Modern Herbal (Grieve), 9
Monarda citriodora, 126, 127
    subsp. *austromontana*, 126
Monarda clinopodia, 126

Phlox divaricata, 206
Phlox paniculata, 206
    'Blue Paradise', 206
    'Bright Eyes', 206
    'Junior Dream', 206
    'Nicky', 206
    'Orange Perfection', 206
    'Tiara Flame', 206
Phlox subulata, 206
phosphorus, 75
Piesse, G. W. Septimus, 14
pineapple sage, 207
pink yarrow, 255
plant height, 59
plant origins, 73
plant shape, 59
poet's daffodil, 208–209
poet's jasmine, 169
Pogostemon benghalensis, 203
Pogostemon cablin, 202–203
Pogostemon heyneanus, 203
Polianthes tuberosa, 242–243
    'The Pearl', 242
Poliomintha incana, 69
pollen, 22
pollinators, 18, 19–20, 22–26, 53
potassium, 74–75
potato beetles, 27
pot marjoram, 190
potpourri, 107–108
potpourri pillows, 32
potted plants, 89–91
potting soil, 84, 85, 87
powdered herbs, 102
'Powis Castle' wormwood, 253
predators, 16, 18, 19–20, 26, 68
preserving/storing, 99–100, 106
primrose, 36, 210
Primula florindae, 210
Primula sikkimensis, 210
Primula veris, 210
Primula vialli, 210
Primula vulgaris, 210
propagation, 84–88
Prostanthera rotundifolia, 195
Proust phenomenon, 34
purple basil, 19, 123
purple giant hyssop, 121

puzzalina, 192
puzzola, 192
Pycnanthemum virginianum, 69

Q

quighaosu, 252

R

rainfall, 78
raised beds, 60
ratkirani, 242
red angel's trumpet, 240
Redouté, Pierre-Joseph, 44
regional natives gardens, 68–69
religious gardens, 38
Reseda odorata, 194
rhizomes, 88, 96
Rhododendron canescens, 69
Ribes odoratum, 69
Rimmel, Eugene, 14
R. K. Bliss & Sons, 44
rockrose, 211
rockwork, 60, 61
Roman chamomile, 62, 134, 135
Roman gardens, 39, 40
root development, 75, 86, 87, 88
root division, 88
rooting hormone powder, 87
rooting mix, 86–87
Rosa centifolia, 148, 149
Rosa ×damascena, 148–149
    var. *semperflorens*, 149
Rosa moschata, 148
rose, 29, 34, 39, 42. *See also* damask
    rose
rose (aromatic compound), 18
rose geranium, 212–213
rosemary, 9, 33, 50, 53, 105,
    215–217
Rosmarinus officinalis, 215–217
Royal Horticultural Society's
    Award of Garden Merit
    Chimonanthus praecox 'Grandi-
      florus', 251
    Chimonanthus praecox 'Luteus',
      251

    Choisya ×dewitteana 'Aztec
      Pearl', 193
    Choisya ternata 'Sundance', 193
    Clerodendrum trichotomum 'Far-
      gesii', 160
    Daphne odora 'Aureomargina-
      ta', 150
    Lilium candidum, 198
    Prostanthera rotundifolia, 195
    Santolina chamaecyparissus
      'Nana', 223
rue, 218–219
Ruff, Emily, 68
rustic sphinx, 184
Ruta graveolens, 218–219

S

sachets, 108–109
sacred basil, 122
sage, 13, 86, 220–221
sagebrush, 252
salvia, 53
Salvia 'Betsy Clebsch', 220
Salvia apiana, 220, 221
Salvia clevelandii, 220, 221
Salvia discolor, 207
Salvia dorisiana, 207
Salvia elegans, 207
    'Tangerine', 207
Salvia lavandulifolia, 220
Salvia melissodora, 207
Salvia officinalis, 220–221
    'Berggarten', 220
Salvia sclarea, 138–139
sambac jasmine, 169
San Francisco Botanical Garden, 67
santolina, 222–223
Santolina chamaecyparissus, 222–223
    'Nana', 223
Santolina rosmarinifolia, 223
Santolina virens, 223
Sarcococca confusa, 226–227
Sarcococca hookeriana var. *humilis*, 226
Sarcococca ruscifolia, 226
scarlet bee balm, 126
scent. *See* fragrance